Review of Rad 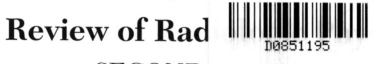 cs
SECOND EDITION

Review of Radiologic Physics
SECOND EDITION

Walter Huda, PH.D.
Professor of Radiology
Director of Radiologic Physics
State University of New York Upstate Medical University
Syracuse, New York

Richard M. Slone, M.D.
Countryside Hospital
Safety Harbor, Florida
Mease Hospital
Dunedin, Florida
Celestial Imaging, PA and
Advanced Imaging Consultants, LLP
Clearwater, Florida

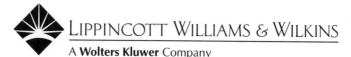
LIPPINCOTT WILLIAMS & WILKINS
A **Wolters Kluwer** Company
Philadelphia · Baltimore · New York · London
Buenos Aires · Hong Kong · Sydney · Tokyo

Acquisitions Editor: Joyce-Rachel John
Developmental Editor: Grace R. Caputo
Production Editor: Emmeline A. Parker
Manufacturing Manager: Timothy Reynolds
Cover Designer: Christine Jenny
Compositor: Maryland Composition
Printer: Data Reproductions Corporation

© 2003 by LIPPINCOTT WILLIAMS & WILKINS
530 Walnut Street
Philadelphia, PA 19106 USA
LWW.com

Printed in the USA

Library of Congress Cataloging-in-Publication Data

Huda, Walter.
    Review of radiologic physics / Walter Huda, Richard M. Slone.— 2nd ed.
      p. ; cm.
    Includes bibliographical references and index.
    ISBN 0-7817-3675-7
      1. Radiology, Medical—Outlines, syllabi, etc. 2. Medical physics—Outlines, syllabi, etc.
I. Slone, Richard M. II. Title.
    [DNLM: 1. Health Physics—Examination Questions. WN 18.2 H883r 2002]
    R896.5 .H83 2003
    616.07′54′076—dc21
                                   2002070239

10 9 8 7 6 5 4 3 2 1

To my parents, Stefan and Paraskevia Huda, for their resolute support and encouragement.

—Walter Huda

To my friends and family, especially my son, Logan.

—Richard Slone

Ordinary language is totally unsuited for expressing what physics really asserts, since the words of everyday life are not sufficiently abstract. Only mathematics and mathematical logic can say as little as the physicist means to say.

—Bertrand Russell

X-rays: their moral is this–that a right way of looking at things will see through almost anything.

—Samuel Butler

Contents

Preface

Seven years have passed since the first edition of *Review of Radiologic Physics* appeared. Although the laws of physics do not change, the practice of radiology continues to evolve at a rapid rate. Medical imaging was essentially "film based" in the 20th century, whereas in the 21st century, it will be all-digital. Radiology residents and technologists starting their careers in radiology today can expect to be operating in a digital world during most of their professional careers. To reflect these changes, an updated Chapter 4 now describes analog x-ray imaging, and Chapter 6 covers digital radiography and fluoroscopy, as well as the advent of the all-digital department known as the picture archiving and communications system (PACS).

In the original edition of *Review of Radiologic Physics*, six of the 13 chapters were on physics topics, and the remaining seven related directly to medical imaging. In the revised text, only three chapters relate to physics and one to radiation protection, and eight chapters are now devoted to medical imaging modalities. Material that has been deleted includes obsolete topics such as xeroradiography. Mammography has been expanded to explicitly include details of the Mammography Quality Standards Act (MQSA) requirements for mammographers, technologists, and medical physicists, together with the latest developments in digital mammography and the increasing role of nuclear medicine in breast imaging. Many of the original tables have been simplified so that they illustrate key concepts, rather than attempt to comprehensively list information available in textbooks.

Image quality and patient dose are very important topics and are closely interwoven with each other, thus meriting their own chapter. The new Chapter 5 addresses image quality in terms of the key characteristic of contrast, resolution, and image noise. Also included is a section on the assessment of medical imaging performance by use of receiver operating characteristic (ROC) methods. For imaging modalities that use ionizing radiation, there is often a direct link between the amount of radiation received by the patient, and the corresponding image quality in the resultant image. For example, increasing the radiation exposure in fluoroscopy or computed radiography will generally reduce the amount of quantum mottle in the resultant image.

The format of the chapters pertaining to the advanced imaging modalities of computed tomography (CT), nuclear medicine, ultrasound, and magnetic resonance (MR) has been updated, but we continue to emphasize the basic physics of these modalities, rather than addressing in detail the latest advances. Regarding CT, we have expanded coverage to include the exciting developments of multislice CT. In nuclear medicine, it is clear that positron emission tomography (PET) imaging is playing an increasingly important clinical role, so coverage of this topic has been expanded. We have expanded coverage of several ultrasound advances of recent years, including contrast agents, harmonic imaging, and power Doppler. We have expanded the MR section to include imaging modes that are commonly used in clinical practice, such as diffusion-weighted imaging.

A number of changes have been made in the 600 questions used in this book. The question format has now been standardized to offer a best answer from five options, and all true/false and matching questions have been eliminated. This brings the question format in line with current practices in most professional examinations, such as those of the American Board of Radiology. In addition, more difficult questions have replaced many of the easier ones, making the questions a greater challenge. The number of questions in each of the 12 chapters has been fixed at 30. Moreover, the two practice examinations each contain 130 questions, and have been reorganized so that the first 10 questions (i.e., 1 to 10) specifically refer to the topic addressed in Chapter 1, the second set of 10 questions (i.e., 11 to 20) refers to Chapter 2, and so on. In this manner, students taking the practice examinations should be able to readily identify specific sections in which they are weaker (or stronger) and devote more (or less) time to these topics in studying for examinations.

The topic of radiologic physics undoubtedly covers a lot of material. There is a wide range of imaging modalities based on x-rays, including radiography, fluoroscopy, CT, and mammography. Additional imaging systems include nuclear medicine, ultrasound, and MR. All of these modes for acquiring medical images are undergoing major advances, and expanding into new applications. Nonetheless, we consider conciseness to be a major virtue, and every effort has been made to limit both the number of chapters and the total length of this review book. Elimination of material is not easy, especially when the book also aims to be comprehensive in covering the whole of radiologic physics. Our focus has been on retaining *essential* material that a radiology resident or radiologic technologist requires to perform their specific tasks.

Acknowledgments

We gratefully acknowledge the assistance of John Aldrich, Ph.D., John Boone, Ph.D., Diane Clark, Ian Cunningham, Ph.D., Geoff Dean, Ph.D., Robert Dixon, M.D., Pat Duffy, R.T., David Feiglin, M.D., Nikolaos Gkantsios, Ph.D., Zhenxue Jing, Ph.D., Ed Nickoloff, Ph.D., Kent Ogden, Ph.D., Terry Peters, Ph.D., Colin Poon, M.D., Dan Rickey, Ph.D., Marsha Roskopf, R.T., John Rowland, Ph.D., Ernest Scalzetti, M.D., Anthony Seibert, Ph.D., and Nikolaus Szeverenyi, Ph.D.

Introduction

I. What Is Radiologic Physics?

Radiology is arguably the most technology-dependent specialty in medicine, and it has seen significant changes during the past decade. Computer integration with constant technical innovations has changed the workplace and influenced the role radiology plays in the diagnosis and treatment of disease. Radiologic physics is not an esoteric subject of abstract equations and memorized definitions, but rather the total process of creating and viewing a diagnostic image. A range of physical principles influences this process of image formation. Radiologists and technologists need to understand the technology and the physical principles that constitute the advantages, govern the limitations, and determine the risks of the equipment they use.

Radiologic physics covers the important medical imaging modalities of radiographic and fluoroscopic x-ray imaging, mammography, computed tomography (CT), magnetic resonance (MR), nuclear medicine, and ultrasound. Radiologic physics provides an understanding of the factors that improve or degrade image quality. Selection of the most appropriate way of generating a medical image is the responsibility of the radiologic imaging team, comprising the radiologist, technologist, medical physicist, and equipment manufacturer. Optimizing medical imaging performance clearly requires a solid understanding of how these images are generated, and of the most important determinants of image quality.

All imaging modalities have a "cost" associated with their use. MR and ultrasound do not have any specific risks, and the "cost" is generally the time required to perform the study. For modalities that employ ionizing radiations, one of the "costs" is the radiation dose to the patient and staff working with these systems. Accordingly, radiation protection principles are important. Radiologists and technologists should understand the magnitude of the radiation dose to the patient and personnel exposed, and ensure that radiation levels are kept as low as reasonably achievable (ALARA principle) and within any relevant regulatory limits.

II. Why Study Radiologic Physics?

Both residents and technologists need to acquire an understanding of the underlying imaging science for each diagnostic modality, and be able to pass their respective radiologic physics examinations. Neither professional will actually practice physics, however, and so there is no need to learn how to generate modulation transfer functions in radiographic imaging, how to write programs to perform filtered back projection algorithms in CT, or how to design radiofrequency pulses in MR imaging.

It is important, nonetheless, for well-rounded radiologists and technologists to have a basic understanding of (1) image quality parameters such as noise, spatial resolution, and contrast; (2) how image quality is affected by radiographic techniques; (3) how to evaluate commercial imaging equipment in terms of its ability to perform the required patient examinations; (4) the radiation dose and risks associated with radiographic exposure; and (5) how to communicate with medical physicists and service personnel regarding imaging problems.

The focus of the text and allied questions is on the physics underlying the creation of clinical images. Special emphasis has been given to the factors that affect image quality, notably image contrast, spatial resolution, and noise. It is important that residents and technologists understand the achievable performance of any imaging equipment, as well as how this equipment should best be used to solve specific patient imaging problems.

III. Structure of this Review Book

This review book is designed to help prepare residents and technologists for the radiological physics portion of their board and registry examinations. It provides a source for comprehensive self-study in the area of diagnostic radiological physics. The text assumes a background of instruction in radiologic physics and is *not* intended to replace the standard radiologic physics texts. This book is designed, rather, to provide a concise yet complete source of review to refresh and reinforce the concepts of radiologic physics expected of residents and technologists.

The text is divided into 12 chapters, each with five or six subsections that cover everything from basic physics to image quality. Each chapter begins with an outline of the "key" information about the area under review. This is followed by 30 questions designed to provide a self-test of the reader's knowledge and comprehension in each area. The philosophy we adopted is that material comprehension, rather than rote memorization, will guarantee success in the examination. Also included are two practice examinations, with questions that reflect the topics covered in this book. At the end of the book is a glossary of key terms commonly used in radiologic physics.

Radiation measurements are generally given in SI (Système International) units, with non-SI units also given in brackets. Use of roentgen units to specify radiation exposure is problematic, and use of the correct conversion factor (i.e., 1 R = 2.58×10^{-4} C/kg) would not have been very helpful. In diagnostic radiology, an exposure of 1 R can be taken to be equal to an air kerma of 8.73 mGy. In the text, exposures are specified as air kerma in SI units and roentgen in non-SI units. For convenience, throughout the text an air kerma of 10 mGy has been taken to be approximately equal to an exposure of 1 R, and the terms *exposure* and *air kerma* are used interchangeably.

IV. Radiology Residents and the ABR Examination

The physics portion of the American Board of Radiology (ABR) written examination is administered in the fall of each year. Board-eligible residents can register a year in advance to take the examination in September of their second, third, or forth year of training. The 4-hour examination contains about 130 single best-response, multiple-choice questions. Most residents comfortably finish the test in the allowed time.

About two thirds of the questions cover diagnostic physics and equipment, including basic principles, x-ray tubes, image intensifiers, recording systems, ultrasound, CT, MR, contrast media, image quality, radiation exposure, and safety. The remaining questions cover nuclear medicine physics, including principles, equipment, dosimetry, measurements, and statistics and radiation biology (cell and tissue kinetics; subcellular, cellular, tissue, and whole-body effects and response). Further information regarding the ABR and the written physics examination can be obtained at the ABR Web site (www.theabr.org).

V. Radiology Technologists and the ARRT Examination

The American Registry of Radiologic Technologists (ARRT) is the credentialing board for radiologic technologists in the United States. The ARRT written examination consists of multiple-choice questions designed to measure the knowledge and cognitive skills underlying the intelligent performance of the major tasks typically required of a radiographer. ARRT examinations are presented in random order. Up to 20% of the test may be pilot questions that are unscored questions for which additional time has been allowed. Data from these pilot questions are used to evaluate new test questions. Calculators are no longer allowed.

The written examination includes questions in five general areas: (1) radiation protection, (2) equipment operation and maintenance, (3) image production and evaluation, (4) radiographic procedures, and (5) patient care. The first three sections make up about 55% of the total examination and are the focus of this book. The total testing time of the radiography examination is 3.5 hours, and an additional 30 minutes is allocated for the exam tutorial and survey after the test has been completed. The results are scaled to take into account the difficulty of a particular test compared with other forms of the same test. Results are reported on a scale that ranges from one to 99, with a score of 75 required to pass the examination. Performance on each section of the test is also reported to provide the examinee with information on their respective strengths and weakness. Pass/fail decisions are *not* based on individual section scores.

Topics that all radiologic technologists need to cover include the biological effects of radiation, techniques to minimize radiation exposure, sources of radiation exposure, methods of protection, basic properties of radiation, units of radiation measurement, dosimeters, personnel monitoring, components of radiographic equipment (including x-ray generators, tubes and transformers, fluoroscopic units, beam restrictors, grids, cassettes, and shielding) as well as image contrast and density, the effect of kVp and mAs, filtration, and screen/film combinations. Technologists planning to specialize in the imaging modalities of nuclear medicine, ultrasound, MR, and CT should find the chapters devoted to these topics of considerable assistance. Radiographic procedures and patient care issues are not addressed in this book. Further information on the ARRT can be obtained at its web site (www.arrt.org).

1

Matter and Radiation

I.   Basic physics

A. Forces

–The **mass** of a body is a measure of its inertia, or resistance to acceleration and is measured in **kilograms** (kg).

–**Velocity** is the constant speed of a body moving in a given direction, and is measured in **meters per second** (m/second).

–**Acceleration** is the rate of change of velocity, and is measured in **meters per second per second** (m/second^2).

–A **force** causes a body to deviate from a state of rest or constant velocity (push or pull).

–**Force = mass × acceleration,** and is measured in **newtons (N).**

–The four physical forces in the universe are **gravitational, electrostatic, strong, and weak.** The relative strength of these four forces is shown in **Table 1.1.**

–**Gravity** pulls objects to Earth; in radiologic physics, the effects of gravity are extremely small and ignored.

–The **electrostatic force** causes protons and electrons to attract each other, and holds atoms together.

–**Strong forces** hold the nucleus of an atom together.

–**Weak forces** are involved in beta decay.

B. Energy and power

–**Energy** is the ability to perform work and is measured in **joules** (J).

–Energy takes on various forms, including electrical, nuclear, mechanical, chemical, and thermal.

–One common form of energy is **kinetic energy,** caused by motion (e.g., a speeding bullet) and given by kinetic energy = $\frac{1}{2} m \times v^2$, where v is velocity and m is mass.

–Another form of energy is **potential energy,** such as a hydroelectric power-generating station, where water falls from a high potential to a low potential.

–Einstein showed that mass and energy are interchangeable and are given by the expression $E = m \times c^2$, where E is energy, m is mass, and c is velocity of light.

–Based on this interconversion of mass and energy, **rest mass energy** is the energy equivalent of a particle.

–In diagnostic radiology, the **electron volt** (eV) is a convenient unit of energy, where 1 eV = 1.6×10^{-19} J.

–**Power** is the rate of performing work.

–Power is the energy used divided by time and is measured in **watts** (W), where 1 W = 1 J/second.

–**Table 1.2** lists the power and energies of a range of sources.

TABLE 1.1. *Relative strength of physical forces*

Type of force	Relative strength	Range of interaction	Force function
Gravitational	1	Infinite	Binds earth to the sum
Weak	$\sim 10^{24}$	$< 10^{-18}$ m	Involved in beta decay
Electrostatic	$\sim 10^{35}$	Infnite	Binds electrons in atoms
Strong	$\sim 10^{38}$	$< 10^{-15}$ m	Binds protons and neutrons in the nucleus

C. Electricity

–The **electric charge** of electrons and protons is 1.6×10^{-19} **coulomb** (C).

–**Electrons** are negatively charged; **protons** are positively charged.

–Any change in voltage in an electrical circuit causes electrons to move.

–The positive region of an electrical circuit is called the **anode,** and the negative region is called the **cathode.**

–Electrons are repelled from the cathode and attracted to the anode.

–Any voltage source in a complete circuit will therefore result in a flow of electrons in the circuit.

–**Electric current,** measured in **amperes** (A), is the flow of electrons through a circuit.

–An ampere is the amount of charge that flows divided by time (1 A = 1 C/second).

–Electrons accelerated through V volts gain a kinetic energy of V electron volts. See **Fig. 1.1.**

–In electric circuits, the **power** (P) dissipated is the product of electric current (I) and voltage (V), or $P = I \times V$ watts.

–If the voltage is 100,000 V (100 kV) and the current is 1 A (1,000 mA), the power dissipated is 100,000 W (100 kW).

–A typical household in North America uses a few kilowatts of electrical power.

II. Matter

A. Atoms

–**Matter** is made up of atoms, which are composed of **protons, neutrons,** and **electrons.**

–**Protons** have a positive charge and are found in the nucleus of atoms.

–**Neutrons** are electrically neutral and are also found in the nucleus.

–The number of neutrons in an atom affects the stability of the nucleus.

–**Electrons** have a negative charge and are found outside the nucleus.

–Electrons are much lighter than protons and neutrons.

–Isolated protons and electrons are **stable,** whereas an isolated neutron is **unstable** and has a half-life of approximately 11 minutes.

TABLE 1.2. *Power and energy associated with a range of sources*

Energy source	Power rating	Energy used in 1 sec (J)
Flashlight	2 W	2
Domestic light bulb	50 W	50
Microwave	500 W	500
Stove burner	2 kW	2,000
X-ray generator	80 kW	80,000
Major power plant	1,000,000 kW (1 GW)	1,000,000,000
[One horsepower]	*[750 W]*	*[750]*

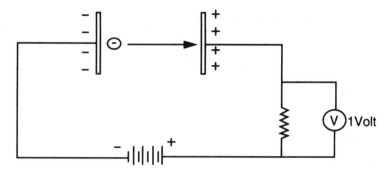

FIG. 1.1. One electron volt (eV) is the kinetic energy gained when a single electron is accelerated between two plates that differ in potential by 1 V. Before leaving the negatively charged plate, the electron has a potential energy of 1 eV.

–The **atomic number** *(Z)* is the number of protons in the nucleus of an atom and is unique for each element.

–The **mass number** *(A)* is the total number of protons and neutrons in the nucleus.

–In the notation ^A_ZX or ^AX, *X* is the unique letter or letters designating the element, *A* is the mass number, and *Z* is the atomic number.

–Electrically neutral atoms have *Z* electrons and *Z* protons.

–Mass on the atomic scale is measured in **atomic mass units** (amu).

  –One atomic mass unit is one twelfth the mass of a carbon atom (^{12}C), or 1.6×10^{-27} kg.

  –Protons and neutrons have a mass of approximately 1 amu.

  –Electrons have a much smaller mass of 9.1×10^{-31} kg, or 0.00055 amu.

–One gram-mole of a substance contains 6×10^{23} atoms, normally expressed as N_o, the **Avogadro number.**

–One gram of an element thus contains N_o/A atoms, where the element has an atomic mass of *A*.

–**Table 1.3** shows the mass, charge, and rest mass of atomic constituents.

B. Electronic structure

–The nucleus of an atom is made up of tightly bound protons and neutrons, which are called **nucleons.**

–The nucleus contains most of the atomic mass.

–In the **Bohr model** of an atom, **electrons surround the nucleus in shells** (e.g., K-shell and L-shell) as shown for tungsten in **Fig. 1.2.**

–Each shell is assigned a principal quantum number (*n*), beginning with one for the K-shell, two for the L-shell, and so on.

–The number of electrons each shell can contain is $2n^2$.

TABLE 1.3. *Mass, charge, and rest mass energy of atomic constituents*

Particle	Relative mass	Charge	Rest mass energy
Electron	1	−1	511 keV
Proton	1,836	+1	938 MeV
Neutron	1,839	0	940 MeV

–The K-shell in tungsten ($n = 1$) has 2 electrons, the L-shell ($n = 2$) has 8 electrons, the M-shell ($n = 3$) has 18 electrons, and so on.

–The number of electrons in the outer shell (**valence electrons**) determines the chemical properties of the atom.

–The **electron density** of a substance is $\rho \times N_o \times (Z/A)$ electrons/cm^3, where ρ is the density measured in **grams per cubic centimeter** (g/cm^3).

  –For most atoms making up humans (e.g., oxygen, carbon, nitrogen, and calcium), Z/A is approximately constant and equal to 0.5.

  –For patients, electron density is generally proportional to the physical density ρ.

C. Electron binding energy

–Atomic electrons are held in place by the **electrostatic pull** of the positively charged nucleus.

–The work that is required to remove an electron from an atom is called the **electron binding energy.**

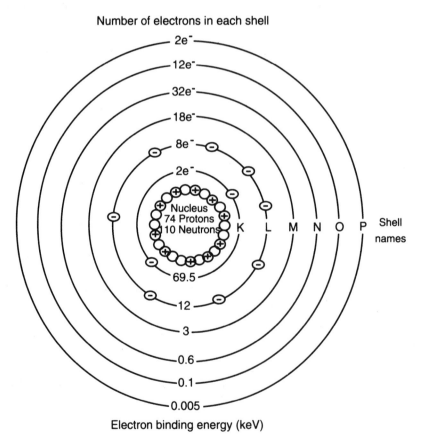

FIG. 1.2. Bohr model of the atom showing tungsten with a total of 74 protons, 74 electrons, and 110 neutrons. The electron binding energy decreases rapidly with electron distance from the nucleus.

TABLE 1.4. *Atomic number, K-shell binding energy, and approximate density of selected elements*

Element	Atomic no.	K-shell binding energy (keV)	Physical density (g/cm^3)
Hydrogen	1	0.01	<0.001
Carbon	6	0.3	1.8–2.3
Nitrogen	7	0.4	0.001
Oxygen	8	0.5	0.001
Calcium	20	4.0	1.6
Copper	29	9.0	8.9
Selenium	34	12.7	4.3–4.8
Molybdenum	42	20.0	10.2
Silver	47	25.5	10.5
Iodine	53	33.2	4.9
Barium	56	37.4	3.5
Tungsten	74	69.5	19.3
Lead	82	88.0	11.3

–The binding energy of **outer-shell electrons** is small and equal to approximately **several electron volts.**

–The binding energy of **inner-shell electrons** is large, that is, **thousands of electron volts** (keV).

–K-shell binding energies increase with atomic number (Z), as listed in **Table 1.4.**

–Energetic particles can knock out inner-shell electrons only if their energy is greater than the electron binding energy.

–A 100 keV electron can eject a K-shell electron from a tungsten atom.

  –A 50 keV electron cannot, as it does not have sufficient energy to overcome the 69.5 keV binding energy.

–A vacancy in the K-shell will be filled by an electron from a higher shell.

–Electrons moving from an outer shell to an inner shell may emit excess energy as **electromagnetic radiation.**

D. Nuclear binding energy

–**Nucleons** are held together by **strong forces.**

–The **total binding energy** of the entire nucleus is the energy required to separate all of the nucleons.

–The binding energy of a single nucleon (i.e., neutron or proton) is the energy required to remove it from the nucleus.

–The **average binding energy** per nucleon is the total binding energy divided by the number of nucleons.

  –The average binding energy per nucleon increases from approximately 1 million electron volts (MeV) for deuterium, with a mass number of 2, to between 7 and 9 MeV for nuclei with mass numbers greater than 20.

–A high binding energy indicates nuclear stability.

–The average binding energy per nucleon increases after radioactive decay, because the daughter is more stable than the parent.

III. Radiation

A. Electromagnetic radiation

–Radiation is the transport of energy through space.

–**Wavelength** (λ) is the distance between successive crests of waves.

–**Amplitude** is the intensity defined by the height of the wave.

–**Frequency** (f) is the number of wave oscillations per unit of time expressed in cycles per second, or in **hertz** (Hz).

–The **period** is the time required for one wavelength to pass ($1/f$).

–For any type of wave motion, velocity (v) = $f \times \lambda$ m/second, where f is measured in hertz and λ in meters.

–Electromagnetic radiation travels in a straight line at the speed of light, c (3×10^8 m/second in a vacuum).

–X-rays are an example of electromagnetic radiation.

–The product of the wavelength (λ) and frequency (f) of electromagnetic radiation is equal to the speed of light ($c = f \times \lambda$).

–Electromagnetic radiation represents a **transverse wave,** in which the electric and magnetic fields oscillate perpendicular to the direction of the wave motion.

–**Fig. 1.3** shows the electromagnetic spectrum from radio waves (long wavelength) to x-rays and gamma rays (short wavelength).

B. Photons

–Electromagnetic radiation is **quantized,** meaning that it exists in **discrete** quantities of energy called photons.

–**Photons** may behave as waves or particles but **have no mass.**

–**Photon energy** (E) is **directly proportional** to **frequency** and **inversely proportional** to **wavelength.**

–The wavelength of an x-ray may be measured in angstroms (Å), where 1 Å is 10^{-8} cm, or 10^{-10} m.

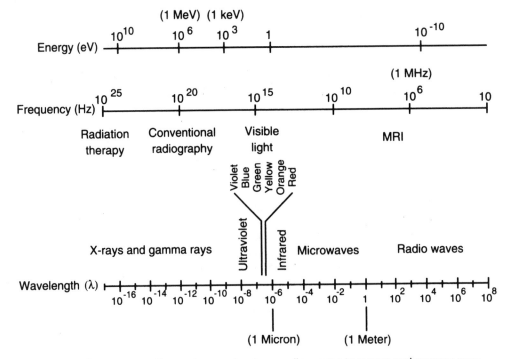

FIG. 1.3. Electromagnetic spectra ranging from radio waves to x-rays and gamma rays.

–Photon energy is $E = h \times f = h \times (c/\lambda) = \mathbf{12.4/\lambda}$, where E is in keV, h is Planck's constant, and λ is the wavelength in angstroms.
  –A 10 keV photon has a wavelength of 1.24 Å, which is equal to the diameter of a typical atom.
  –A 100 keV photon has a wavelength of 0.124 Å.
–By convention, photons are called **x-rays** if produced by electron interactions, and **gamma rays** if produced in nuclear processes.

C. Inverse square law

–X-ray beam intensity decreases with distance from the tube because of the divergence of the x-ray beam.
–The decrease in intensity is proportional to the square of the distance from the source and is an expression of energy conservation.
–This nonlinear fall-off in intensity with distance is called the **inverse square law.**
  –For example, doubling the distance from the x-ray source decreases the x-ray beam intensity by a factor of 4; increasing the distance by a factor of 10 decreases the beam intensity by a factor of 100.
–In general, if the distance from the x-ray source is changed from x_1 to x_2, then the x-ray beam intensity changes by $(x_1/x_2)^2$.

D. Ionization

–**Ionization** occurs when an electron is ejected from a neutral atom, leaving behind a **positive ion.**
–Electromagnetic radiation with sufficient energy to remove electrons is called ionizing radiation.
–**Ionizing radiation** includes x-rays and gamma rays.
–Radiation may be **directly ionizing** (involving charged particles) or **indirectly ionizing** (involving uncharged particles such as neutrons, x-rays, and gamma rays).
–The average amount of energy needed to generate one electron-ion pair in air is approximately 33 eV.
–**Charged particles lose energy** when passing through matter by interacting with electrons in nearby atoms.
–Electrons, positrons, protons, neutrons, and alpha particles are examples of ionizing particles.
–The loss of energy by a charged particle increases with increasing charge.
–The loss of energy by a charged particle increases with increasing mass and decreasing particle velocity.
  –Energy lost from energetic particles can eject electrons from atoms or raise atomic electrons to higher energies.
–**Linear energy transfer** (LET) measures the loss of energy of a charged particle in thousands of electron volts for each micrometer of distance traveled by the particle.
  –**Electrons and positrons** lose approximately 0.5 keV when traveling through 1 μm of soft tissue and are considered to be "low-LET" radiation.
  –**Alpha particles** lose approximately 100 keV when traversing 1 μm of soft tissue and are considered to be "high-LET" radiation.
  –Protons and neutrons (which produce ionization by producing recoil protons) have an LET that is intermediate between these two extremes.
–Ionizing radiation transfers energy to electrons in the absorbing medium.
–The energy deposited in the absorbing medium by ionizing radiation can result in deleterious chemical modifications to molecules such as DNA.

–Energy deposited by radiation is ultimately transformed into increased molecular motion (heat).

–The heating effect of ionizing radiation in radiology is generally negligible.

–For a computed tomography scan of the head, the total amount of energy deposited is approximately 0.2 J, whereas a 500 W microwave oven deposits a total of 5,000 J in 10 seconds.

IV. Radionuclides

A. Introduction

–Nuclei having different numbers of protons, neutrons, or both are called **nuclides.**

–Unstable nuclides are called **radionuclides,** and atoms with unstable nuclei are called **radioisotopes.**

–The mass number *(A)* of a nuclide is the sum of the number of protons *(Z)* and neutrons *(N)*, or $A = Z + N$.

–For example, iodine 131 has 131 nucleons; $Z = 53$ and $N = 78$.

–Nuclides having the same mass number *(A)* are called **isobars.**

–Nuclides having the same atomic number (*protons*) are called **isotopes.**

–Nuclides having the same number of *n*eutrons are called **isotones.**

–An **isomer** is the *e*xcited state of a nucleus.

–**Table 1.5** lists the three isotopes of hydrogen. Hydrogen and deuterium are stable, but tritium is radioactive, with a half-life of 12 years.

B. Nuclear stability

–For common and stable low-mass-number nuclides, the number of neutrons *(N)* is approximately equal to the number of protons *(Z)*. For example, carbon 12 has six protons and six neutrons, and oxygen 16 has eight protons and eight neutrons.

–For stable high-mass-number nuclides, the number of neutrons exceeds the number of protons. For example, tungsten has 74 protons and 110 neutrons.

–**Fig. 1.4** illustrates these relations and shows that stable high-atomic-mass atoms have proportionally more neutrons.

–Very heavy nuclei ($Z > 82$) tend to be unstable.

–The three processes by which an unstable nuclide or radionuclide attains stability are **alpha, beta,** and **gamma decay.**

–The transformation from unstable to stable nuclides is called **radioactive decay.**

–The original nuclide is called the **parent,** and the products are **daughter** nuclei.

–In nuclear transformations, energy, mass number, and electric charge are conserved.

C. Radioactivity

–**Half-life** ($T_{1/2}$) is the time required for half the material to decay.

–**Activity** is the number of transformations per unit of time.

TABLE 1.5. *Isotopes of hydrogen*

Symbol	Protons	Neutrons	Mass no.	Name Nucleus	Atom
^{1}H	1	0	1	Proton	Hydrogen
^{2}H	1	1	2	Deuteron	Deuterium
^{3}H	1	2	3	Triton	Tritium

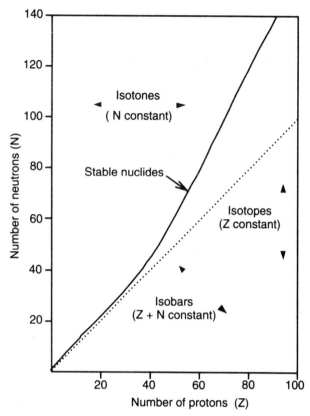

FIG. 1.4. Relation between the number of protons, or atomic number *(Z)*, and the number of neutrons in the nucleus of stable nuclides. As the mass number increases, the ratio of neutrons to protons increases from 1:1 to approximately 1:1.5 for stable nuclides.

–Activity is expressed mathematically as $dN(t)/dt$, where $N(t)$ is the number of atoms at time (t).

–**Lambda** (λ) is the **decay constant,** and $dN(t)/dt = N(t) \times \lambda$.

–Activity is $N \times \lambda$, where N is the number of atoms.

–The relation between λ and the half-life of the radioactivity ($T_{1/2}$) is $\lambda = \log_e(2)/T_{1/2} = 0.693/T_{1/2}$.

–The SI unit of activity is the becquerel (Bq), and the non-SI unit is the curie (Ci). Both units are used to describe a quantity of radioactive material.

 –One **becquerel** is 1 transformation per second.

 –One **curie** is 3.7×10^{10} transformations per second.

 –One mCi = 37 MBq; 1 μCi = 37 kBq.

D. Isomeric transitions

–**Gamma rays** are high-energy photons (electromagnetic radiation) that result from nuclear processes.

–The **ground state** is the lowest energy state of a nucleus and is, therefore, the **most stable** arrangement of nucleons.

–**Excited states** have increased energies, are **unstable,** and have a transient existence before transforming into a more stable state.

–**Metastable states** (isomeric states) are also **unstable** but have relatively long life-times before transforming to another state. To be called metastable, the half-life must exceed 10^{-12} second. The metastable state of an atom is denoted by a lower case "m" after the mass number (e.g., technetium 99m).

–Nuclear transformations to a more stable state (isomeric transitions) release energy in the form of a **gamma ray.**

–After an **isomeric transition,** both parent and daughter nuclei have the same mass number, atomic number, and number of neutrons.

–Rather than emitting gamma rays, energy may be transferred to an orbital electron, which is then emitted from the atom as an **internal conversion electron.**

V. Decay modes

A. Beta-minus decay

–In beta-minus (β^-) decay, a neutron inside the nucleus is converted into a proton, and the excess energy is released as an energetic electron, called a **beta particle,** and an **antineutrino.**

–The **antineutrino** has no rest mass, has no electric charge, and rarely interacts with matter.

–β^- Decay occurs in nuclei with too many neutrons.

–In β^- decay, the atomic number increases by one, but the mass number remains constant.

–The beta particles (electrons) emitted during β^- decay have a range of energies (spectrum), up to a maximum energy (E_{max}).

–The average energy of beta emitters is approximately one third of the maximum.

–^{32}P is a pure beta emitter with a maximum beta particle energy of 1.71 MeV and a mean beta particle energy of approximately 570 keV.

–^{3}H, or tritium, ($E_{max} = 18$ keV) and ^{14}C ($E_{max} = 156$ keV) are low-energy β^- emitters that are ubiquitous in biomedical research.

B. Beta-plus decay

–In beta-plus (β^+) decay (sometimes called positron emission), a proton inside the nucleus is converted into a neutron, and the excess energy is emitted as a positively charged electron, called a **positron,** and a **neutrino.**

–A **neutrino** has no electric charge, has no rest mass, and is similar to an antineutrino.

–β^+ decay occurs in nuclei with too few neutrons.

–In β^+ decay, the atomic number decreases by one, and the mass number stays the same.

–A **positron** is an electron with a positive charge instead of a negative charge and interacts with matter like an electron.

–Energetic positrons lose their energy by ionization and excitation of atomic electrons.

–When the positron loses all of its kinetic energy, it annihilates with an electron.

–The mass (energy) of the positron and electron (511 keV each) is converted into two 511 keV photons that are emitted 180 degrees apart.

–Positron emitters generally have short half-lives (^{11}C, 20 minutes; ^{15}O, 2 minutes; ^{18}F, 110 minutes).

C. Electron capture

–In **electron capture,** a proton inside the nucleus is converted into a neutron by capturing an electron from one of the atomic shells (e.g., K, L, and M).

–A **neutrino** is emitted during **electron capture.**

  –Electron capture is most likely from the K-shell, followed by electron capture from the L-shell, M-shell, and so on.

–Electron capture occurs in nuclei with too few neutrons (too many protons).

–In **electron capture,** the atomic number decreases by one, and the mass number stays the same.

–If the electron is captured from the K-shell (K-shell capture), the resultant K-shell vacancy is filled by an outer-shell electron.

  –The excess energy is emitted as a characteristic x-ray, or **Auger electron.**

  –The energy of the **Auger electron** is equal to the characteristic x-ray energy minus the electron binding energy.

–Electron capture may compete with β^+ decay.

–Important electron capture radionuclides used in nuclear medicine include ^{57}Co, ^{67}Ga, ^{111}In, ^{123}I, ^{125}I, and ^{201}Tl.

D. Alpha decay

–In **alpha decay,** a radionuclide emits an alpha particle consisting of two neutrons and two protons (i.e., helium nucleus).

–Alpha decay is most common in atoms with atomic numbers *(Z)* greater than 82.

–^{226}Ra is a common alpha emitter found in nature, which decays to ^{222}Ra (radon), which is another alpha emitter.

–In alpha decay, the atomic number decreases by two, and the mass number decreases by four.

–Alpha particles have an energy between 4 and 7 MeV.

–Alpha particles can travel from 1 to 10 cm in air, but less than 0.1 mm in tissue.

  –Alpha particles thus pose little risk as an external radiation source but pose a high risk if ingested or injected.

–Table 1.6 summarizes the major modes of radioactive decay.

TABLE 1.6. *R*adioactive decay modes for unstable nuclei containing protons *(Z)*, neutrons *(N)*, and mass number *(A)* [=*Z*+*N*]

| Decay mode | Daughter nucleus value | | | Comments |
	Mass no.	Atomic no.	Neutron no.	
Isomeric transition	*A*	*Z*	*N*	Metastable if half-life $> 10^{-12}$ sec
Beta-minus	*A*	*Z* + 1	*N* − 1	Emits electrons and antineutrinos
Beta-plus	*A*	*Z* − 1	*N* + 1	Emits positrons and neutrinos
Electron capture	*A*	*Z* − 1	*N* + 1	Emits neutrinos and x-rays*
Alpha decay	*A* − 4	*Z* − 2	*N* − 2	Occurs in heavy nuclei (*Z* > 82)

* Characteristic x-rays are emitted as the inner-shell electron vacancies are filled.

Review Test

1. Which of the following is measured in newtons?

(A) Electrons flowing through a medium
(B) Attraction or repulsion between two bodies
(C) Mass
(D) Electric resistance
(E) Energy expended per unit time

2. *Kinetic energy* is the energy associated with the velocity of:

(A) Visible light photons
(B) X-rays
(C) Gamma rays
(D) Mass
(E) Neutrinos

3. Which of the following is uncharged (neutral) particle?

(A) Proton
(B) Neutron
(C) Electron
(D) Positron
(E) Alpha particle

4. The mass number *(A)* of an atom is equal to the number of:

(A) Neutrons
(B) Protons
(C) Protons plus neutrons
(D) Protons plus electrons
(E) Protons plus neutrons plus electrons

5. Which of the following is incorrect regarding the total number of electrons in an electrically neutral atom?

(A) Six for carbon
(B) Seven for nitrogen
(C) Eight for oxygen
(D) Forty for calcium
(E) Fifty-three for iodine

6. The electron density of radiology patients is:

(A) Mass number times density
(B) Inversely proportional to density
(C) Atomic number times Avogadro's number
(D) Number of electrons per cubic centimeter
(E) Density times charge

7. Which of the following is incorrect regarding the K-shell binding energy?

(A) Oxygen is 0.5 keV.
(B) Calcium is 4 keV.
(C) Barium is 20 keV.
(D) Iodine 33 keV.
(E) Lead is 88 keV.

8. The K-shell electron binding energy:

(A) Increases with increasing distance from the nucleus
(B) Decreases with increasing nuclear charge
(C) Is independent of nuclear neutron number
(D) Is 33 eV for iodine
(E) Is generally a few eV

9. The outer-shell electrons in an atom are not:

(A) More loosely bound than are inner-shell electrons
(B) Bound with energies of a few electron volts
(C) Responsible for forming chemical bonds with other atoms
(D) Ejected from the atom by photons and electrons
(E) Unstable

10. Which of the following is not a force?

(A) Electrostatic
(B) Weak
(C) Strong
(D) Gravitation
(E) Electricity

11. Which of the following statements regarding electromagnetic radiation is *false*?

(A) Travel at the speed of light (3×10^8 m/second).
(B) Exhibits particulate properties.
(C) Have a photon energy proportional to frequency.
(D) Travel at a speed proportional to frequency.
(E) The product of frequency and wavelength is constant.

12. Which characteristic increases with increasing *photon energy*?

(A) Wavelength
(B) Frequency
(C) Mass
(D) Charge
(E) Speed

13. What is the minimum wavelength of an x-ray produced at an x-ray tube potential of 80 kV?

(A) 0.0125 Å
(B) 0.155 Å
(C) 1.75 Å
(D) 15.5 Å
(E) 992 Å

14. The difference between a 600 keV x-ray and 600 keV gamma ray photon is the:

(A) Means of production
(B) Position in the electromagnetic spectrum
(C) Wavelength
(D) Modes of interaction with matter
(E) LET

15. If the distance from a radiation source is halved, the radiation intensity will:

(A) Increase by 2%
(B) Increase by 50%
(C) Double
(D) Triple
(E) Quadruple

16. An atom that has lost an outer-shell electron is called:

(A) Unstable
(B) Metastable
(C) An ion
(D) A radioisotope
(E) A radionuclide

17. Which of the following are *not* directly ionizing radiation?

(A) Electrons
(B) Positrons
(C) Neutrons
(D) Alpha particles
(E) Internal conversion electrons

18. Which of the following particles has the highest linear energy transfer (keV/μm)?

(A) Electrons
(B) Positrons
(C) Protons
(D) Neutrons
(E) Alpha particles

19. ^{131}I and ^{125}I have different:

(A) Chemical properties
(B) Z values
(C) Numbers of neutrons
(D) Numbers of protons
(E) K-shell binding energies

20. Of what are ^{15}O and ^{16}O examples of?

(A) Isotopes
(B) Isotones
(C) Isomers
(D) Isobars
(E) Radionuclides

21. Unstable nuclei cannot lose excess energy by emission of:

(A) Beta particles
(B) Electromagnetic radiation
(C) Neutrinos
(D) Alpha particles
(E) Tritium

22. After 10 half-lives, the fraction of activity remaining:

(A) Depends on the initial activity
(B) Is 1/10
(C) Is $(1/10)^2$
(D) Is $(1/2)^{10}$
(E) Is 9/10

23. After 24 hours, the activity of a 100 MBq ^{123}I ($T_{1/2}$ = 13 hours) source will be about:

(A) 50 MBq
(B) 25 MBq
(C) 10 MBq
(D) 5 MBq
(E) 1 MBq

24. An activity of 3.7×10^7 Bq corresponds to:

(A) 1 mCi
(B) 10 mCi
(C) 100 mCi
(D) 1 Ci
(E) 10 Ci

25. In decay by isomeric transition:

(A) The energy remains the same
(B) The atomic number Z decreases by one
(C) The mass number A decreases by one
(D) Only gamma rays are emitted
(E) A and Z remain the same

26. Concerning the radiations emitted in the decay of ^{99m}Tc, which is true?

(A) 140 keV photons are emitted.
(B) Characteristic x-rays and 140 keV gamma rays are emitted.
(C) Characteristic x-rays, Auger electrons, and gamma rays are emitted.
(D) Characteristic x-rays are emitted.
(E) Characteristic x-rays and Auger electrons are emitted.

27. When ^{60}Co ($Z = 27$) decays to ^{60}Ni ($Z = 28$), which of the following is emitted?

(A) Positrons
(B) Electrons
(C) Alpha particles
(D) 140 keV x-rays
(E) Neutrinos

28. Which of the following emits positrons?

(A) ^{3}H
(B) ^{32}P
(C) ^{18}F
(D) ^{99m}Tc
(E) ^{226}Ra

29. Electron capture can result in emission of:

(A) Antineutrinos
(B) High-LET radiation
(C) Characteristic x-rays
(D) Positrons
(E) Neutrons

30. Which of the following decay modes changes the mass number *(A)* of an unstable nucleus?

(A) β^- Decay
(B) β^+ Decay
(C) Alpha decay
(D) Isomeric transition
(E) Electron capture

Answers and Explanations

1–B. Gravitation is an example of attraction between two bodies.

2–D. Kinetic energy is given by $\frac{1}{2} m \times v^2$, where m is the object mass and v is the object velocity; photons have **no** rest mass.

3–B. The neutron has no (net) electric charge.

4–C. Mass number is the number of nucleons (protons and neutrons) in the nucleus.

5–D. Calcium has an atomic number *(Z)* of 20, and an electrically neutral atom of calcium would have only 20 electrons.

6–D. Electron density is the number of electrons per unit volume (cc).

7–C. The K-shell binding energy of barium is 37.4 keV; note that barium ($Z = 56$) must have a higher K-shell binding energy than that of iodine ($Z = 53$).

8–C. K-shell binding energies do not depend on the number of neutrons in the nucleus.

9–E. Outer shell electrons are stable.

10—E. Electriciy is a flow of charge, not a force.

11–D. The speed of light in a vacuum is a *constant* and is independent of frequency ($c = f \times \lambda$).

12–B. Frequency increases with energy ($E = h \times f$, where h is Planck's constant).

13–B. 0.155 Angstrom units (the wavelength is given in angstroms by the formula $12.4/E$, where E is in keV; thus for a photon with an energy of 80 keV, the corresponding wavelength is 0.155 Å).

14–A. X-rays are produced by electrons, whereas gamma rays originate in nuclear transformations.

15–E. The radiation exposure will quadruple according to the inverse square law.

16–C. An ion.

17–C. Neutrons, because they have no charge. All charged particles are directly ionizing; neutrons ionize by producing recoil protons, and photons ionize by generating electrons.

18–E. Alpha particles have an LET of about 100 keV/(μm), whereas electrons and positrons have an LET of about 0.5 keV/(μm).

19–C. All isotopes of iodine have 53 protons *(Z)*, but differing numbers of neutrons (^{125}I has 72 neutrons, and ^{131}I has 78 neutrons).

20–A. Both ^{15}O and ^{16}O have the same number of protons (eight) in the nucleus and are thus isotopes; ^{15}O is unstable (positron emitter), and ^{16}O is stable.

21–E. Unstable nuclei never emit tritium.

22–D. $(1/2)^{10}$ as the activity remaining after one half-live is 1/2, after two half-lives is $(1/2)^2$, and so on; after n half-lives, the remaining activity is $(1/2)^n$.

23–B. After approximately two half-lives (24 hours), there will $(1/2)^2$ of the original activity left.

24–A. 37 MBq is 1 mCi (1 Ci is 3.7×10^{10} Bq).

25–E. In addition to gamma rays, conversion electrons may also be emitted, resulting in both characteristic x-rays and Auger electrons.

26–C. 99mTc decays by an isomeric transition, and approximately 10% of the gamma photons undergo internal conversion producing internal conversion electrons; the resulting vacancies in the K-shells cause emission of characteristic x-rays and Auger electrons.

27–B. In β^- decay, a neutron in the nucleus is converted into a proton, and an energetic electron (beta particle) and antineutrino are emitted.

28–C. ^{3}H and ^{32}P undergo β^- decay, ^{99m}Tc emits a gamma ray, and ^{226}Ra is an alpha emitter.

29–C. In electron capture, an inner-shell electron is absorbed by the nucleus, leaving a vacancy that is subsequently filled by an outer-shell electron, resulting in the emission of characteristic radiation.

30–C. The mass number is reduced by four after the emission of the alpha particle; beta decay, electron capture, and isomeric transitions do not result in any change in mass number *(A)*.

2

X-ray Production

I. Generators

A. Introduction

–An x-ray generator provides power to the x-ray tube.

–X-ray generators also control the x-ray energy, exposure duration, and total exposure required for a particular examination.

–Generators contain high-voltage transformers, filament transformers, and rectifier circuits.

–Generators also include electronic circuits for manual and automatic exposure control, as well as voltage and current meters.

–In the United States, the electric power supply from utility companies is normally 120 volts (V) **alternating current** (AC), which oscillates at a frequency of 60 cycles per second (60 Hz).

–Generators for x-ray systems in radiology use higher voltages (440 V).

–A generator increases the voltage and **rectifies** the waveform from AC to **direct current** (DC).

–Generators permit x-ray operators to control three key parameters of x-ray operation: **x-ray tube voltage** (kilovolts, or kV), which affects the x-ray energy; **tube current** (milliamperes, or mA), which affects the radiation quantity; and **exposure time** (seconds).

–**Voltage** is applied **across** the x-ray tube, and **current** flows **through** the x-ray tube.

–The **power** dissipated equals the product of tube voltage *(V)* in kilovolts and of current in milliamperes *(I),* or $V \times I$, and is measured in **kilowatts** (kW).

–**Typical transformer ratings** in x-ray departments are **100 kV** and **800 mA,** which correspond to a power of 80 kW.

B. Transformers

–One major requirement of a generator is to produce high voltages, which can exceed 100,000 V.

–A transformer changes the size of the input voltage and is used to produce high and low voltages.

–**Step-up transformers** increase the voltage, and **step-down transformers** decrease the voltage.

–If two wire coils are wrapped around a common iron core, current in the primary coil produces a current in the secondary coil by **electromagnetic induction.**

–The voltages in the two circuits (V_p and V_s) are proportional to the number of turns in the two coils (N_p and N_s), expressed mathematically as $N_p/N_s = V_p/V_s$, where "p" refers to the primary and "s" to the secondary coils.

–The product of the voltage *(V)* and current *(I)* is equal to the power and must be equal in the two circuits (conservation of energy) if there are no additional losses.
  –For an ideal transformer, the power in the primary and secondary circuits will be equal, so that $V_p \times I_p = V_s \times I_s$.
–The step-up transformers used in x-ray generators have a secondary coil with many more turns (500:1) to produce a high voltage across the tube.
–Generators also have a step-down transformer with fewer turns in the secondary coil for the x-ray tube filament circuit, which only requires about 10 V.
–An **autotransformer** permits adjustment of the output voltage, using movable contacts to change the number of windings in the circuit.

C. Rectification

–The electric current from an AC power supply flows alternately in both directions, resulting in a voltage waveform shaped like a sine wave.
–**Rectification** changes the AC voltage into DC voltage across the x-ray tube.
–Rectification is achieved using **diodes,** which only permit current to flow in one direction.
  –With **half-wave rectification,** one direction of current is eliminated.
  –In **full-wave rectification** (achieved using a minimum of four diodes), two pulses per cycle are produced.
–**Single-phase generators** use a bridge rectifier circuit that directs the alternating flow of high-voltage electrons so that flow is always from cathode to anode.
–**Single-phase generators** have been replaced by **three-phase generators** for use in diagnostic radiology but may be encountered in dental x-ray units.
–**Three-phase generators** obtain power from three lines of current, each 120 degrees out of phase with the others.
–Diodes are arranged in combinations of **delta** and **wye** circuits to produce six- and 12-pulse outputs.
–Modern high-frequency inverter generators transform AC input into low-voltage DC, then into high-frequency AC, and finally into high voltage AC waveforms that are rectified to yield an approximately constant waveform.
–**High-frequency generators** are smaller and more efficient than are three-phase generators.

D. Voltage waveform

–**Voltage waveform** is a plot of voltage over time.
–A constant high voltage is desired across the x-ray tube for x-ray production, but in practice, there is some variation in the voltage, which is called **ripple.**
–The **peak voltage** or **kilovolt peak** (kVp) is the **maximum** voltage that crosses the x-ray tube during a complete waveform cycle.
–The voltage **waveform ripple** is the maximum voltage minus the minimum voltage per cycle expressed as a percentage of the maximum voltage.
  –Single-phase half- and full-wave rectified systems have 100% ripple.
  –Three-phase six-pulse systems typically have 14% ripple, and 12-pulse systems have approximately 4% ripple.
–High-frequency generators have ripple comparable to that of 12-pulse systems.
–A low ripple is desirable because a more constant voltage is produced.
–**Fig. 2.1** shows the waveforms for different types of generators and their corresponding ripple values.

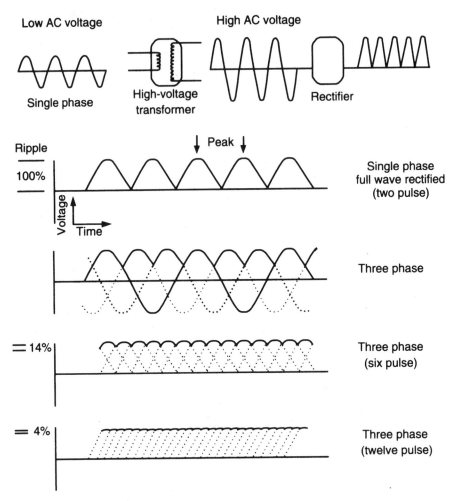

FIG. 2.1. A transformer is used to increase the voltage supplied by the power company to the high voltages (20,000 to 150,000 V) needed for x-ray production. Full-wave rectification with single-phase results in 2 pulses per cycle. Three-phase can be rectified to yield either a six- or 12-pulse waveform, which provides a more constant voltage.

II. X-Ray Production Processes

A. Introduction

–**Diagnostic x-rays** are produced when electrons with energies of 20 to 150 kilo electron volts (keV) are stopped in matter, producing electromagnetic radiation in the form of x-rays.

–Electrons accelerated to the positive anode gain a kinetic energy of V eV, determined solely by the value of the applied voltage *(V)*.

–The kinetic energy of electrons is transformed into heat and x-rays when the electrons strike the anode.

–Electrons only penetrate tens of micrometers (μm) into the anode before losing their energy by ionization and excitation of electrons in the anode material.

–Energetic electrons loose their energy in matter by **excitation,** in which electrons are energized to higher energy states; **ionization,** in which an outer-shell electron is removed; and **radiation,** in which the energy loss is converted directly to a photon.

–X-rays are generated by two different processes known as **bremsstrahlung** (radiation) and **characteristic** x-ray production (ionization).

–Most incident electrons interact with outer-shell electrons (excitation and ionization).

–Energy lost in the form of excitation and ionization appears as heat in the anode.

–The **efficiency** of x-ray production is approximately $\mathbf{kV} \times \mathbf{Z} \times 10^{-6}$ and is approximately 1% for materials with high atomic numbers *(Z)* at 100 kVp.

–A graph of x-ray tube output showing the number of photons at each x-ray energy is called a **spectrum.**

B. Bremsstrahlung radiation

–**Bremsstrahlung** (braking) x-rays are produced when incident electrons interact with nuclear electric fields, which slow them down (brake) and change their direction.

–**Fig. 2.2** shows a bremsstrahlung process in which a fraction of the initial electron kinetic energy is emitted as an x-ray photon.

–Bremsstrahlung x-rays produce a **continuous spectrum** of radiation, up to a maximum energy determined by the maximum kinetic energy of the incident electron.

–The closer the electron passes to the nucleus, the greater the interaction of the incident electron with the nucleus, and the higher the energy of the resulting x-ray.

–Maximum photon energies correspond to minimum x-ray wavelengths.

–The majority of x-rays produced in x-ray tubes are via the bremsstrahlung process.

–Bremsstrahlung x-ray production increases with the accelerating voltage (kV) and the atomic number (Z) of the anode.

C. Characteristic radiation

–**Characteristic radiation** is the result of ionization and is produced when inner-shell electrons of the anode target are ejected by the incident electrons.

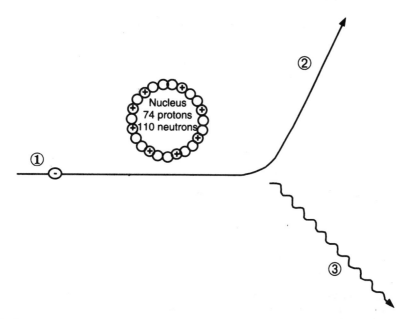

FIG. 2.2. Bremsstrahlung radiation is produced when an energetic electron *(1)* (with initial energy E_1) passes close to an atomic nucleus. The attractive force of the positively charged nucleus causes the electron to change direction and lose energy. The electron *(2)* now has a lower energy (E_2). The energy difference ($E_1 - E_2$) is released as an x-ray photon *(3).*

–To eject a bound atomic electron, the incident electron must have energy greater than the binding energy.

–The resultant vacancy is filled by an outer-shell electron, and the energy difference is emitted as characteristic radiation (e.g., K-shell x-rays, L-shell x-rays), as shown in **Fig. 2.3.**

–Characteristic x-rays occur only at discrete energy levels, unlike the continuous energy spectrum of bremsstrahlung.

–After the ejection of a K-shell electron, the excess energy may also be emitted as an Auger electron.

–Each anode material emits characteristic x-rays of a given energy, as listed in **Table 2.1.**

–K-shell characteristic x-ray energies are always slightly lower than the K-shell binding energy. (**Table 1.4** lists K-shell binding energies).

–K-shell electrons are ejected only if incident electrons have energies greater than the K-shell binding energy.

  –For tungsten, K-shell characteristic x-rays are only produced when the applied voltage exceeds 69.5 kV (K-shell binding energy is 69.5 keV).

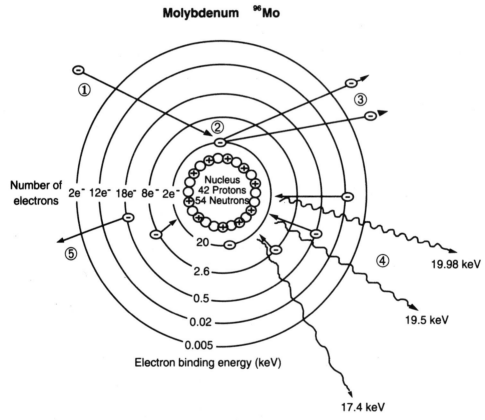

FIG. 2.3. Characteristic radiation is produced when an incoming electron *(1)* interacts with an inner-shell electron *(2)* and both are ejected *(3)*. When one of the outer-shell electrons moves to fill the inner-shell vacancy, the excess energy is emitted as characteristic radiation *(4)*. Sometimes the excess energy is emitted as an Auger electron *(5)* rather than as characteristic radiation.

TABLE 2.1. *Selected characteristic x-ray energies*

| Anode material | Atomic no. | Characteristic x-ray energy (keV) | |
		K-shell	L-shell
Copper (Cu)	29	8.0–8.9	0.9
Molybdenum (Mo)	42	17.4–19.6	2.3–2.6
Tin (Sn)	50	25.0–28.5	3.4–4.1
Tungsten (W)	74	58.0–67.2	8.3–11.3

–For molybdenum, K-shell characteristic x-rays are only produced when the applied voltage exceeds 20 kV.

–L-shell radiation also accompanies K-shell radiation, but because L-shell characteristic x-rays have very low energies, they are absorbed by the glass of the x-ray tube.

–Only K-shell characteristic x-rays are important in diagnostic radiology.

D. Quantity

–**Intensity** refers to the quantity or number of x-ray photons produced.

–Intensity is affected by the generator type, beam filtration, and distance from the beam (inverse square law).

–For conventional radiography with a tungsten target, the characteristic radiation produced accounts for up to 10% of the x-ray beam intensity.

–X-ray output is directly proportional to the current (mA), and to exposure time (seconds).

–The product of the tube current (mA) and exposure time (seconds) is known as the mAs, and the x-ray tube output is proportional to the mAs.

  –Doubling the current at constant exposure time has the same effect as doubling the exposure time at constant tube current.

–Doubling the mAs doubles the number of x-rays emitted but does not change the energy spectrum.

–**Fig. 2.4A** shows how the number of photons at each energy level increases when the tube current is increased, but the spectrum shape does not change.

–The **quantity** of x-rays produced can also be increased by increasing the kVp, but this also changes the quality or shape of the x-ray spectrum, as shown in **Fig. 2.4B**.

  –The quantity (intensity) of x-ray production is approximately proportional to the square of the tube potential.

E. Quality

–X-ray beams in diagnostic radiology are **polychromatic** and consist of a range of photon energies.

–**Quality** refers to effective photon energy of the x-rays produced, and relates to their ability to penetrate the patient.

–The quality of an x-ray beam is obtained from the **effective x-ray energy** of the x-ray spectrum.

–The effective photon energy is taken to be between one third and one half of the maximum photon energy.

  –Increasing the peak voltage (kVp) increases the x-ray tube output, peak energy, and mean energy of the beam.

  –This increases the beam quality as shown in **Fig. 2.4B**.

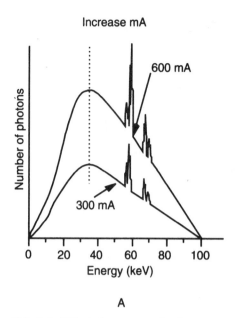 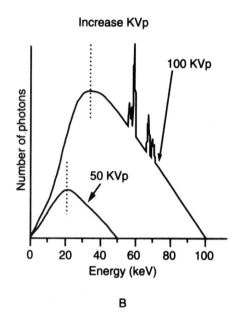

A   B

FIG. 2.4. Effect of current and voltage on x-ray spectra. **(A)** When the mA is increased and the peak voltage and exposure time are constant, the intensity of the x-rays increases but the energy distribution stays the same. **(B)** When peak voltage is increased and the milliamperes and exposure time are constant, the intensity, peak, and mean energy of the x-rays increase.

–Increasing beam quality increases x-ray beam **penetrating power** because the average photon energy is higher.

–A rule of thumb is that increasing the peak voltage by 15% has the same effect on film density as that of doubling the mAs.

–For example, changing tube voltage by 10 kVp (from 65 to 75 kVp) normally has the same effect on film density as doubling the mAs.

–Reducing the voltage waveform ripple increases average photon energy and thus x-ray beam quality.

–Increasing x-ray tube filtration also increases beam quality, as low-energy photons are preferentially removed from the x-ray beam **(beam hardening).**

–**Table 2.2** lists typical x-ray outputs as a function of x-ray tube voltage and filtration.

III. X-Ray Tubes

A. Introduction

–The x-ray tube converts the electric power from the generator into x-ray photons.

–**Fig. 2.5** is a diagram of a radiographic x-ray tube.

TABLE 2.2. *Typical x-ray outputs for a three-phase generator*

Peak voltage (kVp)	X-ray output (mGy/mAs) at 100 cm*	
	2.5 mm Al filtration	3.5 mm Al filtration
80	0.10	0.08
100	0.15	0.12
120	0.20	0.17

* 1 mGy ~ 100 mR.

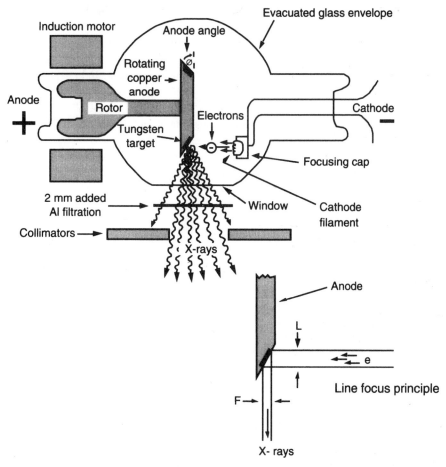

FIG. 2.5. Major components of an x-ray tube. The tube is typically surrounded by an oil bath and lead housing. The magnified view of the target illustrates the line focus principle, whereby the focal spot size *(F)* is smaller than the electron beam *(L)* because of the anode angle.

–X-ray tubes contain a negatively charged **cathode** containing the **filament** that serves as an electron source.

–The **anode** is positively charged and includes the target where x-rays are produced.

–The anode may be stationary or rotating, in which case the tube also contains a rotor and stator.

–The anode and cathode are contained in an evacuated envelope to prevent the electrons from colliding with gas molecules.

–The envelope is contained in a **tube housing** that protects and insulates the tube and provides shielding to prevent leakage radiation.

–The housing contains an oil bath to provide electrical insulation and help cool the tube.

–The primary x-rays exit through a window in the tube housing.

–The x-ray window may be a thinner area in the glass or a different material such as beryllium, which absorbs fewer low-energy x-rays (used in mammography).

B. Filaments

–The **filament** is the source of electrons that are accelerated toward the anode to produce x-rays.

–The filament is usually made of coiled tungsten wire, with modern x-ray tubes having two filaments to allow a choice of two focal spot sizes.

–A **focusing cup** or **cathode block** surrounds the filament and helps direct the electrons toward the target.

–**Typical voltages across** the x-ray tube filament are **10 V,** and **currents through** the cathode filament are **4 A.**

–The power dissipated from the filament $(I \times V)$ is typically 40 W.

–The high resistance in the filament causes temperature to rise (>2200°C), resulting in the thermionic emission of electrons.

–Electrons emitted from a heated filament form a negative cloud around the filament called a **space charge,** which prevents further emission of electrons.

–The **tube current** is the flow of electrons from the filament to the anode; this occurs when a negative potential is applied to the filament (cathode) and a positive potential is applied to the anode.

–Tube current is in the range of 1 to 1,000 mA.

–At low peak voltage, the potential is insufficient to cause all the electrons to be pulled away from the filament, and a residual space charge remains (**space charge limited** operation).

–At the **saturation voltage,** all electrons are immediately pulled away from the filament, and the tube current is maximized.

–Above 40 kVp, the filament current is proportional to and determines the tube current **(emission-limited operation).**

C. Anode

–The **anode** is the positive electrode in the x-ray tube.

–Electrons striking the target, located in the anode, produce heat and x-rays.

–**Tungsten** is the most common target material because of its high atomic number (Z = 74) and melting point.

  –Rhenium is often added to reduce the pitting and cracking caused by overheating.

–Molybdenum (Z = 42) and rhodium (Z = 45) are used for targets in mammography.

–A **stationary anode usually** consists of a tungsten target embedded in a copper block.

  –Although copper is a good heat conductor, heat dissipation is limited.

  –Stationary anodes are used in some C-arm x-ray units.

–A **rotating anode** greatly increases the effective target area used during an exposure and therefore raises the heat capacity.

–To maintain the vacuum required inside the x-ray tube, rotating anodes use an electric induction motor.

–The rotor (inside the envelope) turns in response to the changing electric current in the stator electric windings (outside the envelope).

D. Focal spots

–The **focal spot** is the apparent source of x-rays in the tube.

–Focal spot size is a result of the filament shape, focusing cup, and electric field created between the cathode and anode.

–Focal spots must be small to produce sharp images, but large enough to tolerate a high heat loading without melting the target.

  –The focal spot size enlarges as milliamperes increase owing to the repulsion of adjacent electrons. This effect is called **blooming.**

TABLE 2.3. *Focal spot sizes used in diagnostic radiology*

Nominal focal spot size (mm)	Clinical applications
0.1–0.15	Magnification mammography
0.3	Mammography; magnification radiography
0.6*	Conventional radiography (small focal spot)
1.2	Conventional radiography (large focal spot)

* Also used for fluoroscopy.

–The **line focus principle** is used to permit larger heat loading while minimizing the size of the focal spot by orienting the anode at a small angle to the direction of the x-ray beam irradiating the patient (inset in **Fig. 2.5**).

–The anode angle is the angle between the target surface and the central beam.

–Typical anode angles range from about 7 to 20 degrees.

–Radiation field coverage increases with increased target angle.

–The **focal spot** size is the dimension of the x-ray source as viewed from the image.

–**Focal spot** sizes, as quoted by manufacturers of x-ray tubes, range from about 0.1 to 1.2 mm.

–Focal spot dimensions, as quoted by manufacturers, are nominal values.

–Focal spot sizes can be measured using pinhole cameras, star or bar test patterns, or slit cameras.

–Measured **focal spot** sizes may be up to 50% larger than the nominal values listed in **Table 2.3**.

–A large focal spot is favored when a short exposure time is the priority.

–A small focal spot is preferred when spatial resolution is a priority.

IV. Tube Loading

A. X-ray techniques

–In manual mode, the operator selects the x-ray tube voltage, x-ray tube current, and exposure time on the generator control panel.

–In **automatic exposure control** (AEC) mode, the operator selects the x-ray voltage and the desired film density, and the generator circuits control the exposure time and current (mAs).

–The x-ray tube output is directly proportional to the x-ray tube current.

–A typical current for radiography is 100 to 1,000 mA.

–Typical radiographic exposure times are between tens and hundreds of millisecond.

–Typical tube current exposure times in radiography are tens of mAs.

–In fluoroscopy, tube currents are typically between 1 and 5 mA.

–For small body parts, such as the extremities, x-ray tube voltages are generally 55 to 65 kVp.

–Most radiographic and fluoroscopy imaging is performed at x-ray tube voltages between 70 and 90 kVp.

–Higher voltages may be used for larger patients.

–Chest radiography is often performed at higher x-ray tube voltages of about 120 kVp.

–High voltages (>100 kVp) are also used in some fluoroscopy performed with barium contrast agents to provide sufficient penetration.

B. Energy deposition

  –Only about 1% of the electric energy supplied to the x-ray tube is converted to x-rays.

  –Approximately 99% of the electrical energy supplied to an x-ray tube is converted to heat.

  –The amount of heat energy deposited during an x-ray exposure is known as **the tube loading.**

  –X-ray tube loading depends on the tube voltage, voltage waveform, tube current, exposure time, and number of exposures.

    –For a constant x-ray tube voltage *(V)* and current *(I)*, the energy deposited during an x-ray exposure is $V \times I \times t$ joules, where t is the exposure time measured in seconds.

    –This energy is temporarily stored in the anode, which has a heat capacity of several hundred thousand joules.

  –X-ray tube loading is assessed by using an x-ray tube rating chart and an anode thermal characteristics chart.

  –If the voltage is not constant, the calculation of energy deposition in joules is more complicated.

  –For systems with single-phase power supplies and full-wave rectification, the quantity *kVp* $\times$ *mA* $\times$ *time* is termed **heat units.** One heat unit = 0.74 J (1 J = 1.35 heat units).

C. Tube rating

  –The **rating** of an x-ray tube is based on maximum allowable kilowatts (kW) at an exposure time of 0.1 second.

    –For example, a tube with a rating of 80 kW (80,000 W) tolerates a maximum exposure of 80 kVp and 1,000 mA at 0.1 second.

  –Typical x-ray tube ratings are between 5 and 100 kW and depend on focal spot size.

  –The loading on the focal spot, anode, and x-ray tube housing must be considered to ensure none of these components overheats.

  –In radiography, power loadings are typically 80 to 100 kW for a large focal spot size and 20 kW for the small focal spot size

  –In fluoroscopy, power loadings are very low and typically between 100 to 500 W.

  –Increasing the exposure time or using a larger focal spot size may be required to achieve the required x-ray tube output without overheating.

D. X-ray tube heat dissipation

  –X-ray tubes are designed to efficiently dissipate heat.

  –Modern anodes are circular and rotated at high speeds (3,000 to 10,000 rpm) to spread heat loading over a large area.

  –Heat is transferred from the focal spot by **radiation** to the tube housing and **conduction** into the anode.

    –Radiation is the primary way that anodes transfer heat from the anode to the housing, as the anode gets white hot during the x-ray exposure.

  –X-ray tubes are usually immersed in oil for electrical insulation and for aiding heat dissipation by **convection.**

  –Air fans are sometimes used to increase the rate of heat loss.

  –Cooling of the anode and housing are described by thermal characteristics charts.

  –Taking a large number of radiographs, or a prolonged acquisition in computed tomography, can result in the tube overheating.

–An x-ray tube that has reached the maximum anode heat loading may require several minutes to cool down before additional use.

–In fluoroscopy, the rate at which heat is deposited into the anode (100 to 500 W) is low enough that the heat dissipation rate will always prevent overheating.

–Fluoroscopy can normally be performed without the risk of tube overheating.

V. Diagnostic X-Ray Beams

A. Filters

–The x-ray beam emerging from the x-ray tube may contain a high number of low-energy photons.

–Low-energy photons have a negligible chance of getting through the patient, thereby contributing to patient dose but adding nothing to the image.

–Some of the very low energy x-rays are stopped as they exit the x-ray tube by the glass window, which acts as an inherent x-ray beam filter.

–Beryllium provides very little filtration and is often used as a window in mammography x-ray tubes, which use low-energy photons.

–Filters are also added to the x-ray tube window to increase the filtration effect, as listed in **Table 2.4.**

–Filters are designed to preferentially absorb low-energy photons.

–Added filtration does not affect the maximum energy of the x-ray beam spectrum.

–Added filtration will *always* reduce the x-ray tube output.

B. Beam hardening

–**Beam hardening** refers to the **preferential loss** of lower-energy photons from a polychromatic beam with filtration.

–Beam hardening results in a change in x-ray spectrum shape but not in maximum photon energy.

–The x-ray beam output is decreased with increased filtration (**Table 2.2**), but the average x-ray energy is increased.

–The x-ray beam becomes **more penetrating** as mean photon energy increases.

–Filtered beams with higher mean photon energies are called **harder** x-ray beams.

–Beam hardening does not occur with monochromatic x-ray beams.

–**Hard beams** are produced at high peak voltages using heavy filtration.

–**Soft beams** are produced at low peak voltages using less filtration.

–**Fig. 2.6** shows the effect of filtration on an x-ray spectrum in which low-energy photons are preferentially lost when passing through a filter (or any absorber).

C. Heel effect

–At typical energy levels used in radiography, x-rays are produced within the anode that travel equally in all directions (isotropic).

TABLE 2.4. *Representative filtration values*

Technique	Filtration value (kVp)	Typical added filtration
Screen/film mammography	25–30	30 μm molybdenum
Radiography	~80	>2.5 mm aluminum
High-voltage studies (chest)	>100	Copper/aluminum
High-energy imaging	>200	Tin/copper/aluminum*

* Thoraeus filter.

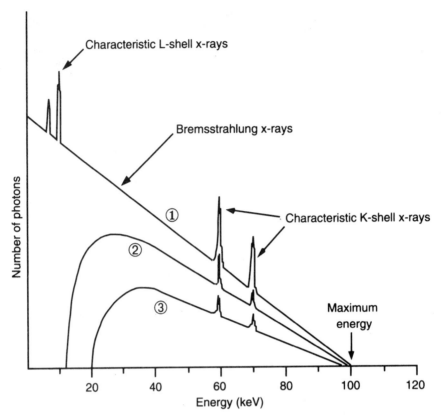

FIG. 2.6. X-ray emission spectra from a tungsten target produced at 100 kV. Curve *1* is the theoretical spectrum without any filtration. Curve *2* is the typical spectrum with the inherent filtration of the x-ray tube and added filtration. Curve *3* shows the effect of additional filtration.

–However, x-rays produced within the anode must pass through a portion of the target and are attenuated as they pass out of the anode material.

–This attenuation is greater in the anode direction than in the cathode direction because of differences in the path length within the target.

–This is known as the **heel effect** and results in higher x-ray intensity at the cathode end and in lower x-ray intensity at the anode end of the beam.

–The magnitude of the heel effect depends on the anode angle (**Fig. 2.5**), source-to-image detector distance, and field size.

  –To reduce the heel effect, the anode angle should be increased, source-to-image detector distance increased, and field size decreased.

–The heel effect can be taken advantage of by placing denser parts of the body at the cathode side and thinner parts at the anode side of the beam.

  –In mammography, for example, the more intense cathode side is used to irradiate the denser chest wall region.

D. Unwanted radiation

  –X-ray tubes are surrounded by lead to absorb unwanted radiation.

  –**Leakage radiation** is radiation that is transmitted through the x-ray tube housing.

–Federal regulations require the leakage radiation at 1 m to be no more than 1 mGy/hour (100 mR/hour).

–**Scattered radiation** has been deviated in direction after leaving the tube.

–The intensity of scattered radiation is typically 0.1% of the intensity incident on a patient, when measured 1 m from the patient.

–**Stray radiation** is the sum of the leakage and scattered radiation.

Review Test

1. The power loading on a target operated at 80 kV and 100 mA:

(A) Is 8 kJ
(B) Is 8 kW
(C) Is 8 kW/second
(D) Is 8 keV
(E) Cannot be determined

2. Transformers in an x-ray machine:

(A) Work on the principle of electromagnetic induction
(B) Need a filament as a source of electrons
(C) Are used to transform electron energy into x-rays
(D) Use thermionic emission
(E) Cannot be used to generate low voltages

3. Alternating electric current sources produce:

(A) Static electric fields
(B) Static magnetic fields
(C) Unidirectional flow of electrons
(D) Oscillatory flows of electrons
(E) Stationary electrons

4. Which high-voltage generator results in the *longest* exposure time?

(A) Constant potential
(B) High-frequency
(C) Three-phase (12-pulse)
(D) Three-phase (six-pulse)
(E) Single-phase

5. Electrons passing through matter lose energy primarily by:

(A) Production of bremsstrahlung radiation
(B) Photoelectric interactions
(C) Collision with atomic electrons
(D) Compton interactions
(E) Thermionic emission

6. The continuous x-ray spectrum obtained from an x-ray tube is caused by:

(A) Transition of electrons between atomic energy levels
(B) Deceleration of electrons in the target
(C) Target heating by the electrons
(D) Ejection of K-shell electrons
(E) Ionization of target atoms

7. The maximum photon energy in a x-ray beam is determined by:

(A) Atomic number of the target
(B) Atomic number of the x-ray beam filter
(C) Voltage across the x-ray tube
(D) Total exposure time (seconds)
(E) Current flowing through the x-ray tube

8. Characteristic x-rays are characteristic of the:

(A) Mass number *(A)* of the target atoms
(B) Energy of the projectile electrons
(C) Electron shell structure of the target atom
(D) X-ray tube voltage
(E) material used for the x-ray filament

9. X-ray production with a tungsten anode at 100 kVp is primarily:

(A) Bremsstrahlung radiation
(B) Characteristic radiation
(C) Compton scatter
(D) Photoelectric
(E) Coherent scatter

10. Changing the x-ray tube current (mA) is most likely to modify the x-ray beam:

(A) Maximum energy
(B) Characteristic x-ray energy
(C) Quantity
(D) Quality
(E) Patient penetration (%)

11. X-ray tube output is increased *most strongly* by increasing the:

(A) Voltage across the tube (kVp)
(B) Anode diameter
(C) Atomic number *(Z)* of the target
(D) Tube current (mA)
(E) Filtration

12. All are true of the *average* photon energy in a x-ray beam except:

(A) Is less than the maximum energy
(B) Increases with increasing voltage
(C) Increases with x-ray beam filtration
(D) Is independent of the mAs
(E) Decreases with increasing distance

13. X-ray beam quality is determined primarily by:

(A) Focal spot size
(B) Filament current

(C) X-ray tube current
(D) Filament voltage
(E) X-ray tube voltage

14. The x-ray tube output increases when what is reduced?

(A) mA
(B) Filament current
(C) Voltage
(D) Filtration
(E) Exposure time

15. The number of electrons accelerated across an x-ray tube is determined by:

(A) Anode speed
(B) Focal spot size
(C) Filament current
(D) X-ray tube filtration
(E) X-ray tube voltage

16. The typical current in a x-ray tube filament is:

(A) 4 mA
(B) 40 mA
(C) 0.4 A
(D) 4 A
(E) 40 A

17. Targets for production of x-rays have:

(A) Low atomic numbers *(Z)*
(B) Air cooling
(C) Beryllium covering
(D) High heat capacities
(E) Good insulation

18. All are true of the small focal spot in radiographic x-ray tubes except:

(A) The origin of x-rays
(B) Typically 0.6 mm
(C) Used in fluoroscopy
(D) Used to get good resolution
(E) Increases power loading

19. The line focus principle may be explained as:

(A) Apparent focus is smaller than exposed target region
(B) Another name for the heel effect
(C) X-ray intensity falls as square of distance
(D) Reduction in intensity at anode edge
(E) Image magnification

20. All are true of the size of an x-ray tube focal spot except:

(A) Larger than the nominal value by up to 50%
(B) Dependent on applied milliamperes (blooming)

(C) Smaller for magnification radiography
(D) Measured using pinhole cameras
(E) Increases with additional filtration

21. Which of the following is *not* typical of a chest x-ray technique factor?

(A) 120 kVp
(B) 500 mA
(C) 20 millisecond exposure time
(D) 0.1 mm focal spot
(E) 3 mm Al filtration

22. The ratio of heat to x-rays produced in a x-ray tube is about:

(A) 1:99
(B) 10:90
(C) 50:50
(D) 90:10
(E) 99:1

23. The formula mA $\times$ kV $\times$ time for a constant potential x-ray generator is:

(A) Heat units deposited
(B) The total energy deposited
(C) The exposure level at 1 m
(D) The focal spot loading (power)
(E) Filament heating

24. Heat generated in an anode is primarily dissipated by:

(A) Convection
(B) Conduction
(C) Combustion
(D) Air cooling
(E) Radiation

25. Filters remove mainly what type of radiation from an x-ray beam?

(A) Scatter
(B) Low-energy
(C) High-energy
(D) Leakage
(E) Stray

26. Increasing the filtration of a 120 kV x-ray beam from 2 to 3 mm Al will not:

(A) Reduce the intensity
(B) Keep the maximum x-ray energy the same
(C) Increase the effective x-ray energy
(D) Result in a shorter exposure time
(E) Harden the beam

27. Beam hardening is affected primarily by:

(A) Filament current
(B) Tube current

(C) Exposure time
(D) Filtration
(E) Distance from x-ray tube

28. The heel effect is more pronounced:

(A) At larger distances from the focal spot
(B) With a larger target (anode) angle
(C) With a smaller anode angle
(D) At the cathode edge of the x-ray field
(E) Perpendicular to the anode-cathode axis

29. Radiation transmitted through the *tube housing* of a x-ray tube is called:

(A) Transmitted beam
(B) Primary radiation
(C) Stray radiation
(D) Leakage radiation
(E) Scattered radiation

30. Stray radiation is the sum of:

(E) Primary and transmitted
(B) Primary and scatter
(C) Scatter and leakage
(D) Primary and leakage
(E) Transmitted and leakage

Answers and Explanations

1–B. Power is the product of the voltage (kV) and current (mA), and is expressed in watts (1 W = 1 J/second).

2–A. Transformers are used to generate high (or low) voltages and operate according to the laws of electromagnetic induction.

3–D. In North America, voltage changes direction 60 times per second (60 Hz), resulting in an oscillating flow of electrons in the circuit.

4–E. Single-phase waveforms produce fewer lower-energy nonpenetrating x-rays as the waveform drops toward 0 kVp during each pulse, which results in longer exposure times.

5–C. Up to 99% of the electron energy is lost by collisions with outer-shell atomic electrons (i.e., ionizations and excitations), which will appear as heat in the x-ray tube target.

6–B. The continuous x-ray spectrum (bremsstrahlung) occurs when an electron undergoes rapid deceleration in the nuclear electric field.

7–C. The voltage across the x-ray tube determines the maximum photon energy. (Doubling the current will double the x-ray tube output but have no effect on the x-ray spectrum shape.)

8–C. The electron shell structure of the atoms in the target determines the characteristic x-rays emitted.

9–A. Bremsstrahlung. Characteristic x-ray production only accounts for a few percent of a typical x-ray beam produced at 100 kVp.

10–C. The x-ray beam quantity (intensity) is directly proportional to the x-ray tube current.

11–A. Increasing tube current and atomic number *(Z)* of the anode increases the x-ray output approximately linearly; the largest increase is from the peak kilovolts, for which the output is approximately the square of voltage.

12–E. Distance does not affect the average x-ray energy.

13–E. The x-ray tube voltage determines the x-ray beam quality; the higher the voltage, the higher the average x-ray energy and the more penetrating the x-ray beam.

14–D. Reducing filtration permits more x-rays to emerge from the x-ray tube.

15–C. The filament current determines the filament heating and the corresponding rate of release of electrons, which determines the x-ray tube current.

16–D. A typical filament operates at 4 A and 10 V (40 W), which is a power rating comparable to a common domestic light bulb.

17–D. Anodes need high heat capacities to prevent their melting when subjected to high power loadings.

18–E. Power loading is lower for small focal spot sizes.

19–A. The line focus principle results in an apparent focal spot that is smaller than the area of the anode irradiated by the x-ray tube current, and depends on the anode angle (Fig. 2.5).

20–D. Focal spot size in chest radiography is 1 mm, not 0.1 mm..

21–E. All the techniques given are representative values for a chest x-ray examination performed on a dedicated chest x-ray unit.

22–E. Ninety-nine percent of the energy appears as heat in the anode.

23–B. This expression for a constant potential generator gives the total energy deposited in the anode.

24–E. Heat dissipation occurs primarily by radiation through the x-ray tube vacuum into the housing (anodes get white hot during prolonged exposures).

25–B. Filters are used to remove the low-energy photons that increase patient dose but do not contribute to the image.

26–D. Exposure times will be increased, because additional filtration reduces the exposure rate, which needs to be offset by using a longer exposure time.

27–D. Only filtration affects the average photon energy (quality) in the x-ray beam, whereas the other four factors affect the beam quantity (intensity).

28–C. The heel effect is more pronounced with smaller target (anode) angles.

29–D. Leakage radiation, which should be less than 1 mGy/hr at 1 meter.

30–C. Stray radiation is the sum of the leakage and scattered radiation.

3

X-ray Interactions

I. Absorption and Scattering

A. Introduction

–X-rays traveling through matter can be transmitted, absorbed, or scattered.

–**Attenuation** is the removal of x-ray photons, as a result of tissue absorption and scatter, from the x-ray beam as it passes through matter.

–**X-ray photons** may **pass through** matter unaffected (i.e., penetrate), **be absorbed** (and transfer their energy to the tissue), or **be scattered** (i.e., change direction and possibly lose energy).

–**Compton scatter** and the **photoelectric (PE) effect** are the two most important x-ray interactions in diagnostic radiology.

–**Coherent scatter** is of minor importance in diagnostic radiology.

–**Pair production** and **photodisintegration** do not occur in a diagnostic radiology environment.

–The arrangement of atoms in the molecule (i.e., molecular structure) has a negligible effect on photon interactions.

–X-ray photons transfer energy to electrons, normally in substantial amounts, which are measured in kiloelectron volts (keV).

–These energetic electrons, in turn, lose energy by interacting with the orbital electrons from other atoms and producing additional ionizations.

–An energetic electron may produce several hundred additional ion pairs.

–The approximate maximum distances, or ranges, traveled by energetic electrons are listed in **Table 3.1**.

B. Coherent scatter

–**Coherent scatter** occurs when a low-energy **x-ray photon excites an atom but then passes through** without any net energy transfer to the atom.

–Coherent scatter is sometimes referred to as Rayleigh or classical scatter.

–Coherent scatter does not result in any energy deposition in the patient (i.e., dose).

–The scattered x-ray photon is usually emitted from the atom in a forward direction.

–Coherent scatter is generally present in diagnostic radiology but is of minimal concern.

–Coherent scatter typically accounts for only 5% of all photon interactions at diagnostic energies.

C. Pair production and photodisintegration

–**Pair production** occurs when a high-energy photon interacts with the nucleus of an atom and is converted to matter and antimatter.

–In pair production, the photon disappears, and the energy is converted into an **electron** and a **positron**.

TABLE 3.1. *Distances traveled by energetic elections in media of different effective atomic number and physical density*

Electron energy (keV)	Air* (cm)	Water† (μm)	Bone‡ (μm)
10	0.25	3	2
30	1.7	18	12
50	4.1	43	28
100	13.5	140	94
150	26.5	280	180

* Atomic number, 7.8; physical density, 0.0012 g/cm^3.
† Atomic number, 7.5; physical density, 1.0 g/cm^3.
‡ Atomic number, 12.3; physical density, 1.7 g/cm^3.

–Pair production has a photon energy threshold of 1.02 MeV, which is the energy required to produce an electron (511 keV) and positron (511 keV) pair.
  –The positron eventually combines with an electron, producing two 511 keV photons that are emitted at 180 degree to each other (annihilation radiation).
–**Photodisintegration** occurs when a high-energy photon is absorbed by a nucleus, resulting in **immediate disintegration** of the nucleus.
–The **energy threshold** for photodisintegration is approximately **15 MeV.**
–Photodisintegration and pair production are important only at the high-photon energies encountered in megavoltage radiotherapy.

D. Image formation

–The information captured by image receptors in diagnostic radiology is a result of the interaction, or lack of interaction, of the x-ray beam with patient tissues.
–Important factors affecting these photon interactions include the **incident photon energy** and the **density, thickness,** and **atomic number** *(Z)* of the medium.
–Scatter results in some energy deposited in the patient (dose).
–Scatter contributes to image degradation (loss of image contrast).
–Absorption contributes to image contrast but will increase the dose to the patient.
  –Understanding these x-ray interactions permits operators to change the x-ray tube voltage and thereby change image quality and patient dose.
–An important goal of selecting radiographic techniques is to optimize image quality and minimize patient dose.

II. Photoelectric and Compton Effects

A. Photoelectric effect

–The **PE effect** occurs between tightly bound (**inner-shell) electrons** and incident x-ray photons.
–The PE effect occurs when a photon is totally absorbed (PE absorption) by an inner-shell electron and an electron is ejected (**photoelectron is emitted).**
  –As a result of the photoelectron emission, a positive atomic ion is formed.
–The energy of the emitted photoelectron equals the difference between the incident photon energy and the electron binding energy.
–The photoelectron loses energy by ionizing other atoms in the tissue and contributes to patient dose.
–Outer-shell electrons then fill the inner-shell electron vacancies to stabilize the atom, and the excess energy is emitted as **characteristic radiation** or Auger electrons.

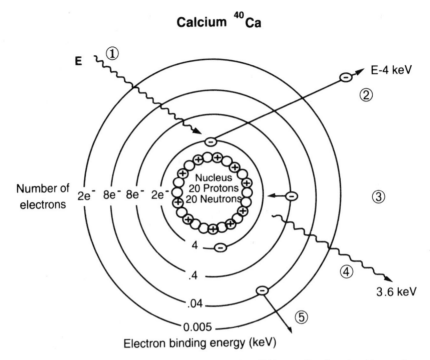

FIG. 3.1. The PE effect occurs when an incident x-ray *(1)* is totally absorbed by an inner-shell electron, which is ejected as a photoelectron *(2)*. The vacancy *(3)* is filled by an outer-shell electron, and the energy difference is emitted as characteristic radiation *(4)* or as an Auger electron *(5)*.

–An **Auger electron** is an outer-shell electron with a binding energy less than the energy difference of the electron transition.

–The alternative to an Auger electron is the emission of a characteristic x-ray.

–**Fig. 3.1** shows a PE interaction.

B. Probability of photoelectric effect

–For the PE effect to occur, the incident x-ray must have energy at least equal to or greater than the binding energy of the inner-shell electron.

   –The absorption of photons increases markedly as the x-ray photon energy is increased from below to above the binding energy of the K-shell electrons (K-edge).

   –The binding energy of the K-shell electrons (K-edge) in iodine is 33 keV, and a sharp increase in the interaction of photons occurs when the x-ray photon energy exceeds 33 keV.

–However, the probability of PE absorption decreases rapidly as the photon energy *(E)* further increases above the k-edge, and is **proportional to $1/E^3$**.

–The PE effect predominates at energies just above the k-edge of the absorber.

–The probability of PE absorption increases significantly with atomic number and is **proportional to Z^3**.

–The more tightly bound an electron is, the greater is the probability of the PE effect, if *E* is greater than the binding energy.

   –Photoelectric absorption is thus highest for K-shell electrons, which are most tightly bound in an atom, followed by the L-shell, and so on.

–The PE effect is important if the atomic number *(Z)* is high and the photon energy is just above the K-edge.

–Important K-shell binding energies are as follows: oxygen ($Z = 8$), 0.5 keV; calcium ($Z = 20$), 4 keV; iodine ($Z = 53$), 33 keV; barium ($Z = 56$), 37 keV; and lead ($Z = 82$), 88 keV.

C. Compton scatter

–In **Compton scatter,** incident photons interact with loosely bound valence **(outer-shell) electrons.**

–A Compton interaction results in a **scattered photon** that has less energy than that of the incident photon, and that travels in a new direction.

–The scattered photon may participate in additional tissue interactions, or reach the image receptor and degrade image quality.

–The higher the incident photon energy, the more likely that the direction of scatter will be in a forward direction.

–A **scattered (ejected or recoil) electron** carries the energy lost by the incident photon.

  –This electron loses energy by excitation and ionization of other atoms in the tissue, thereby contributing to the patient dose.

–As a result of the Compton interaction, a positive atomic ion, which has lost an outer-shell electron, remains.

–Compton interactions occur most commonly with electrons with a low binding energy.

  –Outer-shell electrons have binding energies of only a few electron volts, which is negligible compared with the high energy (30 keV) of a typical diagnostic energy x-ray photon.

–**Fig. 3.2** shows a Compton interaction.

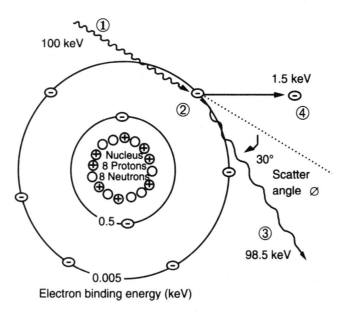

FIG. 3.2. Compton scattering occurs when an incoming x-ray photon *(1)* interacts with an outer-shell electron *(2)*. The x-ray photon loses energy and changes direction *(3)*. The Compton electron carries away the energy lost by the scattered photon *(4)*.

TABLE 3.2. *Energies of Compton-scattered photons deflected through 90 and 180 degrees**

	Photon energy (keV)	
Incident	Scattered 90 degrees	Scattered 180 degrees
60	54	49
80	69	61
100	84	72
120	97	82

* Energy difference between incident and scattered photons is transferred to the Compton-scattered electron.

–Compton interactions account for most scattered radiation encountered in diagnostic radiology.

D. Probability of a Compton interaction

–The **probability** of a Compton interaction is **proportional to the number of outer-shell electrons** available in the medium (electron density).

–Compton interactions are **inversely proportional to the photon energy (1/E).**

–Scattered photons may move in any direction, including 180 degrees to the direction of the incident photon (**backscattered**).

–As the angle of deflection decreases, the energy retained by the scattered x-ray increases.

–Energy transfer to the electron is maximized when the photon is backscattered.

–The incident and Compton-scattered x-ray energies at different scatter angles are listed in **Table 3.2.**

–For soft tissue, the PE and Compton effects are equal in magnitude, at 25 keV.

III. Attenuation of Radiation

A. Linear attenuation coefficient

–The **linear attenuation coefficient** (μ) is the fraction of incident photons removed from the beam in traveling unit distance, expressed in inverse centimeters (cm^{-1}).

–The attenuation coefficient accounts for all possible x-ray interactions, including coherent scatter, the PE effect and Compton scatter.

–The attenuation coefficient generally increases with atomic number.

–Attenuation also increases with increasing physical density of the absorbing medium.

–In diagnostic radiology, attenuation decreases with increasing photon energy (except at K-edges).

–**Monochromatic** (monoenergetic) x-rays are absorbed according to the **exponential formula** $N = N_0 e^{-\mu t}$, where N_0 is the initial number of photons incident on an absorbing medium of thickness t (cm), N is the number of photons transmitted, and μ (cm^{-1}) is the attenuation coefficient.

–An attenuation coefficient of 0.01/cm (0.01 cm^{-1}) means that 1% of the incident photons are lost (absorbed or scattered) in traveling 1 cm, with the remaining 99% being transmitted.

–Attenuation coefficients are a function of photon energy; the value of soft tissue μ is 0.38 cm^{-1} at 30 keV, but is 0.21 cm^{-1} at 60 keV.

–Bone μ is 1.6 cm^{-1} at 30 keV and 0.45 cm^{-1} at 60 keV.

B. Mass attenuation coefficient

  –The probability of an x-ray photon interacting with matter depends on the number of atoms encountered.

  –The linear attenuation coefficient normally depends on the density of the absorbing material.

  –For any absorbing medium, however, the attenuation is the same with only half the thickness but double the density.

   –For example, compression of lung has no effect on photon transmission because the amount of absorbing material (i.e., total number of atoms) remains the same.

   –However, the values of *both* the attenuation coefficient (μ) and density (ρ) change as the lungs are expanded or compressed.

  –The **mass attenuation coefficient** is the linear attenuation coefficient (μ) divided by density (ρ).

  –Use of the mass attenuation coefficient allows attenuation to be described as a function of the mass of the material traversed rather than the physical distance.

   –The mass attenuation coefficient is independent of the density of the material.

   –The thickness of the absorbing medium must be specified using the **mass thickness g/cm^2, or $\rho \times t$.**

  –X-ray attenuation is determined by the product of the mass thickness and mass attenuation coefficient, that is, $(\rho \times t) \times (\mu/\rho)$.

   –This product equals $\mu \times t$, giving the attenuation factor $e^{-\mu t}$ because the densities (ρ) cancel out.

  –**Fig. 3.3** shows the mass attenuation coefficient for different materials as a function of x-ray energy.

C. Half-value layer

  –Linear and mass attenuation coefficients can be used with monoenergetic beams of x-rays.

  –The **half-value layer (HVL)** is normally used to quantify polyenergetic beams.

  –The HVL quantifies the ability of an x-ray beam to penetrate tissue.

  –The HVL is the thickness of material that attenuates an x-ray beam exposure by 50%.

  –The thickness of material that attenuates an x-ray beam by 90% is called the **tenth-value layer** because it transmits only one tenth of the incident intensity.

  –At average diagnostic x-ray beam energies, the HVL for soft tissue typically ranges from 2.5 to 3.0 cm.

  –Approximate values for transmission of the primary beam through a patient is 10% for chest radiographs, 1% for skull radiographs, and 0.5% for abdominal radiographs.

  –At the low energies (28 kVp spectra) used in mammography, the HVL for soft tissue is about 1 cm.

  –The relation between the linear attenuation coefficient (μ) and HVL is HVL $= \log_e[2]/\mu = 0.693/\mu$.

  –**Table 3.3** shows typical HVLs and tenth-value layers for a range of monoenergetic x-ray beams.

D. X-ray beam half-value layer

  –The **quality** of an x-ray beam can be specified as the **thickness of aluminum** (mm) that reduces the x-ray beam exposure by 50% (i.e., HVL).

  –At 80 kVp, the legal minimum x-ray beam HVL in many states is 2.5 mm of aluminum.

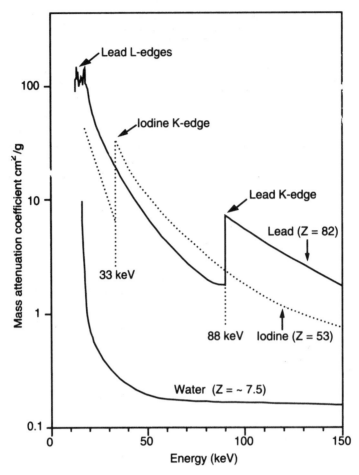

FIG. 3.3. Mass attenuation coefficient as a function of photon energy. The sharp increase at the K-edge of lead and iodine is caused by the photoelectric effect at the K-edge of these materials.

–A lower HVL means that the beam has proportionally more low-energy photons.
–A typical HVL is 3 mm of aluminum for conventional radiography at 80 kVp.
–**Table 3.4** gives typical values of x-ray beam HVL for a three-phase generator as a function of peak voltage and beam filtration, showing that HVL increases with increasing filtration.
–After filtration by one HVL, a greater thickness of material is required to further reduce the more penetrating beam intensity by an additional 50%.

TABLE 3.3. *Selected half-value layer and tenth-value layer data for monoenergetic photons*

Energy (keV)	Muscle (cm)		Bone (cm)		Lead (mm)	
	HVL	TVL	HVL	TVL	HVL	TVL
30	1.8	6.1	0.4	1.5	0.02	0.07
50	3.0	9.9	1.2	4.0	0.08	0.26
100	3.9	13.0	2.3	7.7	0.11	0.37
150	4.5	14.8	2.8	9.3	0.31	1.0

HVL; half-value layer; TVL, tenth-value layer.

TABLE 3.4. *Representative half-value layers showing the effect of filtration on beam quality*

Peak voltage (kVp)	Half-value layer (mm Al)	
	2.5 mm Al filtration	3.5 mm Al filtration
60	2.2	2.6
80	2.7	3.2
100	3.3	3.9
120	4.0	4.6

–This means that the **second HVL** is always **greater than** the **first HVL** for polychromatic x-ray beams.

IV. Radiation Units

A. Exposure

–**Exposure** is used to express the intensity, strength, or amount of radiation in an x-ray beam based on the ability of radiation to ionize air.

–Exposure is related to the **total charge of electrons** liberated per unit mass of air by the x-ray photons.

–Exposure is measured in **coulombs per kilogram (C/kg)** in the SI system or in **roentgens (R)** in non-SI units: $1\ R = 2.58 \times 10^{-4}\ C/kg.$

–Exposure is only defined for photons with energies less than 3 MeV and cannot be used for electrons, neutrons, or protons.

–Exposure from an x-ray source obeys the **inverse square law** and decreases with the square of the distance from a source.

–**Entrance skin exposure** is a measure of exposure at the skin surface but is a poor metric for assessing radiation risk.

–Skin exposures do not take into account the penetration and area of the x-ray beam, or the sensitivity of the tissues irradiated.

B. Kerma

–**Kerma** stands for the *kinetic energy released in media* and may replace the roentgen as a measure of exposure in the SI system.

–Kerma is the **kinetic energy transferred** from uncharged particles (photons and neutrons) to charged particles (electrons and protons).

–Kerma is specified in units of **joules per kilogram (J/kg).**

–For practical purposes, an exposure of 1 R may be taken to be (approximately) equal to an air kerma of 10 mGy, as used in this book.

–Scientifically, an exposure of 1 R corresponds to an air kerma of 8.7 mGy.

C. Absorbed dose

–**Absorbed dose** *(D)* measures the amount of radiation energy *(E)* absorbed per unit mass *(M)* of a medium: $D = E/M.$

–Absorbed dose is specified in **grays (Gy)** in the SI system and **rad** (radiation absorbed dose) in non-SI units.

–One gray is equal to 1 J of energy deposited per kilogram, and 1 rad is equal to 100 ergs of energy deposited per gram: $1\ Gy = 100\ rad;\ 1\ rad = 10\ mGy.$

–For practical purposes, an air kerma of 1 mGy may be taken to approximately equal to an absorbed dose of 1 mGy in soft tissue.

–The absorbed dose in a radiation field depends on the particular material or tissue in the radiation field.

–Therefore, the absorbing medium (e.g., air, soft tissue, bone) and its location (e.g., entrance skin, thyroid, spleen) should always be specified.

–Absorbed dose is the preferred metric in radiobiology.

–The organ absorbed dose is normally required to estimate the corresponding radiation risk in diagnostic radiology.

  –For example, the risk to a pregnant patient will require an estimate of the absorbed dose to the embryo or fetus.

D. f-Factor

–The **f-factor** is the conversion factor between exposure and absorbed dose that accounts for the photon energy of the x-rays and characteristics of the medium irradiated.

–The relation between absorbed dose *(D)* and exposure *(X)* is $D = f \times X$, where f is the roentgen-to-rad conversion factor, or **f-factor.**

–At diagnostic x-ray energies, the f-factor for air, muscle, and other soft tissue is close to one, so that absorbed dose (rad) is numerically approximately equal to exposure measured in roentgen.

–The f-factor for bone ranges from about four, at diagnostic x-ray photon energies, to one, for the very high photon energies used in radiotherapy (MeV).

–**Table 3.5** lists the f-factor for a range of photon energies and absorbing media.

V. Radiation Detectors

A. Ionization chambers

–**Ionization chambers** detect ionizing radiation by measuring the charge (electrons) liberated when x-ray photons ionize the gas inside.

–The exposure *(X)* corresponds to a measurement of the total charge *(Q)* liberated *(X = Q/M)*, where *M* is the mass of air in the chamber.

–Ionization chambers need a positive voltage at the collecting electrode (anode), which attracts the liberated electrons.

–The applied voltage should be high enough to collect all the liberated electrons.

–During radiography, a total charge of *Q* coulombs liberated in the chamber is collected and used to determine the radiographic exposure, which is expressed in roentgens (R) or coulombs per kilogram (C/kg).

–During fluoroscopy, there is a flow of charge liberated every second that corresponds to a current *(I = Q/t)* detected at the collecting electrode.

–A measurement of the rate of charge being liberated, which is equal to an electric current *Q/t*, corresponds to an exposure rate expressed in roentgens per second, minute, or hour.

TABLE 3.5. *f-Factor values for converting exposure to absorbed dose (rad/R)*

Photon energy (keV)	Fat $\bar{Z} = 6.5$	Muscle $\bar{Z} = 7.6$	Bone $\bar{Z} = 12.3$
30	0.53	0.92	4.4
50	0.66	0.94	3.6
100	0.91	0.96	1.5
150	0.96	0.96	1.1

$\bar{Z}$, effective atomic number.

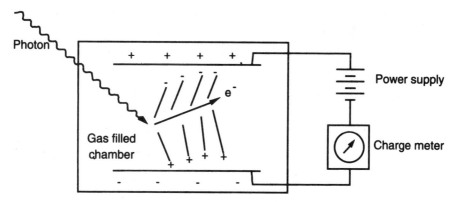

FIG. 3.4. Exposure measured by an ionization chamber. The radiation ionizes air. The ions produced are attracted to the oppositely charged plates, where they are detected and counted.

–**Fig. 3.4** shows a typical ionization chamber used for measuring x-ray exposures.

–Ionization chambers are accurate dosimetry devices and are frequently used to measure the output of x-ray tubes.

–Ionization chambers are used as **phototimers** in automatic exposure controls and as **dose calibrators** in nuclear medicine.

B. Pocket ionization chamber

–Pocket ionization chambers are shaped like large pens.

–As a result of the ionization produced in the chamber, a charged capacitor is discharged when exposed to radiation.

–Pocket ionization chambers can provide immediate readings.

–The typical range of a pocket ionization chamber is 0 to 2 mGy (200 mrad).

–Pocket ionization chambers are easily recharged and reused but are not very accurate because of their mechanical fragility (e.g., they may be damaged if dropped on the floor).

C. Geiger counters

–A Geiger counter is an **ionization chamber** with a high voltage across the chamber.

–An incident photon interacting in this chamber produces a small number of **free electrons.** These electrons are accelerated by the large positive potential and **gain energy.**

–These energetic electrons result in more electrons being ejected from the gas atoms in the chamber.

–As a result, there is an **electron avalanche,** or large amplification of the charge liberated by the incident electron.

–The large amplified output results in the "click" heard when using the Geiger counter.

–**Quenching gases** are added to Geiger counters to improve stability by minimizing the production of secondary discharges.

–Geiger counters are sensitive and are used to detect low levels of radioactive contamination.

–Geiger counters are too sensitive to measure diagnostic x-ray beams, which may have more than 10^7 photons/mm^2.

D. Film dosimetry

–Film may be used to measure the radiation exposure of radiation workers.

–Film badges are the most common and least expensive monitoring device.

–The sensitivity of film to x-rays depends on photon energy.
  –The response of film at 60 kVp is as much as 100 times higher than the response of film at 1 MeV (cobalt 60 energy levels) for the *same* exposure.
  –This enhanced sensitivity arises at the K-edge of the silver in film at 25 keV.
–Personnel monitoring devices are worn to ensure that workers receive doses below the appropriate dose limit and to monitor radiation safety practices.
–Film badges consist of a small case with a piece of film placed between filters.
–An estimate of photon energy is needed because the film response is energy dependent and is obtained by the use of three filters in front of the film.
  –The filters assess the penetrating power of the radiation source, thus permitting the energy to be estimated.
–The film is processed and the optical density measured to estimate dose based on the average photon energy.
–The minimum dose that a film badge can detect is approximately 0.2 mGy (20 mrad).
–Personal film badges provide a permanent record of operator exposure.
–Film badges have limited accuracy because of their strong energy dependence.
–The accuracy of the reading can also be affected by heat and chemicals, which may blacken a film.

E. Thermoluminescent dosimetry

–Solid-state materials can store some of the absorbed x-ray beam energy in electron traps.
–In **thermoluminescent dosimeters (TLDs),** these electrons are released by the application of heat.
–The released electrons result in the emission of visible light.
  –Heating TLDs after exposure results in a light output that is proportional to the radiation exposure.
–Lithium fluoride (LiF) is the TLD used in diagnostic radiology because its low atomic number ($Z = 8.3$) makes it reasonably tissue equivalent.
–The response of a TLD as a function of photon energy is reasonably constant and is much better than that of film.
–TLDs also have high dynamic ranges and can measure doses as low as 0.01 mGy (1 mrad) or as high as 10 Gy (1,000 rad).
–TLDs are frequently used to measure patient exposures during radiographic examinations and can be used for **personnel dosimetry** (e.g., ring dosimeters).
–Because the energy response of TLDs is generally close to one, TLDs do not generally require an estimate of the energy of the radiation source.
–The detection limit for a TLD is approximately 0.2 mGy (20 mrad).

Review Test

1. Coherent scatter:

(A) Cannot occur at diagnostic x-ray energies
(B) Is more important than Compton scatter
(C) Involves no energy loss
(D) Increases patient dose
(E) Depends on the K-edge energy

2. The threshold energy for pair production is:

(A) 1.022 keV
(B) 5.11 keV
(C) 511 keV
(D) 1.022 MeV
(E) There is no threshold

3. Which of the following is *not* an example of x-ray interactions with matter?

(A) Coherent scatter
(B) PE effect
(C) Compton scatter
(D) Bremsstrahlung radiation
(E) Pair production

4. PE interactions cannot produce:

(A) Characteristic x-rays
(B) Auger electrons
(C) Photoelectrons
(D) Positive ions
(E) Scattered photons

5. A 30 keV photon incident on an iodine atom can produce:

(A) No photoelectrons
(B) 30 keV photoelectrons
(C) K-shell photoelectrons
(D) L-shell photoelectrons
(E) K-characteristic x-rays

6. The energy *(E)* and atomic number *(Z)* dependence of the PE effect varies approximately as:

(A) Z^3/E^3
(B) E^3/Z^3
(C) Z/E
(D) E^2/Z
(E) $Z^3 \times E^3$

7. All the following are true of the PE effect in diagnostic radiology except:

(A) Is most important at low photon energies
(B) Is affected by absorption edges

(C) Occurs with inner-shell (bound) electrons
(D) Accounts for visualization of iodine contrast
(E) Accounts for lung visualization in chest x-rays

8. In a Compton interaction:

(A) The photon is totally absorbed
(B) No energy is lost by the incident photon
(C) A Compton electron can be back-scattered
(D) A photon of reduced energy can be back-scattered
(E) Characteristic x-rays are produced

9. A 51 keV photon interacting with an atom and emitting a 55 keV electron is an example of:

(A) Coherent scatter
(B) Compton scatter
(C) PE effect
(D) Pair production
(E) This is energetically impossible

10. Which interaction dominates for 45 keV photons in water?

(A) PE effect
(B) Coherent scatter
(C) Compton scatter
(D) Photodisintegration
(E) Pair production

11. The attenuation coefficient for diagnostic x-ray photons in soft tissue:

(A) Decreases continuously with increasing energy
(B) Decreases to about 25 keV, then rises again
(C) Increases continuously with increasing energy
(D) Exhibits discontinuities at 69.5 keV
(E) Depends on the molecular structure

12. For an absorbing medium with thickness *t*, the quantity $e^{-\mu t}$ is independent of:

(A) Incident photon intensity
(B) Photon energy
(C) Absorbing medium density
(D) Absorbing medium atomic number
(E) Mass attennation coefficient

13. The mass attenuation coefficient is independent of:

(A) PE effect
(B) Compton scatter

45

(C) Coherent scatter
(D) Density of material
(E) Photon energy

14. An x-ray beam intensity attenuated by three HVLs, is reduced by a factor of:

(A) 2
(B) 4
(C) 8
(D) 16
(E) 32

15. The HVL for a material with a linear attenuation coefficient of 0.1 cm^{-1} is approximately:

(A) 1 cm
(B) 1.4 cm
(C) 7 cm
(D) 10 cm
(E) 20 cm

16. Adding a 1 mm filter to a x-ray beam would result in all of the following except:

(A) Lower the patient skin exposure
(B) Increase the HVL
(C) Increase the exposure times
(D) Increase the mAs
(E) Reduce the focal spot size

17. The x-ray beam HVL does not depend on the:

(A) Radiation intensity
(B) Tube voltage
(C) Voltage waveform
(D) Anode angle
(E) Filtration

18. All of the following could affect the HVL of an x-ray beam except:

(A) Tube voltage
(B) Voltage ripple
(C) Tube current
(D) Anode angle
(E) Tube filtration

19. Exposure is:

(A) The energy deposited from a photon beam to any material
(B) Defined for charged particles below 3 MeV
(C) The absorbed dose multiplied by the quality factor
(D) The number of photons crossing unit area
(E) The electrical charge liberated by photons in a mass of air

20. Kerma is the energy per unit mass:

(A) Deposited in soft tissue
(B) Deposited in air

(C) Transferred from photons to charged particles
(D) Transferred from charged particles to photons
(E) Radiated away from the interaction site

21. Five rad equals:

(A) 5 μGy
(B) 50 μGy
(C) 500 μGy
(D) 5 mGy
(E) 50 mGy

22. The difference between exposure and dose is the difference between:

(A) The rad and the gray
(B) Absorption and temperature increase
(C) Photons and charged particles
(D) Ionization in air and absorption in a medium
(E) Ionizing and nonionizing radiation

23. Conversion of exposure to absorbed dose requires:

(A) Absorber thickness
(B) Absorber atomic number
(C) Absorber density
(D) f-Factor
(E) Radiation LET

24. The f-factor in diagnostic radiology:

(A) Is the roentgen-to-rad conversion factor
(B) Is generally 1.0 for bone
(C) Increases with photon energy
(D) Is 20 for alpha particles
(E) Is proportional to x-ray intensity

25. Ionization chambers measure:

(A) Charge
(B) Mass
(C) Density
(D) Power
(E) Voltage

26. What type of dosimeter could be given to a parent who holds a child during an x-ray examination?

(A) Ionization chamber
(B) Geiger counter
(C) TLD
(D) Film badge
(E) Pocket ionization chamber

27. Geiger counters:

(A) Can detect individual photons
(B) Are used to measure the output of x-ray tubes
(C) Emit light after absorption of radiation
(D) Require full-wave rectification
(E) Use filters to estimate photon energy

28. Quenching gases are used in:

(A) Ionization chambers
(B) Pocket chambers
(C) TLDs
(D) Film badges
(E) Geiger-Müller counters

29. Film badges:

(A) Cannot distinguish between low- and high-energy x-rays

(B) Can measure doses of 0.01 mGy
(C) Are insensitive to heat
(D) Estimate the dose from the film optical density
(E) Can be reused

30. When heated, TLDs emit:

(A) X-rays
(B) Photoelectrons
(C) Characteristic x-rays
(D) Alpha particles
(E) Light

Answers and Explanations

1–C. Coherent scatter results in scattered photons but *no transfer of energy,* and typically accounts for less than 5% of x-ray interactions in diagnostic radiology.

2–D. In pair production, a positron and electron are created, each of which has a rest mass energy of 511 keV.

3–D. Bremsstrahlung is a process whereby an electron interacts with matter, loses energy, and results in the production of a photon.

4–E. Because the incident photon is absorbed, scattered photons are not produced.

5–D. Only L-shell photoelectrons can be produced, because the photon does not have enough energy to knock out the tightly bound (33 keV) K-shell electrons of iodine.

6–A. The probability of the PE effect increases rapidly as Z increases (Z^3) and decreases rapidly as E increases ($1/E^3$).

7–E. Chest x-rays are taken at high voltages (120 kV) and Compton scatter dominates soft tissue (lung) interactions.

8–D. A photon of reduced energy (i.e., longer wavelength) can be backscattered.

9–E. A scattered electron cannot have an energy greater than that of the incident photon.

10–C. Only the PE and Compton scatter are important in radiology. The PE and Compton effects

are equal at 25 keV, with the PE more important at lower energies and vice versa.

11–A. Attenuation decreases with energy (note the K-edge discontinuity for oxygen is at 0.5 keV, which is *much* lower than the energies encountered in diagnostic radiology).

12–A. The term measures the fractional transmission, which is independent of incident x-ray intensity.

13–D. The mass attenuation coefficient is independent of density.

14–C. Each HVL reduces the intensity by half, so the total intensity reduction is $(1/2)^n$ for n HVLs, and three HVLs reduce intensity by a factor of 8.

15–C. The HVL is given by the expression $\ln_e 2/\mu$ (0.693/0.1 cm, or approximately 7 cm).

16–E. Filtration has no direct effect on focal spot size; increasing the mA could also require the focal spot size to be increased to cope with increased focal spot power loading.

17–A. The HVL expressed in mm Al depends only on the x-ray spectrum; it is thus independent of the intensity of the beam as measured by the exposure.

18–C. The HVL is independent of the tube current.

19–E. Exposure is given by the charge liberated in air by photons per unit mass and is expressed in coulomb per kilogram.

20–C. Kinetic energy released in media; the kinetic energy refers to charged particles released by incident photons.

21–E. 50 mGy (1 Gy = 100 rad; 1 rad = 10 mGy).

22–D. Exposure is ionization in air, and dose is energy absorbed in a medium.

23–D. The f-factor, the value of which will depend on the absorbing material and photon energy, is all that is required to convert exposure to absorbed dose.

24–A. The f-factor converts exposure (roentgen) into absorbed dose (gray or rad). At diagnostic x-ray energies, f is approximately one for soft tissue but about four for bone.

25–A. Ionization chambers measure charge liberated during an exposure.

26–E. A pocket ionization chamber is most likely, as these can be read out immediately after the examination has been completed.

27–A. Each ionization event in a Geiger counter generates a single large pulse, making it very sensitive to low levels of radiation.

28–E. Quenching gases are used in Geiger-Müller detectors to minimize the production of secondary discharges.

29–D. Film badge doses are obtained using film optical densities values.

30–E. TLDs emit light when heated, with the light intensity proportional to the absorbed x-ray dose.

4

Analog X-ray Imaging

I. Film

A. Emulsions

–Analog radiography uses film to capture, display, and store radiographic images.

–Film consists of an approximately 10 μm thick **emulsion** supported by a 150 to 200 μm thick polyester (Mylar) base.

–Most films have an emulsion layer on both sides of the base.

–Additional layers on radiographic film can include a protective coating, antistatic, or anti-crossover layer.

–The emulsion contains **silver halide** (iodobromide) **grains,** which can be sensitized by radiation or light to hold a latent image.

–Silver halide grains are typically about 1 μm in diameter and contain between 10^6 and 10^7 silver atoms.

–There are about 10^9 grains per cubic centimeter.

–Several light photons must be absorbed to sensitize each grain.

–A grain may also be sensitized by absorbing a single x-ray photon.

–Absorbed light photons liberate electrons in the grain, which combine with positively charged silver ions (Ag^+), forming a latent image of silver.

–After exposure, grains have a few neutral silver atoms in the speck along with millions of Ag^+ ions.

B. Film development

–The film development process converts the invisible latent image to a permanent visible image.

–Sensitized grains are **reduced** in the alkaline developer solution by the addition of electrons, which converts the positive silver ions to silver atoms.

–A **developed grain** results in a speck of silver that appears black on the film.

–The unexposed grains with no latent image are also developed, but at a much slower rate.

–Film speed, contrast, and base and fog levels are all affected by developer chemistry and temperature.

–Increasing the developer temperature or time increases the film contrast and density and also fog.

–The development process is one of the most important aspects in producing good quality images.

C. Film processors

–Modern **film processors** automatically run film sequentially through the **developer, fixer,** and **washing solutions,** using a series of rollers to transport the film.

–Developer temperatures typically range from 31° to 35°C.

–Film is washed to remove all developer before proceeding to the fixing solution.

–The fixing solution contains acetic acid to inhibit further development and remove unexposed silver halide grains.

  –Fixing makes the image stable and prevents any further effects by light.

  –Inadequate fixation can result in a milky appearance to the film.

–After fixing, the film is washed again to eliminate all chemicals and is then dried by heaters or infrared lamps.

–Incomplete removal of the fixer causes the film to turn brown.

–The total **processing time** is typically **90 seconds** (developer time, 25 seconds; fixer time, 21 seconds, and washing and drying time, 44 seconds).

–Dirty, uneven, or maladjusted rollers can leave lines or other artifacts (e.g., π lines) on the film.

  –Static electricity can also cause severe film artifacts.

–Film processor quality control is essential in maintaining film image quality at a high level.

–Processor quality control involves measuring developer temperature and monitoring the density and contrast of film exposed to a light source in a **sensitometer.**

–Silver removed from the film during processing can be recovered for recycling.

D. Film density

–After processing, the blackening on the film reflects the pattern of x-rays reaching the cassette.

–Film blackening is directly related to the number of photons that reach the film.

–Film blackening is normally measured using **optical density (OD).**

  –**OD = $\log_{10}(I_0/I_t)$,** where I_0 is the light intensity incident on the film, and I_t is the light transmitted through the film.

  –OD can be measured using a densitometer.

–**Transmittance** is the fraction of incident light passing through the film (transmittance = I_t/I_0).

–As OD increases, transmittance decreases.

–The useful range of film ODs is from about 0.3 (50% transmittance) to two (1% transmittance). Densities above about 2.2 require the use of a hot (bright) light.

–A logarithmic scale permits large density difference to be expressed on a small scale.

–The physiologic response of the eye to brightness is logarithmic.

–The OD of superimposed films is additive, so two films with an OD of one (10% transmittance) superimposed would have an OD of two and would transmit 1% of the incident light.

–**Table 4.1** shows the relationship between OD and transmittance.

TABLE 4.1. *Percentage transmittance and resultant value of film optical density*

Transmittance (%)*	Optical density†	Comments
50	0.3	Base plus fog has a density of about 0.2
25	0.6	Lowest useful density in radiology
10	1.0	Relatively light region
5	1.3	Normally the region with good film contrast
1	2.0	Higher densities require use of hot light
0.1	3.0	Typical maximum film density

* Transmittance = $100 \times (I_t/I_0)$%.

† Optical density = $\log_{10}(I_0/I_t)$.

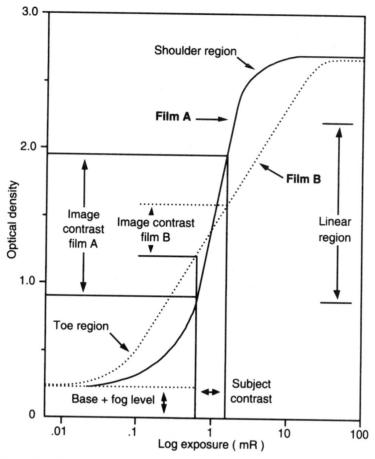

FIG. 4.1. Characteristic curve showing relation between exposure and optical density for two different films. Film A has a higher contrast; film B has a wider exposure latitude.

E. Characteristic curves

–The characteristic curve represents the relation between exposure and resultant film OD, as shown in Fig. 4.1.

–Characteristic curves are also known as **H and D curves,** named after Hurter and Driffield, who first generated these types of curve in 1890.

  –The **toe** is the low-exposure region, and the **shoulder** is the high-exposure region of the curve.

–**Base plus fog** level is the film density in the absence of any radiation exposure and typically ranges from 0.1 to 0.2 OD units.

  –Fog is the level of blackening caused by a few grains being developed in the absence of any radiation exposure.

  –**Base** refers to the density of the film base alone, which will absorb a small faction of any incident light.

–The maximum possible OD for exposed film ranges up to 3.5 OD units.

  –Fast films require less exposure to achieve a given film density; slow films require more exposure.

II. Intensifying Screens

A. Screens

-**Intensifying screens** contain phosphor crystals that absorb x-ray photons and emit many more visible light photons, which expose the film as shown in **Fig. 4.2.**
  -The screen therefore converts the x-ray pattern to a light pattern, which is recorded on film.
-Intensifying screens improve the efficiency of radiographic imaging over use of film alone.
  -The use of intensifying screens decreases the mAs required for a given film density, resulting in a lower patient dose.
  -Shorter exposure times also decrease x-ray tube loading and image blur caused by patient motion.
-Intensifying screens are typically made of a polyester base for support with a 40 to 200 μm thick phosphor layer.
  -About 50% of the radiation incident on a cassette containing a pair of screens will be absorbed.
-**Absorption efficiency** refers to the percentage of x-ray photons absorbed in a screen and is typically 25%.

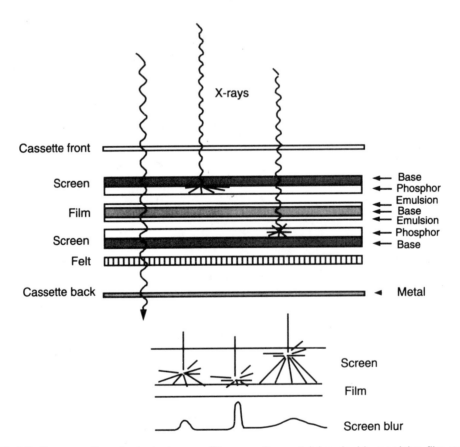

FIG. 4.2. Cross-section of a typical screen/film cassette containing double-emulsion film and two screens.

TABLE 4.2. *Elements used in screens*

Element	Atomic no.	K-shell binding energy (keV)
Yttrium (Y)	39	17
Barium (Ba)	56	37
Lanthanum	57	39
Gadolinium (Gd)	64	50
Tungsten (W)	74	70

–**Conversion efficiency** refers to the percentage of the absorbed x-ray energy that is converted into light energy and is typically 10%.

–The **intensification factor** is the ratio of exposures, without and with intensifying screens, required to obtain a given film density.

–Intensification factor depends on the absorption and conversion efficiency of the screen.

–Typical intensification factors are 30 to 50.

B. Screen materials

–Screens contain high atomic number materials to maximize the absorption of x-rays.

–**Calcium tungstate (CaWO$_4$)** was used in intensifying screens until about 1970.

–Tungsten has a high K-shell binding energy (69.5 keV) compared with the mean photon energy levels normally used in diagnostic radiology; therefore, absorption was less than optimal.

   –For example, an examination performed at 100 kVp corresponds to a mean photon energy level of about 40 keV, which is well below the K-shell binding energy in the screen.

–**Rare earth screens** are "faster" than calcium tungstate because they have a higher absorption efficiency at the mean x-ray energies normally used in radiology.

–Rare earth screens also have a higher conversion efficiency and produce more light for a given amount of deposited x-ray energy.

–**Table 4.2** summarizes the K-shell binding energy levels of the rare earth elements used in screens.

–Gadolinium oxysulfide (Gd$_2$O$_2$S) emits mainly green light, and lanthanum oxybromide (LaOBr) and CaWO$_4$ emit mainly blue light.

–The light output—that is, wavelength (λ) or color—of a screen and the light sensitivity of the film must be matched (**spectral matching**).

   –Conventional film is sensitive to ultraviolet and blue light.

   –Orthochromatic film is also sensitive to green light.

C. Cassettes

–The film and screens are held in a light-tight cassette.

–Screens are usually permanently mounted inside the cassette.

–A thin layer of resilient foam holds the screen tightly against the film when the cassette is closed.

–The front of the cassette is made of a minimally attenuating material, such as aluminum or carbon fiber.

–Dual-screen, dual-emulsion systems are frequently used to improve x-ray absorption.

–Intensifying screens can be significant sources of image artifact.

   –Scratches, stains, hair, dust, cigarette ash, and talcum powder are all potential sources of image artifacts.

TABLE 4.3. *Screen characteristics and common clinical applications*

Screen classification	Typical composition	Limiting resolution (lp/mm)	Clinical uses
Mammography (Min-R)	$Gd_2O_2S{:}Tb$	~20	Mammography
Detail (80)	$La_2O_2S{:}Tb$	~12	Extremity radiography
Medium (200)	$La_2O_2S{:}Tb$	~7	Chest imaging
Fast (600)	$BaPbSO_4$	~5	Abdominal imaging

–As part of a quality control program, all screens should be regularly cleaned.

–Cassettes should also be evaluated for good screen/film contact.

　–Screen/film contact is evaluated by taking an image of a wire mesh and ensuring that the resultant image permits visualization of the mesh.

D. Screen/film speed

–The **speed of a screen/film combination** is inversely related to the exposure required to produce a given density.

–As the speed increases, the exposure required decreases.

–The speed of a screen/film combination used in radiology ranges from approximately 50 to 800.

–Screen/film speed is normally expressed relative to a $CaWO_4$ standard assigned a speed of 100.

–Screen speed increases with increasing screen thickness, absorption, and conversion efficiency.

–Both screen and film must be specified when assigning speed to any screen/film combination.

–**High-speed screens** are generally thicker and have decreased spatial resolution.

　–Thick screens increase image blur because of increased diffusion of light in the screen before striking the film.

–**Detail screens** are thinner and therefore slower, but they have better spatial resolution.

–Fast screen/film combinations are used for abdominal studies; slow films are used for extremity examinations.

–Single-emulsion single-screen systems are used for bone detail and mammography.

–An exposure of 5 µGy (0.5 mR) will produce a satisfactory image for a screen/film combination with a speed of 200.

–To ensure the correct film density, phototiming systems are generally used.

–A phototimer measures the actual amount of radiation incident on the screen/film and terminates the exposure when the correct amount has been received.

–**Table 4.3** lists a range of screen types used in radiology, as well as their clinical applications.

III. Scatter Removal

A. Scatter

–**Scattered radiation** is undesirable in diagnostic radiology because it **reduces subject contrast.**

–Of paramount significance are the scattered photons resulting from **Compton scatter.**

–The ratio of scatter to primary radiation exiting a patient can easily be 5:1 or greater.

　–Scatter increases with increased field size (i.e., area of x-ray beam) and increased patient thickness.

–**Collimation** reduces the total patient mass irradiated and therefore reduces scatter.
–At low voltages (kVp), there is more absorption because of the photoelectric effect and less Compton scatter.
–However, lowering the x-ray tube voltage reduces patient penetration and increases dose; therefore, it is not a practical method for reducing scatter.

B. Air gaps

–Air gaps between the patient and cassette reduce scatter, because the scattered photons are less likely to reach the screen/film receptor.
–However, by moving image receptors away from patients, magnification is introduced.
–Magnification also requires a larger x-ray tube output and results in additional focal spot blurring.
–Air gaps are used for magnification radiography in **neuroradiology** and **mammography.**
–Air gaps are sometimes used in chest radiography.
–A long source-to-patient distance (3 m) helps to compensate for loss of sharpness caused by focal spot size and minimizes magnification.

C. Grids

–**Antiscatter grids** are the most effective and practical method for **removing scatter** in diagnostic radiology.
–Grids are made up of many narrow parallel bars of lead or other highly attenuating material.
–X-rays pass between the strips, which are filled with low-attenuation material.
–Grids are placed between the patient and the film.
–**Fig. 4.3** shows how grids reduce the amount of scatter radiation reaching the screen/film combination.

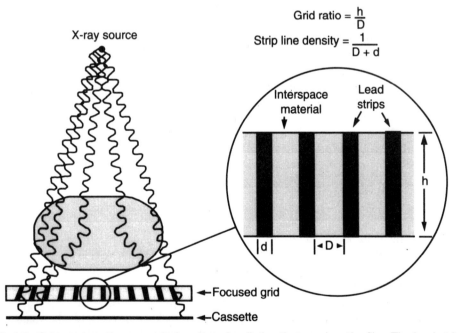

FIG. 4.3. Grids reduce the amount of scattered radiation that reaches the film. The lead strips of a focused grid are designed to be aligned to the incoming beam.

TABLE 4.4. *Common radiography grid characteristics*

Grid ratio	Increase in mAs (relative to no grid)*	X-rays transmitted at 80 kVp (%)	
		Scattered	Primary
5:1	× 2	~18	~75
6:1	× 3	~14	~72
8:1	× 4	~10	~70
12:1	× 5	~5	~68

* Bucky factor.

–The **grid ratio** is defined as the ratio of the strip height *(h)* along the x-ray beam direction to the gap *(D)* between the lead strips; that is, grid ratio is *h/D*.

–The **strip line density** is $1/(D + d)$ lines per unit length, where *d* is the strip thickness.

–Grid ratios typically range from four to 16, and strip line densities range from 25 to 60 lines per centimeter.

–**Focused grids** have diverging strips and must be used at specified focal distances.

–Most grids are **reciprocating grids,** in which the grid moves during the exposure, spreading the image of the gridlines over the film and rendering them invisible.

–The device that moves the grid is called a Bucky, after its inventor.

D. Grid characteristics

–**Primary transmission** is the percentage of incident primary radiation (not scattered) that passes through the grid.

–The **Bucky factor** is the ratio of radiation incident on the grid to the transmitted radiation.

–The Bucky factor is also an indicator of the increase in patient dose owing to the use of a grid.

–Typical values for the Bucky factor are two to six.

–The **contrast improvement factor** is the ratio of contrast with a grid to contrast without a grid.

–A typical contrast improvement factor is approximately two.

–Artifacts such as **grid cutoff** may be caused by improper alignment, the wrong focal spot to film distance for focused grids, and inverted grids.

–Increasing the grid ratio by either increasing the height of the lead strips or reducing the space between the lead strips increases image contrast.

–Increasing the grid ratio also increases x-ray tube loading and patient exposure.

–**Table 4.4** lists the principal radiographic characteristics of several common grids.

E. Clinical applications

–A **12:1** (30 lines/cm) ratio is common in a **reciprocating grid.**

–**Stationary grids** with low ratios of **6:1** and about 45 lines/cm are used with mobile x-ray units because a low grid ratio tolerates beam misalignments.

–A high strip line density is used for stationary grids to reduce the visibility of gridlines on resultant radiographs.

–Grids are generally used for body parts greater than 12 cm thick or techniques above 70 kVp.

–Portable chest radiography is generally performed at lower x-ray tube voltages to minimize scatter, because using grids at the bedside is very difficult.

–Grids are generally not used for extremity radiographs in which scatter is negligible.

IV. Image Intensifiers

A. Image intensifiers

–An **image intensifier** converts incident radiation into an amplified light image to be viewed, recorded, or photographed.

–An image intensifier consists of an evacuated glass, aluminum, or nonferromagnetic envelope that contains **input phosphor, photocathode, electrostatic focusing lenses, accelerating anodes, and output phosphor (Fig. 4.4).**

–Image intensifiers have diameters that range up to 57 cm.

  –Large image intensifiers cover large areas, such as the chest and abdomen.

  –Small image intensifiers achieve high resolution in small regions, such as the heart.

–The **input phosphor** absorbs x-ray photons and re-emits part of the absorbed energy as a large number of light photons.

  –The input phosphor is typically a 200 to 400 μm thick **cesium iodide** (CsI) **screen.**

–Light photons emitted by the input phosphor are absorbed by a **photocathode,** which emits photoelectrons.

–The photoelectrons are accelerated across the image intensifier tube by the anode (25 to 35 kV potential) and focused onto the **output phosphor** by an electrostatic lens.

–These electrons, which now have energies of 25 to 35 keV, are absorbed by the output phosphor (ZnCdS:Ag) and emit a large number of light photons.

–Imaging a smaller patient area results in a magnified image (image zoom).

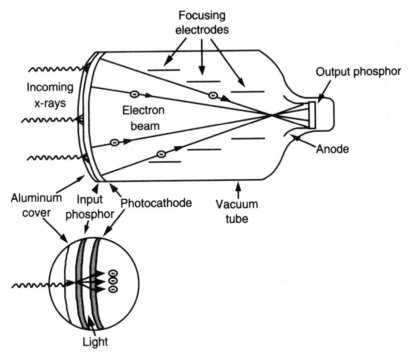

FIG. 4.4. Incoming x-ray photons pass through the thin aluminum cover of the image intensifier and strike the input phosphor to produce light. The light strikes the photocathode, producing electrons, which are accelerated toward the anode by a 25 kV potential. Light is produced when the electrons strike the output phosphor.

–Magnification is accomplished electronically using electrostatic focusing that projects part of the input layer onto the output phosphor.

B. Image intensification

–The image intensifier converts the pattern of incident x-ray intensities at the input phosphor into an intense pattern of visible light at the output phosphor.

–The light image on the output of an image intensifier is brighter than that on the input phosphor by several thousand-fold.

–The increase in brightness at the output phosphor relative to the brightness at the input phosphor is the **brightness gain (BG).**

–The BG of an image intensifier equals the product of the **minification gain** and **flux gain.**

–**Minification gain** is the increase in image brightness that results from reduction in image size from the input phosphor to the output phosphor: minification gain $= (d_i/d_0)^2$, where d_i is the input diameter and d_0 is the output diameter.

–The output phosphor is typically 2.5 cm in diameter; thus, for a 25 cm image intensifier, minification gain $= (25/2.5)^2$, or 100.

–**Flux gain** is the increased number of light photons emitted from the output phosphor compared to the input phosphor.

–The flux gain is typically 50 to 100, so for each light photon emitted at the input phosphor, there are 50 to 100 light photons emitted at the output phosphor.

C. Conversion factor

–The conversion factor is a modern method of measuring performance of an image intensifier.

–The **conversion factor** is the ratio of the **luminance** of the output phosphor, measured in candela per square meter (cd/m^2), to the input exposure rate, measured in μGy/second (mR/second).

–A **candela** is a measure of luminance intensity or light brightness.

–The conversion factor of modern image intensifiers is approximately 10 to 30 $cd/m^2/\mu$Gy/second (100 to 300 cd/m^2/mR/second).

–To maintain a constant brightness level at the image intensifier output phosphor, the exposure to the input phosphor must be increased when the field size is reduced.

–Reducing the image intensifier size by a factor of two reduces the exposed region by a factor of four.

–As a result, a four-fold increase in radiation exposure would be required to maintain a constant brightness at the output of the image intensifier.

–The brightness of an image intensifier decreases with age.

D. Image intensifier performance

–As with intensifying screens, absorption is greater as the input phosphor thickness increases, but resolution is poorer because of light diffusion.

–The central portion of an image intensifier image has a limiting **spatial resolution** of between 4 and 5 line pairs per millimeter (lp/mm).

–The resolution is reduced at the edges of the image intensifier.

–**Table 4.5** gives typical values of resolution and light conversion factors for different-sized image intensifiers.

–The image intensifier **contrast ratio** is the ratio of periphery to central light intensities (output) when imaging a fully absorbing lead disc that is one tenth of the area of the image intensifier input phosphor.

TABLE 4.5. *Representative values of spatial resolution and conversion gain for cesium iodine-based image intensifiers*

Image intensifier diameter (cm)	Resolution (lp/mm)	Conversion gain (cd/m^2/μGy/sec)*
57	3	60
33	4	20
23	5	10

* 1 cd/m^2/μGy/sec $\equiv$ 10 cd/m^2/mR/sec.

–The light appearing behind the image of the lead disk is called **veiling glare.**

–A typical image intensifier contrast ratio is 20:1.

   –Loss of contrast occurs because some x-ray photons pass through the input phosphor and photocathode, strike the inside of the II, and are scattered back to the input phosphor.

–Contrast is also reduced by light scattered and reflected within the image intensifiers and output window.

E. Image intensifier artifacts

   –**Lag** is the continued luminescence at the output phosphor after x-ray stimulation has stopped.

   –Modern CsI tubes have a low lag time of about 1 millisecond, which is of little concern.

   –**Pincushion distortion**, in which straight lines appear curved, is produced by all image intensifiers.

   –**Pincushion distortion** is about 3% for 23 cm image intensifiers.

   –**Vignetting** is a fall-off in brightness at the periphery of the image intensifier field.

   –**Vignetting** is typically less than 25%.

   –The curvature of the image intensifier faceplate give rise to both **pincushion distortion** and **vignetting.**

      –Imperfections in electron focusing and associated optical lens system also contribute to **pincushion distortion** and **vignetting.**

   –Pincushion distortion and vignetting both improve with smaller field sizes (i.e., less minification).

V. Television

A. Introduction

   –Fluoroscopy uses closed-circuit television (TV) systems to view the image output of the image intensifier, which allows for multiple observers.

   –A beam splitter allows two recording techniques, such as fluoroscopy and cine, to be used simultaneously.

   –A diaphragm (camera aperture) between the lenses controls the light intensity.

   –Output images from image intensifiers are focused onto the photoconductive target in the TV camera by use of optical lenses.

   –**TV cameras** convert light images into electric (video) signals that can be recorded or viewed on a monitor.

   –The TV target is scanned with an electron beam in a series of horizontal lines (raster scanning) to read the image light intensity.

–The display monitor converts video signals back into the "original" image for direct viewing.

B. Television scan modes

–In conventional TV systems, 262.5 odd lines (**1 field**) are first scanned, then 262.5 even lines (1 field) are **interlaced** to generate a full **frame** (sum of 2 fields) totaling 525 lines.
  –Interlacing prevents **flickering,** even though only 30 full frames are updated every second.
–In North America, conventional TV systems and display monitors read 30 frames per second, which corresponds to 60 fields per second.
–European TV systems generally use 625 lines and 25 frames per second (50 fields per second).
–European TV is not compatible with North American TV.
–Modern radiographic equipment generally uses 1,000 line TV systems that may improve resolution by a factor of two.
–Raster scanning may be progressive or interlaced.
–If TV cameras are operated in a **progressive scan mode** rather than an interlaced mode, then each line is read sequentially.
–Progressive scan modes are used in digital systems and reduce motion artifacts.

C. Television camera types

–TV systems are classified as Vidicon or Plumbicon camera systems.
–**Vidicon TV cameras** reduce contrast by a factor of about 0.8, and TV monitors enhance the contrast by a factor of two.
  –Vidicon systems improve the contrast of a fluoroscopy system compared with the contrast at the image intensifier output.
  –Vidicon systems have high image lag, which improves image quality by "averaging" sequential image frames.
–**Plumbicon TV cameras** have much less lag than that of Vidicon cameras.
  –Low lag permits motion to be followed with minimal blur, but quantum mottle is increased.
  –Vacuum tube type TV cameras are currently being replaced by charged coupled device (CCD) TV cameras.
  –CCDs TV cameras have virtually no lag.

D. Television performance

–The theoretical vertical resolution for a 525 line TV system, and a 23 cm image intensifier is about 1 lp/mm.
  –Only approximately 70% of this theoretical limit is achieved in practice.
  –The ratio of measured to theoretical vertical resolution is called the **Kell factor,** which is normally taken to be about 0.7.
–Horizontal resolution is determined by the **bandwidth** of the TV system and is normally equal to the vertical resolution.
–Use of a 500 line TV system limits the achievable fluoroscopy spatial resolution to about 1 lp/mm.
  –Use of a 1,000 line TV system can improve the spatial resolution of fluoroscopy by a factor of two.
–Fluoroscopy resolution may be improved by use of magnification modes, but it is generally markedly inferior to radiographic imaging.

VI. Fluoroscopy

A. Introduction

–Fluoroscopy allows real-time observation and imaging of dynamic activities such as barium moving through the gastrointestinal tract or the flow of contrast through blood vessels.

–**Fig. 4.5** is an overview of the complete fluoroscopic imaging system.

–Modern fluoroscopy systems use closed-circuit TV systems for real-time observation.

–Fluoroscopy systems also provide several options for image recording, including video, spot film and film changers, cine and photospot cameras, and digital capture.

–Fluoroscopy is performed at low doses, which means that relatively few x-rays are used to produce the image, and this results in high **quantum mottle** (noise) levels.

–Fluoroscopy tube currents are low, between 1 and 5 mA, and x-ray tube voltages are normally between 70 and 90 kVp.

–The x-ray pulse width or duration can also be varied when pulsed exposures are used, such as in cardiac cine.

–Fluoroscopy systems use grids to remove scatter radiation, with a typical grid ratio of 10:1, and use collimation to match the x-ray beam to the image intensifier size.

–Portable fluoroscopy systems are C-arm devices, with 18 and 23 cm diameter image intensifiers being most common.

B. Automatic brightness control

–The **automatic brightness control** regulates the amount of radiation incident required to maintain a constant TV display.

–The amount of radiation is changed by adjusting the technique factors to maintain a constant light level at the image intensifier output phosphor.

–Most modern systems use a combination of tube current and voltage variability to control image brightness.

–The light output of an image intensifier is proportional to the input area of the image intensifier and the radiation exposure.

  –Reducing the image intensifier size thus requires the radiation exposure to be increased if the image brightness is to be kept constant.

  –A reduction of the image intensifier input from 25 to 18 cm normally requires the radiation level to be nearly doubled (i.e., $25^2/18^2 = 1.9$).

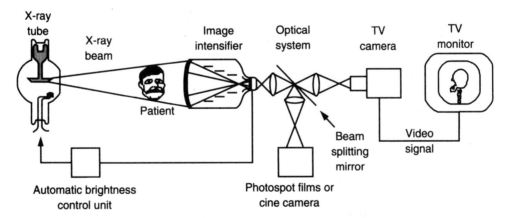

FIG. 4.5. A typical fluoroscopy imaging system.

–An ionization chamber between the grid and cassette is used for taking spot films (phototiming).

C. Spot films and photospot films

–**Spot film** refers to direct film recording in which a radiograph is taken using a screen-film cassette moved in front of the image intensifier for the exposure.

–Fluoroscopy is interrupted during the exposure of the spot film.

–Various film changer devices may be used for rapid acquisition of serial radiographs, such as in vascular imaging.

–**Photospot films** are a method of indirect image recording in which the output of an image intensifier is recorded onto 70 and 105 mm roll film or onto 100 mm cut film.

–A series of mirrors and lenses (optical distributor) focuses the image from the image intensifier output phosphor onto the film **(Fig. 4.5).**

–Photospot films have an exposure of about 1 μGy (100 μR) per frame at the receptor, about five times lower than that required for conventional screen/film combinations.

–Other advantages of photospot film include the following:

–There is no need to change the film as there would be to change a cassette.

–The short exposure time (50 milliseconds) reduces patient motion artifacts.

–Rapid sequences up to 12 frames per second are possible.

–The small size of photospot films results in a substantial film cost savings (80%).

D. Cine fluorography

–A **cine film** is a series of photospot images obtained in rapid sequence.

–Cine studies require the use of a grid-controlled x-ray tube, an optical distributor, and a synchronization circuit.

–Cine uses 35 mm film and images are 18×24 mm.

–The x-ray pulses and cine shutter are synchronized.

–Framing frequency is in fractions or multiples of 30 (15, 30, 60, or 90 frames per second; 30 frames per second is the most common).

–**Fig. 4.6** shows how the area of the rectangular film (35 mm) and the circular image intensifier output phosphors are used in two framing modes.

–With **exact framing,** the image intensifier circle fits exactly within the film frame.

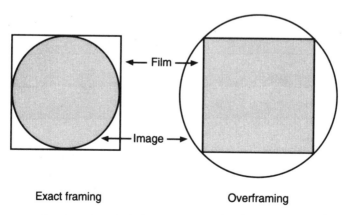

Exact framing   Overframing

FIG. 4.6. With exact framing, the whole image is recorded, but only 79% of the film is used. With overframing, the entire film is used, but only 64% of the image is recorded.

–With **total overframing,** the film frame fits within the image intensifier circle, and the outer part of the image intensifier image is lost.

E. **Exposure rates in fluoroscopy**

–Entrance skin exposure rates in fluoroscopy typically range from 10 to 100 mGy/minute (1 to 10 R/minute).

–Because fluoroscopy exposure times are much longer than in those in radiography, total patient radiation doses are much higher in fluoroscopy.

–The U.S. **maximum legal limit** for entrance skin exposure is generally **100 mGy/minute (10 R/minute).**

–**High-dose fluoroscopy** can be performed to maintain image quality in large patients.

　–High-dose fluoroscopic options require special activation mechanisms and visible/audible indicators to show that the option is being used.

　–The maximum exposure rate in high-dose fluoroscopy is 200 mGy/minute (20 R/minute).

–There are no regulatory exposure rate levels when a fluoroscopy imaging system is **acquiring images** for diagnostic purposes (e.g., cine imaging, DSA imaging, digital photo spot acquisitions).

–Indiscriminate use of high-dose fluoroscopy may result in very high doses and induce skin erythema or epilation.

Review Test

1. The sensitive layer in an x-ray film contain an emulsion of gelatin and crystals of:

(A) $CaWO_4$
(B) Silver bromide
(C) LaOBr
(D) Silver nitrate
(E) CsI

2. The developer converts sensitized silver halide crystals to:

(A) Bromine
(B) Acidic halide
(C) Silver alkalide
(D) Individual silver atoms
(E) Metallic silver specks

3. Increasing which temperature is most likely to result in a high fog level?

(A) Anode
(B) Developer
(C) Fixer
(D) Dryer
(E) Radiographic room

4. In film processing, the fixer is used to:

(A) Modify the developer pH
(B) Remove unexposed silver halide
(C) Fix the silver to the emulsion
(D) Remove the bromine
(E) Reduce unexposed silver halide

5. Which is *incorrect* for an automatic film processor for x-ray film?

(A) A common temperature for the developer solution is 32°C
(B) Total processing time is typically 90 seconds
(C) It contains developing solution, fixing solution, and clean water
(D) The fixing solutions contain acetic acid to inhibit development
(E) Chemical replenishment is not required

6. OD is defined as:

(A) Ratio of transmitted to incident light
(B) Ratio of incident to transmitted light
(C) Logarithm of ratio of transmitted to incident light
(D) Logarithm of ratio of incident to transmitted light

(E) Exponential of ratio of transmitted to incident light

7. When a film with an OD of 0.3 is placed on top of a film with an OD of 0.5, the resultant OD will be:

(A) 0.2
(B) 0.8
(C) 1.0
(D) 1.5
(E) Unable to be determined

8. When a screen-film system replaces film with no screen:

(A) Patient dose is reduced
(B) Resolution is improved
(C) Motion artifacts increase
(D) Scatter increases
(E) Exposure time increases

9. Compared with $CaWO_4$, rare earth screens generally result in a decrease of:

(A) Number of light photons per absorbed x-ray
(B) Screen mottle
(C) Speed
(D) Patient dose
(E) Film processing time

10. A screen with a higher conversion efficiency but the same x-ray absorption and screen thickness, will likely result in:

(A) Increased patient dose
(B) Constant image noise
(C) Reduced image noise
(D) Loss of image detail
(E) Faster screen-film system

11. All of the following are true of poor screen/film contact except:

(A) Can be caused by poor cassette construction
(B) Can result from trapped dirt
(C) Will result in blurred images
(D) Can be tested by radiographing wire mesh
(E) Result in markedly lighter radiographs

12. The speed of an imaging system cannot be increased by using:

(A) Larger focal spot sizes

(B) Faster films
(C) Phosphors with a higher conversion efficiency
(D) Thicker phosphors
(E) Higher developer temperatures

13. The radiation exposure at the cassette required to correctly expose a 200 speed system is:

(A) Less than 0.5 μGy (50 μR)
(B) 0.5 μGy (50 μR)
(C) 5 μGy (0.5 mR)
(D) 50 μGy (5 mR)
(E) More than 50 μGy (5 mR)

14. For thick body parts, the scatter-to-primary ratio of photons leaving the patient is about:

(A) 0.3
(B) 0.5
(C) 1.0
(D) 2.0
(E) 5.0

15. The number of scattered photons reaching a screen/film decreases with increasing:

(A) Field size
(B) Patient thickness
(C) Kilovolt peak
(D) Filtration
(E) Grid ratio

16. High ratio grids increase all the following except:

(A) Required mAs
(B) Image contrast
(C) Patient dose
(D) Removal of scatter
(E) Screen/film speed

17. The reason 12:1 grids are seldom used with portable radiography is because:

(A) Output of portable x-ray units is too low
(B) Low voltage used is unable to penetrate grids
(C) Accurate grid alignment is too difficult
(D) Scatter is not important in portable x-rays
(E) Air gaps are preferred to eliminate scatter

18. The image intensifier input phosphor is made of:

(A) NaI
(B) ZnCdS
(C) TLD
(D) CsI
(E) PbI

19. Which of the following is not a component of an image intensifier?

(A) Anode
(B) Input phosphor
(C) Photocathode
(D) Photomultiplier tube
(E) Output phosphor

20. The BG of an image intensifier tube does *not* depend on the:

(A) Patient dose
(B) Efficiency of the photocathode
(C) Voltage across the image intensifier tube
(D) Ratio of input to output screen sizes
(E) Output phosphor conversion efficiency

21. Changing the image intensifier magnification mode from 30 to 15 cm will normally increase:

(A) Entrance skin exposure rate
(B) Distortion
(C) Vignetting
(D) Image brightness
(E) Scatter radiation

22. Typical values for modern image intensifiers do *not* include:

(A) Minification gains of 100
(B) Flux gains of 50
(C) Contrast ratios of 2:1
(D) BGs of 5,000
(E) Spatial resolutions of 5 lp/mm

23. Fall off in brightness at the periphery of a fluoroscopic image is called:

(A) S distortion
(B) Pincushion distortion
(C) Barrel distortion
(D) Vignetting
(E) Edge packing

24. The reason for interlacing two fields to form one frame in a TV system is to reduce the:

(A) Patient dose
(B) Motion artifacts
(C) Input phosphor lag
(D) Quantum mottle
(E) Flicker

25. A Plumbicon TV camera is used in cardiac imaging to:

(A) Reduce patient dose
(B) Increase the frame rate
(C) Reduce image flicker
(D) Reduce image lag
(E) Improve spatial resolution

26. The *vertical* resolution of a TV system is primarily determined by the:

(A) Image brightness
(B) TV Bandwidth
(C) Number of TV lines
(D) Radiation exposure level
(E) Focal spot size

27. The *horizontal* resolution of a TV system is determined primarily by the:

(A) Image brightness
(B) TV bandwidth
(C) Number of TV lines
(D) Radiation exposure level
(E) Focal spot size

28. Fluoroscopic spatial resolution is most limited by the:

(A) Radiation scatter
(B) Grid
(C) Image intensifier tube
(D) Optical system
(E) TV system

29. Automatic brightness control in fluoroscopy maintains a constant:

(A) Kilovolt peak
(B) Milliamperes
(C) Exposure time
(D) Patient dose
(E) Image intensifier output brightness

30. Patient doses in fluoroscopy can exceed 100 mGy/minute (10 R/minute) if:

(A) High kilovolt peak values are used
(B) Exposure time does not exceed 5 minutes
(C) Visible/audible indicators are activated
(D) Contrast agents have been administered
(E) Magnification (zoom) is used

Answers and Explanations

1–B. Silver bromide crystals.

2–E. The sensitized grains, containing about 10^6 to 10^7 atoms, are reduced to specks of metallic silver, which is black in appearance.

3–B. Increasing the developer temperature generally increases the observed film fog level.

4–B. The fixer removes unexposed silver halide.

5–E. Developer and fixer needs replenishing as films are processed.

6–D. Film density, D, is given by $\log_{10}(I_0/I_t)$, where I_0 is the incident light intensity, and I_t is the transmitted light intensity.

7–B. One of the advantages of the logarithmic scale is that film ODs are additive.

8–A. The patient dose is reduced, with the reduction in patient exposure being about a factor of 50 (this also permits shorter exposures to minimize patient motion artifacts).

9–D. Rare earth screens are faster because they absorb more x-rays and are more efficient at producing light, which allows the same film density to be obtained with less radiation; thus, the patient dose decreases.

10–E. Higher conversion efficiency results in more light, so that less radiation is needed to blacken the film (i.e., faster system).

11–E. Poor screen/film contact will not have any significant effect on film density.

12–A. The focal spot size is irrelevant to the speed of a screen/film combination.

13–C. 5 μGy (0.5 mR) exposure at the cassette is typical in radiography.

14–E. The scatter-to-primary ratio for thick body parts such as the abdomen is about 5:1.

15–E. Higher grid ratios reduce the amount of scatter reaching the screen/film combination.

16–E. The speed of the screen/film system has nothing to do with the grid characteristics.

17–C. 12:1 grids are sensitive to misalignment problems; grids used for portable examinations are commonly about 6:1.

18–D. Virtually all image intensifiers have input phosphors made from CsI.

19–D. A photomultiplier tube is a light detector used in a nuclear medicine gamma camera.

20–A. BG is independent of exposure (i.e., patient dose) but is a measure of how much light you get out of the image intensifier for a given light level at the input phosphor.

21–A. Entrance skin exposure rate will increase by a factor of four because only one fourth of the image intensifier will be absorbing x-rays, and the light level at the output phosphor has to remain constant.

22–C. Contrast ratios are typically 20:1; all the other values are representative of modern image intensifiers.

23–D. Vignetting typically results in a 20% fall in intensity at the edge compared with the central (max) value.

24–E. When fields are displayed at a rate of 60/second (30 frames/second), there is no perception of flicker.

25–D. Cardiac imaging uses Plumbicon TV cameras, which have lower lag and improve temporal resolution of the moving heart.

26–C. The number of TV lines is the primary determinant of the vertical TV resolution (525 lines in the United States; 625 lines in Europe).

27–B. The bandwidth determines the horizontal TV resolution.

28–E. The limiting resolution of the TV system for a 15 cm image intensifier size is about 1 lp/mm; for the image intensifier itself, the limiting resolution is about 4 lp/mm.

29–E. Automatic brightness control in fluoroscopy modifies the kilovolt peak/milliampere rate to ensure the image at the image intensifier output has a constant intensity (brightness).

30–C. For large patients, exposure rates of up to 200 mGy/minute (20 R/minute) are allowed only if visible/audible indicators show that the high dose fluoroscopy option has been selected.

5

Image Quality and Patient Dose

I. Contrast

A. Object and subject contrast

–Object and lesion depiction in radiography is the result of the differential attenuation of the x-ray beam as it passes through the patient.

–**Object contrast** refers to the attenuation characteristics of a lesion in comparison to those of the adjacent tissue that contains the lesion.

–Increasing the lesion thickness increases object contrast.

–Object contrast depends on lesion density and atomic number.

  –Increasing the difference in density or atomic number between the lesion and the adjacent structure increases object contrast.

–Object contrast is essential for any lesion to be visualized in an image.

–**Subject contrast** is the difference in x-ray intensities **transmitted** through a lesion and the adjacent structures.

–Subject contrast requires object contrast, but the reverse is not true.

  –For example, if there is negligible patient penetration by the x-ray beam, object contrast will *not* result in any subject contrast.

B. Contrast and photon energy

–For a given lesion, subject contrast is affected primarily by the photon energy.

–Low photon energies result in high subject contrast because the photoelectric effect is sensitive to the atomic number of the absorbing medium.

  –High subject contrast, however, can be difficult to record on a radiograph because of the limited dynamic range of film.

  –Very low kilovolt peak x-ray beams are rarely used in radiology because of limited penetration through patients.

–High kilovolt peak x-ray beams have high mean x-ray energies and are more penetrating.

–However, Compton scatter becomes more important as kilovolt peak is increased, and reduces contrast.

–**Fig. 5.1** shows how subject contrast depends on the x-ray tube voltage, with increasing voltage generally reducing subject contrast.

C. Image contrast

–Image contrast is the difference in intensity of a lesion in the image, in comparison to the intensity of the adjacent tissues.

–Image contrast is the result of subject contrast, together with the effect of the recording device and image display characteristics.

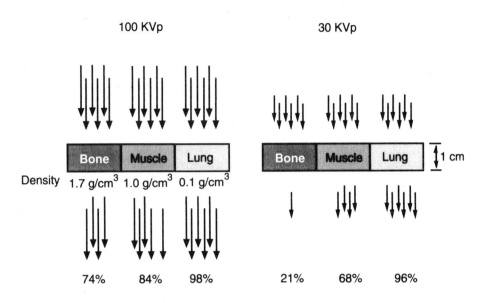

Percent transmitted

FIG. 5.1. Subject contrast decreases with increasing photon energy. As energy increases, so does the ability of the x-ray to penetrate, resulting in less difference in x-ray attenuation between air and bone at high energies.

–In screen/film radiography, image contrast is primarily dependent on film density.
–Underexposed (and overexposed) films have very little image contrast.
  –Correct exposure in screen/film imaging is achieved using phototiming, with the x-ray duration terminated by a radiation sensor at the detector.
–In any digital imaging modality, image contrast can be adjusted by the operator.
–Digital modalities, therefore, should never be "contrast limited."
–Object and subject contrast are essential prerequisites for image contrast.
–The presence of object/subject contrast, however, does not guarantee image contrast because the image can be overexposed/underexposed or incorrectly displayed.

D. Contrast and latitude

–**Film contrast** relates to the observed density difference measured on the film for a given exposure difference incident on the film.
–Film contrast is determined by the **slope** of the characteristic curve **(Fig. 5.1).**
–**Film gamma** is the **maximum slope** of the linear portion of the characteristic curve and is primarily determined by film type and processing.
–The **film gradient** is the **mean slope** between two specified film densities (normally 0.25 and 2.0 optical density units).
–A high gradient (greater than 1.0) means that subject contrast is amplified.
–**Film latitude** is the **range of exposure levels** over which the film may be used.
–Film latitude and contrast are inversely related.
  –The higher the gradient, the narrower the range of exposure (latitude) that will result in a discernible density difference on the film.
  –A wide latitude film has a low gradient and low contrast.
–**Dynamic range** is the ratio of highest to lowest exposure that can be usefully detected by the image capture system and is approximately 40:1 for a typical film.

–Exposures outside this range are in the toe or shoulder region of the characteristic curve and therefore result in very low image contrast.

–Wide latitude films are used for chest radiographs, in which there is a wide dynamic range of exposures (high subject contrast) between the lungs and mediastinum.

–High-contrast films are used in mammography because of the low subject contrast of mass lesions.

E. Contrast agents

–Contrast agents, including air, barium, and iodine, are used to improve subject contrast.

–Barium is administered as a contrast agent for visualization of the gastrointestinal tract on radiographic examinations.

–The attenuation of barium is high because of its high atomic number (Z = 56; K-edge = 37 keV) and physical mass density, which increase photoelectric absorption.

–The barium K-edge energy matches the mean photon energies used in fluoroscopy.

–Iodine (Z = 53; K-edge = 33 keV) is also an excellent contrast agent for similar reasons to those for barium.

–Iodinated contrast agents can be injected intravenously or intraarterially.

–Dilution and the osmolar limitations of intravascular fluids limit the achievable iodine concentration.

–Air is a negative contrast agent and increases subject contrast because it is less attenuating than tissue.

–Carbon dioxide is also sometimes used as a contrast agent in angiography.

II. Resolution

A. Introduction

–**Spatial resolution** is the ability of an imaging system to resolve two adjacent **high-contrast** objects as discrete entities.

–Spatial resolution may also be described by the terms **high-contrast resolution, blur,** and **modulation transfer function (MTF).**

–**Focal spot size, screen thickness,** and **patient motion** are the most important factors that affect resolution in radiography.

–Resolution is often expressed in **line pairs per millimeter** (lp/mm), which is a measure of spatial frequency.

–A **line pair** includes an opaque line and radiolucent space.

–Large objects may be represented by low spatial frequencies and small structures by high spatial frequencies.

–**High-contrast resolution** is estimated using a parallel line bar phantom.

–One line pair per millimeter has 0.5 mm lead (Pb) bars separated by 0.5 mm of radiolucent material.

–Two line pairs per millimeter has 0.25 mm lead bars separated by 0.25 mm of radiolucent material, and so on.

–The **limiting spatial resolution** is the maximum number of line pairs per millimeter that can be recorded by the imaging system.

–The human eye can resolve a maximum of 30 lp/mm on close inspection and only about 5 lp/mm at a viewing distance of approximately 25 cm.

–The best spatial resolution is achieved when film is exposed directly without using a screen, with up to 100 lp/mm being achievable.

–Each image recording system has an inherent limit on spatial resolution; **Table 5.1** summarizes representative values in x-ray imaging.

TABLE 5.1. *Representative values of limiting spatial resolution*

Imaging technique	Resolution (lp/mm)
Mammography	15–20
Screen/film (400 speed)	5–8
Photospot	~4
35 mm cine	~3.5
Digital subtraction angiography	~2
Conventional fluoroscopy	~1

B. Screen blur

–With intensifying screens, the film is exposed by a cone of light photons produced in the screen when the x-ray photon is absorbed.

–**Screen blur** (lack of sharpness) is caused by light diffusion in the intensifying screen **(Fig. 4.2).**

–**Thick screens** have greater light diffusion in the screen and therefore more blur.

 –Thicker screens (fast screens) also have improved x-ray absorption efficiencies and require decreased exposure times and reduced patient doses.

–**Thin screens** (slow screens) have poor x-ray absorption efficiencies but excellent spatial resolution (detail screens).

–Spatial resolution can improve with increasing magnification, because the image is spread out over a large area.

–In magnification, the amount of screen blur remains the same, but the actual image is bigger, so the relative importance of screen blur is reduced.

–In screen/film radiography, screen blur is an important limiting factor in the imaging chain.

–Separation of the film from the screen by poor film-screen contact in a damaged cassette will also increase blur.

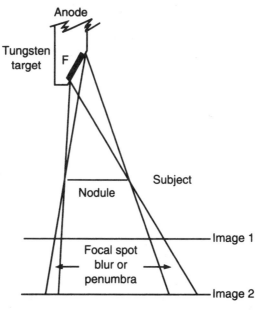

FIG. 5.2. Focal spot blur increases as an object moves farther from the film and as focal spot size increases.

–Screen-film contact can be tested by radiographing a sheet of wire mesh; poor contact is recorded as a local area of reduced contrast and blurring of the wire.

C. Focal spot blur

–The blurred margin at the edge of objects is called the **penumbra.**

–The penumbra is the result of x-rays arriving from slightly different locations in the focal spot, because the focal spot is not a true point source but has a finite area.

–The resultant unsharpness is called **focal spot blur** or **geometric unsharpness.**

–Focal spot blur increases with magnification and focal spot size, as shown in **Fig. 5.2.**

  –Reducing the focal spot size increases the sharpness and definition of object edges by minimizing the penumbra.

–In magnification radiography, it is important to have very small focal spot sizes.

  –Magnification in mammography improves visibility of microcalcifications, but needs a 0.1 mm focal spot to minimize geometric unsharpness.

–Magnification is sometimes used in angiograms to improve the visibility of very small blood vessels and makes use of a 0.3 mm focal spot.

D. Motion blur

–**Patient motion** introduces blur into a radiograph by smearing out the object in the exposed film.

–Organ movement such as the heart, as well as gross movement of the patient, contribute to patient motion.

–Increasing the x-ray tube current to reduce the exposure time will minimize motion blur.

  –Increasing the x-ray tube current may not be possible, however, because of limits on the focal spot loading of the x-ray tube.

–Faster screen-films decrease motion blur by allowing a shorter exposure.

–Motion blur is independent of image magnification.

–Patient motion can be reduced by the use of immobilization devices such as the compression paddle in mammography.

E. Measures of resolution

–The image of a narrow line source is called a **line spread function (LSF)** and its width may be taken as a measure of resolution.

  –Normally, width is measured at half the maximum value, termed **full-width half maximum.**

–A wide LSF implies a low limiting spatial resolution and vice versa.

–The limiting spatial resolution in line pairs per millimeter may be estimated as 1/(2 × FWHM).

  –An LSF with a full-width half maximum of 0.1 mm can thus be taken to have a limiting resolution of about 5 line pairs per mm.

–The **MTF** is a curve based on a Fourier analysis that describes the resolution capability of an imaging system.

  –The **MTF** is the ratio of output to input modulation (signal amplitude) in an imaging system at each spatial frequency.

  –At **low spatial frequencies,** the MTF is close to **one** and corresponds to excellent visibility of relatively large features.

  –At **high spatial frequencies,** the MTF falls to **zero,** which corresponds to the poor visibility of small features.

–The MTF of the imaging system is the product of the MTFs of the respective subcomponents.

–If for a given spatial frequency, the MTF due to the focal spot is 0.9, due to motion is 0.8, and due to the screen is 0.7, then the **imaging system MTF** at this spatial frequency is the product of the individual components: $0.9 \times 0.8 \times 0.7 = 0.5$.

III. Noise

A. Radiographic mottle

–**Noise** is the random fluctuation of image intensity about some mean value following uniform exposure.

–Noise degrades image quality and limits the ability to visualize low-contrast objects.

–**Radiographic mottle** describes the noise present in film images and has three distinct components: **screen mottle, film mottle,** and **quantum mottle.**

–**Screen mottle** (structure mottle) is caused by nonuniformities in screen construction but is usually negligible in modern screens.

–**Film mottle** (graininess) is caused by the grain structure of emulsions and is normally of little importance in screen/film radiography.

–**Quantum mottle** is caused by the discrete nature of x-ray photons and is the most important source of noise in radiography.

–In diagnostic radiology, the number of x-ray photons used to create a radiographic image is typically $10^5/mm^2$.

–In conventional photography, the corresponding number of light photons required to expose a film is 10^9 to $10^{10}/mm^2$.

–This difference in photon intensity explains why noise is generally negligible in conventional photography but is of paramount importance in radiology.

B. Quantum mottle

–For a *uniform* x-ray exposure, adjacent areas of the film (measured in mm^2) have photon counts that randomly differ from the mean value N.

–The distribution of the number of photons in each square millimeter is described by **Poisson statistics.**

–For a **Poisson distribution,** the mean is equal to the **variance (σ^2),** and is generally asymmetrical for low mean values (less than 10).

–In Poisson statistics, the **standard deviation (σ)** is given by the square root of the mean number of counts ($\sigma = \sqrt{N}$).

–Sixty-eight percent of the regions contain counts within one standard deviation of N ($N \pm \sqrt{N}$).

–Ninety-five percent have counts within two standard deviations of N ($N \pm 2\sqrt{N}$).

–Ninety-nine percent have counts within three standard deviations of N ($N \pm 3\sqrt{N}$).

–For example, for a uniform object imaged with an average of 100 photons per square millimeter [mean (N) = 100; $\sigma = \sqrt{N} = 10$], 68% of sampled areas are in the 90 to 110 range, 95% are in the 80 to 120 range, and 99% are in the 70 to 130 range.

–This random variation of photons incident on a radiation detector is known as **quantum mottle.**

–Quantum mottle depends only on the number of photons used to produce an image.

–Doubling the radiation exposure will reduce the *relative* fluctuations about the mean value (quantum mottle) by $2^{1/2}$, or 41%.

–A Gaussian distribution **(Fig. 5.3)** is a good approximation to the Poisson distribution if the mean number of events is greater than 10.

C. Screen speed versus noise

–For screen/film combinations, there is normally a trade-off between speed and noise.

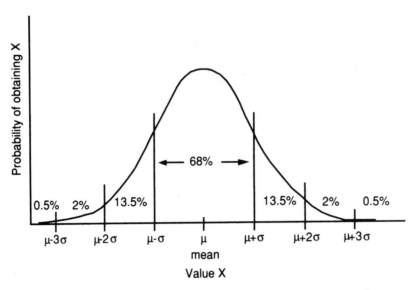

FIG. 5.3. Gaussian probability distribution (normal curve). The percentage values correspond to the areas between the specified limits.

–Noise is determined by how many x-ray photons are absorbed by the screen to produce the image.

–Screen/film speed can be increased either with the same number of detected x-ray photons or with fewer detected x-ray photons.

–If the number of detected photons is constant, then noise remains the same.

–If the number of detected photons is lower, noise increases.

–If screens are made thicker (faster), the resultant image noise remains the same, because the same number of x-ray photons must be absorbed in the screen to produce the desired optical density **(Fig. 5.4).**

–Image noise also remains the same if the x-ray absorption of the screen increases.

–If a phosphor emits more light per absorbed x-ray photon (i.e., higher conversion efficiency), fewer x-ray photons need to be absorbed in the screen to produce the desired optical density, and noise increases **(Fig. 5.4).**

–Similarly, if speed is increased by the use of a faster film, fewer photons are required and noise increases.

D. Mottle in radiology

–For screen-film imaging, the typical exposure required to produce a radiograph is 5 μGy (0.5 mR), which defines the amount of quantum mottle present.

–In fluoroscopy, the amount of radiation used to generate a single frame is more than a hundred times lower.

–The amount of mottle in fluoroscopy is therefore much larger than that in radiography, because the number of photons used to create an image is hundreds of times lower.

–**Table 5.2** provides a summary of the exposures at the imaging receptor required to produce satisfactory radiographic images.

–Cine exposures at the image intensifier input are between screen/film and fluoroscopy.

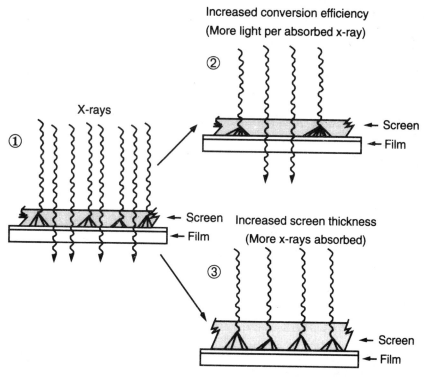

FIG. 5.4. Relation between screen speed and noise. **(1)** A single-emulsion film and screen with an absorption efficiency of 50%. **(2)** A screen with a higher conversion efficiency produces more light photons for each absorbed x-ray, and dose is decreased. The resulting image is noisier because fewer x-rays are used to produce the same film blackening. **(3)** A thicker screen has a higher absorption efficiency, stops more of the incoming x-rays, and reduces dose. Noise is not increased because the same number of absorbed x-rays is used to produce the image.

–Cine mottle in a single cardiac frame is intermediate between fluoroscopy and radiography.

–For a quantum noise–limited system, there is a direct trade-off between the patient radiation exposure, and the corresponding amount of mottle in the resultant image.

–Most radiographic imaging systems are designed to be quantum noise limited and have minimal additional sources of noise.

E. Contrast-to-noise ratio

–To detect a lesion, the image contrast must be large in comparison to image noise (mottle).

TABLE 5.2. *Representative values of image receptor exposures required to produce a satisfactory radiographic image*

Imaging modality	Receptor exposure
Fluoroscopy	0.01–0.02 μGy (1–2 μR)
Cine	0.15–0.30 μGy (15–30 μR)
Photospot film	1 μGy (100 μR)
Screen/film (200 speed)	5 μGy (500 μR)
Detail screen/film	20 μGy (2 mR)
Mammography	100–200 μGy (10–20 mR)

–Improving the contrast is one way of increasing the visibility of a lesion.

–The object contrast can be increased by the administration of a contrast agent.

–Image contrast can also be improved by reducing the x-ray photon energy or by reducing the amount of scatter.

–Reducing the amount of noise is another way of improving lesion visibility.

–Quantum mottle can be reduced by increasing the number of photons used to make the radiographic image.

–Image processing (filtering) can also be used to numerically reduce noise in digital images, but at the price of loss of spatial resolution.

–It is the relative size of lesion contrast to image noise that ultimately determines lesion visibility.

–Image contrast-to-noise ratio is therefore often used as a general descriptor of image quality.

–Improving contrast-to-noise ratio will generally improve lesion detectability and vice versa.

–Signal-to-noise ratio is similar to contrast-to-noise ratio and is another general term used to describe image quality.

IV. Diagnostic Performance

A. Data analysis

–**Mean** is the arithmetic average of a group of data.

–**Median** is a measure of the central tendency and is the value that separates the data in half and defines the 50th percentile.

–**Mode** is the most common data point.

–**Range** is the difference between the highest and lowest values and is a measure of dispersion of the data distribution.

–**Standard deviation** (defined for a population) is used to describe the spread or distribution of a data set and is the square root of the average of the square of all the sample deviations.

–**Bias** is the presence of systematic error.

–**Precision** is the reproducibility of a result but does not imply accuracy.

–**Accuracy** refers to how close a measured value is to the true value.

B. Diagnostic tests

–Excellent diagnostic performance is the primary objective of any radiological imaging system.

–One measure of good diagnostic performance is to maximize true positives and true negatives.

–**True-positives (TPs)** are positive test results in patients who have the disease.

–**True-negatives (TNs)** are negative test results in patients who do not have the disease.

–Another goal of good diagnostic performance is to minimize false-positives and false-negatives.

–**False-positives (FPs)** are positive test results in patients who do not have the disease.

–**False-negatives (FNs)** are negative test results in patients who have the disease.

C. Test results

–**Table 5.3** is a truth table that can be applied to any diagnostic test.

–**Sensitivity** is the ability to detect disease and is TP/(TP + FN), also known as the **true-positive fraction.**

TABLE 5.3. *Truth table for any diagnostic test*

Patient Status	Diagnostic test result	
	Positive	Negative
Disease present	True-positive (TP)	False-negative (FN)
Disease absent	False-positive (FP)	True-negative (TN)

–A **sensitive test** has a low false-negative rate.

–**Specificity** is the ability to identify the absence of disease and is TN/(TN + FP), also known as the **true-negative fraction.**

–A **specific test** has a low false-positive rate.

–**Accuracy** is the fraction of correct diagnosis and is (TP + TN)/(TP + FP + TN + FN).

–**Positive predictive value** is the probability of having the disease given a positive test and is TP/(TP + FP).

–**Negative predictive value** is the probability of not having the disease given a negative test and is TN/(TN + FN).

–Diagnostic performance will generally depend on the disease prevalence.

–**Prevalence** of the disease is [TP + FN]/[TP + FP + TN + FN].

D. Receiver operator characteristic curve

–A **receiver operator characteristic (ROC) curve** is used to compare the performance (sensitivity and specificity) of diagnostic tests at various thresholds of interpreter confidence.

–**Fig. 5.5** shows a typical ROC curve.

–An ROC curve is a plot of the **true-positive fraction** (sensitivity) against the **false-positive fraction** (1-specificity) as the threshold criterion is relaxed.

–Threshold criteria for accepting a positive diagnosis range from the most strict, which corresponds to underreading, to the most lax, which corresponds to overreading.

  –At the most restrictive threshold criterion, both sensitivity and the false-positive fraction are zero.

  –At the most lax threshold criterion, both sensitivity and the false-positive fraction are one.

–Choice of a threshold criterion represents a compromise between the need to increase sensitivity while minimizing the number of false-positives.

E. Area under the receiver operator characteristic curve

–As the threshold criterion is relaxed, both the sensitivity and the false-positive fraction increase from zero to one.

–The area under an ROC curve is a measure of overall imaging performance and is commonly called A_Z.

–The maximum area under the curve is one (100%).

–For random guessing, the ROC curve is a straight line through the points 0,0 and 1,1, and the area under the curve is 0.5 (50%).

–As the imaging performance improves, the ROC curve moves toward the upper left-hand corner, and the area under the ROC curve increases.

–ROC analysis is generally considered a good scientific way of comparing two imaging modalities.

–For any imaging modality, the ROC curve generally moves to the upper left-hand corner as image quality improves.

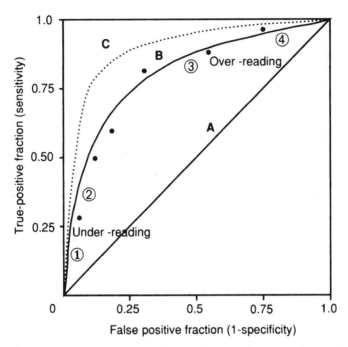

FIG. 5.5. ROC curves. Curve *A* represents the results of random guessing and has no predictive value. Curve *B* represents a typical result; curve *C*, an improved performance. Location *1* represents an area of high specificity where the interpreter is certain the test is normal. Location *2* represents underreading by the interpreter with specificity remaining high. Location *3* has increased sensitivity caused by overreading. Location *4* is the point of greatest sensitivity, in which most results are called positive.

–One difficulty of ROC analysis is determination of the clinical truth, which is needed to compute sensitivity and specificity.

V. Patient Doses

A. Patient skin doses

–The radiation exposure incident on a patient in a radiologic exam is the **entrance skin exposure.**

–The resultant radiation absorbed by the skin is the **entrance skin dose.**

–**Table 5.4** gives typical skin doses in radiographic imaging.

–Skin doses are generally easy to measure or calculate, but they are poor indicators of patient risk.

–Skin doses do not take into account the exposed area, penetrating power of the x-ray beam, or the radiosensitivity of the exposed region.

TABLE 5.4. *Typical values of patient skin doses*

Examination	Skin dose
Chest radiograph (anterior-posterior)	0.1–0.2 mGy (10–20 mrad)
Skull radiograph (anterior-posterior)	1.5 mGy (150 mrad)
Abdominal radiograph	3 mGy (300 mrad)
Lumbar spine (lateral)	10 mGy (1 rad)

–Entrance skin doses are generally lower than are threshold doses (i.e., about 2 Gy/200 rad) for deterministic effects such as epilation and skin erythema.

–At increased voltages, less x-ray tube output is needed to achieve a given level of patient penetration to result in a satisfactory radiographic image.

–Increasing voltages allows the x-ray output values (mAs) to be reduced and produce the same film density with *reduced* entrance skin exposures.

B. Organ doses

–For a given entrance skin dose, it is possible to estimate individual organ doses for many common radiologic examinations.

–Organ doses will be substantially less than the skin dose.

–Organs which are not in the direct field of view are only subject to scatter radiation and will generally receive very low radiation doses.

–For an anterior-posterior projection, the embryo dose will be between one third and one fourth the entrance skin dose (in the direct beam).

–For a posterior-anterior projection, the embryo dose will be about one sixth of the entrance skin dose (in the direct beam).

–For a lateral projection, the embryo dose will be about one twentieth of the entrance skin dose (in the direct beam).

C. Gonadal doses

–Gonad doses are only significant if the gonads are in the direct beam, and gonad shields are not used.

–The **genetically significant dose** (GSD) is a dose parameter that is an index of potential genetic damage.

–The GSD takes into account the dose received by the gonads and the number of offspring an individual is likely to produce.

–If the whole population received a gonad dose equal to the GSD, the genetic harm would be equal to that resulting from current medical exposures of the gonads.

–The GSD from medical exposures is currently estimated to be 0.2 to 0.3 mGy (20 to 30 mrad) per year.

–The GSD from medical exposure is thus about a quarter of natural background radiation.

–The natural rate of occurrence of serious birth defects is about 5%.

–The genetic doubling dose is the dose that would bring about an additional 5% of such defects.

–Current estimates of the genetic doubling dose is of the order of several Gy (several hundred rad)

D. Integral dose and dose-area product parameters

–The **integral dose** measures the total amount of energy (in mJ) imparted to a patient and may be considered a crude estimate of patient risk.

–Approximately 1 mJ of energy is imparted for a chest x-ray.

–Approximately 100 mJ of energy is imparted for a head CT examination.

–Another measure of patient exposure is the **dose-area product,** which is the product of the entrance skin dose and cross-sectional area of the x-ray beam (exposed area).

–For example, the entrance skin dose for chest x-rays is approximately 0.1 mGy (10 mrad) and the x-ray beam area is approximately 1,000 cm^2, resulting in a dose-area product of approximately 100 mGy-cm^2 (10,000 mrad-cm^2).

–Integral dose and **dose-area** product are a useful means of providing relative risks to patients undergoing similar types of radiographic examination.

–Dose-area product devices also permit an estimate to be made of the skin dose if the cross-sectional area of the x-ray beam is known.

E. Effective dose

–Most medical radiologic exposures result in a nonuniform dose distribution within the patient.

  –An anterior-posterior abdominal x-ray results in a entrance skin dose of approximately 3 mGy (300 mrad), exit skin dose of about 0.03 mGy (3 mrad), and (scatter) thyroid dose below 0.003 mGy (less than 0.3 mrad).

–The **effective dose** *(E)* adds the dose of all exposed organs to give an estimate of the total risk to a patient exposed during a radiographic procedure.

–*E* is a weighted sum of the doses to all the exposed organs and tissues in the body.

–In diagnostic radiology $E = \sum_i w_i \times D_i$, where D_i is the dose to organ *i*, which has a radiation weighting factor of w_i.

–The radiation weighting factor w_i is a measure of the relative radiosensitivity of each organ *i* for the induction of stochastic effects (fatal cancer).

  –Radiosensitive organs include the red bone marrow, colon, lung and stomach which have a w_i of 0.12.

  –The bladder, breast, liver, esophagus, and thyroid are moderately radiosensitive and have a w_i of 0.05.

  –Skin and bone are relatively insensitive and have a w_i of 0.01.

–*E* is the uniform whole-body dose, resulting in the same risk of stochastic effects of radiation as a given nonuniform dose.

–Effective doses are expressed in terms of equivalent dose and use **mSv (mrem)**, which are numerically equal to **mGy (mrad)** (see Chapter 10, section I.D).

–**Table 5.5** shows the effective doses received by the patient for common radiological examinations.

–There are likely to be large variations for any individual depending on the technique, factors used, total number of films taken, total fluoroscopy time, and so forth.

TABLE 5.5. *Representative values of patient effective doses in radiographic imaging*

Examination type	Effective dose
Chest	0.02–0.05 mSv (2–5 mrem)
Skull	0.1–0.2 mSv (10–10 mrem)
Abdominal	0.5–1.5 mSv (50–150 mrem)
Upper gastrointestinal	2–4 mSv (200–400 mrem)
Barium enema	3–7 mSv (300–700 mrem)

Review Test

1. The object contrast does not depend on the lesion's:

(A) Thickness
(B) Density
(C) Atomic number
(D) Background composition
(E) Temperature

2. Subject contrast depends on:

(A) Focal spot to film distance
(B) mAs
(C) Tube voltage
(D) Developer temperature
(E) Film gradient

3. *Film* contrast, as opposed to subject contrast, is affected primarily by:

(A) Tube voltage
(B) Iodine contrast
(C) Use of grid
(D) Differences in *Z*
(E) Optical density

4. The *maximum slope* of the characteristic curve is also known as:

(A) Density
(B) Gamma
(C) Transmittance
(D) Opacity
(E) Lambda

5. Which of the following features cannot be determined from the film characteristic curve?

(A) Speed
(B) Gamma
(C) Base plus fog level
(D) Average gradient
(E) Mottle

6. In chest x-ray examinations, one should choose a film with:

(A) High gradient
(B) High gamma
(C) Slow speed
(D) Wide latitude
(E) Low fog level

7. Gastrointestinal tract contrast could be improved by all of the following *except:*

(A) Infusion of barium
(B) Reduced tube voltage
(C) Increased tube current
(D) Increased grid ratio
(E) Reduced field size

8. Spatial resolution *cannot* be assessed using:

(A) Line pair phantom
(B) LSF image
(C) Full-width half maximum
(D) MTF curve
(E) Pixel standard deviation

9. Screen-film resolution can be best improved by changing to:

(A) Lower tube voltage
(B) Slower film
(C) Higher grid ratio
(D) Thinner screens
(E) Green sensitive film

10. Compared with a regular screen, a detail screen of the same phosphor will have a lower:

(A) Spatial resolution
(B) Speed
(C) Noise level
(D) Conversion efficiency
(E) Linear attenuation coefficient

11. Poor screen/film contact will primarily result in a significant loss of:

(A) Contrast
(B) Magnification
(C) Image detail
(D) X-ray absorption efficiency
(E) Conversion efficiency

12. A limitation of geometric magnification is due to:

(A) Increased screen/film dose
(B) Focal spot blurring
(C) Need for focused grids
(D) Increased quantum mottle
(E) Longer processing times

13. Which of the following factors would have the least effect on image sharpness?

(A) Film type
(B) Focal spot size
(C) Motion
(D) Screen thickness
(E) Screen/film contact

14. The MTF is *not:*

(A) A description of any imaging system resolution performance
(B) The ratio of image to subject contrast at each spatial frequency
(C) Equal to the unity when the spatial resolution is perfect
(D) Usually lower at high spatial frequencies
(E) Fifty percent at half the limiting spatial resolution

15. Which of the following is *not* true for Poisson distributions?

(A) They are used to describe radioactive decay
(B) They are used to describe quantum mottle
(C) The variance is equal to the mean
(D) They are always symmetrical
(E) They are approximate to a Gaussian for means greater than 10

16. Quantum mottle is determined primarily by which one of the following factors?

(A) X-ray beam filtration
(B) X-ray photons absorbed in screen
(C) X-ray photon energy
(D) Screen conversion efficiency
(E) Screen thickness

17. The speed of a screen/film can be increased *without* increasing noise by:

(A) Using a faster film
(B) Using phosphor with a higher conversion efficiency
(C) Increasing the processor developer temperature
(D) Increasing the phosphor absorption efficiency
(E) Decreasing screen thickness

18. The major contributor to noise in a fluoroscopic image is variations in the:

(A) Input phosphor thickness
(B) Accelerating tube voltage
(C) Output phosphor thickness
(D) Display screen brightness
(E) Quantum mottle

19. Image contrast-to-noise ratio could not be increased by using:

(A) Lower tube voltages
(B) Higher-ratio grids
(C) Larger x-ray beam areas
(D) Screens with lower conversion efficiency
(E) Slower films

20. The mode is:

(A) The arithmetic average
(B) The 50th percentile value
(C) The most common value
(D) Standard deviation
(E) Variance

21. Sensitivity is given by the:

(A) False positive fraction
(B) True positive fraction
(C) False negative fraction
(D) True negative fraction
(E) Area under ROC curve

22. Specificity is given by:

(A) The true-negative fraction
(B) The true-positive fraction
(C) (1 − true-positive fraction)
(D) (1 + true-negative fraction)
(E) Area under the ROC curve

23. A ROC curve is used to measure diagnostic imaging:

(A) Performance
(B) Accuracy
(C) Specificity
(D) Sensitivity
(E) Cost benefit ratio

24. In 35 mm cardiac cine, patient entrance skin dose is *reduced* by increasing the:

(A) Acquisition frame rate
(B) Tube voltage
(C) Tube current
(D) Grid ratio
(E) Focal spot size

25. In screen/film radiography, raising the kilovolt peak will increase all of the following *except:*

(A) Half-value layer
(B) Scatter
(C) Patient transmission (%)
(D) Subject contrast
(E) Grid penetration

26. The dose to the fetus after 2 minutes of pelvic fluoroscopy is:

(A) Less than 1 mGy (0.1 rad)
(B) 1 mGy (0.1 rad)
(C) 10 mGy (1 rad)
(D) 100 mGy (10 rad)
(E) More than 100 mGy (10 rad)

27. The patient integral dose does not depend on the:

(A) Skin dose
(B) Beam area
(C) Beam quality
(D) Patient thickness
(E) Organ sensitivity

28. The GSD does *not* depend on the patient's:

(A) Weight
(B) Age
(C) Sex
(D) Gonad dose
(E) Likelihood of having children

29. The skin dose for a chest x-ray examinations is:

(A) Less than 0.05 mGy (3 mrad)
(B) About 0.05 mGy (3 mrad)
(C) About 0.15 mGy (15 mrad)
(D) About 0.5 mGy (50 mrad)
(E) More than 0.5 mGy (50 mrad)

30. The effective dose for a chest x-ray examination does not take into account:

(A) Mean organ doses
(B) Radiation LET
(C) Organ sensitivity
(D) All exposed organs
(E) Patient age

Answers and Explanations

1–E. Temperature has no effect on object contrast.

2–C. Developer temperature and film gradient affect image contrast.

3–E. At very low and very high film densities, the contrast will be very low, whereas the optimal contrast will be produced at a film density of about 1.2 to 1.8.

4–B. The maximum slope of the characteristic curve is the film gamma.

5–E. Mottle is the random fluctuation in density for uniform x-ray exposure.

6–D. Wide-latitude film is required to capture the low exposures through the mediastinum *and* the high exposures through the lungs.

7–C. Increasing tube current has no effect on the contrast per se. Lower tube voltage, increase in the grid ratio, and tighter collimation also serve to reduce scatter and increase the subject contrast.

8–E. Pixel standard deviation would be used to estimate image noise, not spatial resolution.

9–D. Changing to thinner screens will generally improve spatial resolution performance.

10–B. Detail screens are thinner and therefore have a reduced speed.

11–C. The gap between the screen and film will increase diffusion of light reaching the film and increase image blur.

12–B. Blurring because of focal spot size increases because of the increase in geometric penumbra.

13–A. There is no loss of detail owing to a film per se. In practice, the MTF of a film alone is 1.0 at all spatial frequencies of interest in radiological imaging.

14–E. There is nothing magical about the 50% MTF value.

15–D. A Poisson distribution is not symmetrical at low mean values (below 10) but is approximately symmetrical for large means (over 10).

16–B. The primary factor is the number of x-ray photons used to create the image.

17–D. Increasing the phosphor absorption efficiency will require the same number of absorbed photons to create an image, so that noise remains the same. Fewer photons will be incident on the patient, however, which means that the system speed has increased.

18–E. Variation in input x-ray photons (quantum mottle) is the dominant noise source in fluoroscopy.

19–C. A larger x-ray beam area will increase scatter and lower image contrast, thereby reducing the contrast-to-noise ratio.

20–C. The mode is the most common data point.

21–B. Sensitivity is TP/(TP + FN), or the true-positive fraction.

22–A. Specificity is the true-negative fraction.

23–A. Performance is obtained from the area under the ROC curve. (Both sensitivity and specificity change with threshold criterion.)

24–B. Increasing tube voltage increases the patient penetration and therefore reduces entrance skin doses for a constant image intensifier input dose level.

25–D. Subject contrast generally falls with increasing photon energy achieved by raising the kilovolt peak.

26–C. Ten mGy (1 rad), because the entrance skin dose after 2 minutes of fluoroscopy will be about 2 (minutes) $\times$ 20 mGy/min or 40 mGy; the fetus dose will be about one fourth the entrance skin dose.

27–E. The integral dose is the total energy deposited in the patient and takes no account of the sensitivity of exposed organs.

28–A. The patient weight per se is irrelevant when computing the GSD; it is only the gonad dose that counts.

29–C. A typical skin dose for a chest x-ray is 0.15 mGy, whereas the resultant effective dose would be much lower (0.03 mSv).

30–E. Patient age is not taken into account when computing effective doses.

6

Digital X-ray Imaging

I. Computers

A. Basics

–**Computers** use the **binary system** (base 2).

–A **bit** *(bi*nary dig*it)* is the fundamental information element used by computers and can be assigned one of two discrete values.

  –One bit can code for two values, or two shades of gray, which correspond to white and black.

  –*n* bits can code for 2^n values, or gray levels.

–The American Standard Code for Information Exchange (ASCII) uses 8 bit groups (designated a byte) to represent common letters and symbols.

–**Eight bits = 1 byte; 2 bytes = 1 word** (16 bits).

  –A total of 256 shades of gray (2^8) can be coded for by 1 byte (8 bits).

  –A total of 4,096 shades of gray (2^{12}) can be coded for by 12 bits.

–Memory and file storage requirements for computers are normally specified using kilobytes (kB; 1,024 bytes) or megabytes (MB) (1,024 kB).

  –Large storage requirements are specified using gigabytes (1 GB = 1,024 MB).

  –Radiology storage is huge and measured in terabytes (1 TB = 1,024 GB).

B. Computer hardware

–Computer hardware refers to the physical components of the system, including the central processing unit, memory, and data entry and export devices.

–Computer memory stores the various bit sequences and is either **random access memory (RAM)** or **read-only memory (ROM)**.

  –**RAM** is temporary (volatile) memory that stores information while the software is used. It is the primary memory component in most computers.

  –**ROM** is for permanent storage and cannot be overwritten. Important central processing unit (CPU) instructions for system operation are stored in ROM.

–**Buffer memories** are normally considered a part of RAM and are used for video displays.

–**Cache memory** provides transitional memory storage and is often built into CPU chips to provide a buffer between RAM and disc memory.

–**Address** refers to the location of bit sequences in memory.

–A **CPU** performs calculations and logic operations by manipulating bit sequences under the control of software instructions.

  –A Pentium 4 microprocessor is an example of a CPU.

–**Parallel processing** occurs when several tasks are performed simultaneously.

–**Serial processing** refers to performing tasks sequentially.

–**Array processors** are hard-wired devices dedicated to performing one type of rapid calculation.

–Array processors are used in computed tomography and magnetic resonance imaging, where large numbers of calculations are needed to convert data into images.

–A **bus** is a local pathway linking components.

C. Computer software

–Computers use **operating systems** to perform internal system bookkeeping activities such as storing files.

–A file is a collection of data treated as a unit.

–Examples of operating systems are Windows (for IBM personal computers), UNIX (for SUN computers and others), and VMS (for many mainframe computers).

–Macintosh computers use a proprietary operating system.

–**Computer software** instructs the computer where input data are stored, how these data are to be manipulated, and where the results are to be placed.

–Most **computer programs** are written using high-level languages such as C, Pascal, COBOL, dBase, FORTRAN, or Basic.

–**Object code,** or **machine language,** is the machine-specific binary code instructions used by the CPU.

–High-level machine-independent languages are called **source code.**

–**Java** is a platform-independent programming language designed to run in a network environment.

–A **compiler** is a software program used to convert high-level language (source code) to machine language (object code).

D. Computer peripheral devices

–**Input devices** include keyboards, joysticks, light pens, trackballs, and touch screens.

–**Output devices** include cathode ray tubes, laser film printers, and paper printers.

–**Data storage devices** include hard disks, floppy disks, optical disks, optical jukeboxes, and magnetic tapes.

–**Table 6.1** summarizes the capabilities of various data storage devices.

–**RAID** (*r*edundant *a*rray of *i*nexpensive *d*isks) provides redundant, inexpensive, readily accessible local storage.

–Computers communicate via coaxial cables, telephone lines, magnetic tape transfers, microwaves, and fiber-optic links.

–A **modem** (*mo*dulator/*dem*odulator) is used to transmit information over telephone lines.

–**Fig. 6.1** shows the peripheral devices associated with computers.

TABLE 6.1. *Typical storage capacities and access times for computer storage media*

Media	Storage capacity	Access time
Floppy disk	1.4 MB	~0.5 sec
Zip drive	100–250 MB	~0.5 sec
Hard disk	20 MB–50 GB	10 msec
Magnetic tape	600 MB–50 GB	10 sec–4 min
Optical disk	600 MB–10 GB	16 msec
Optical jukebox	500 GB–3 TB	10–60+ sec

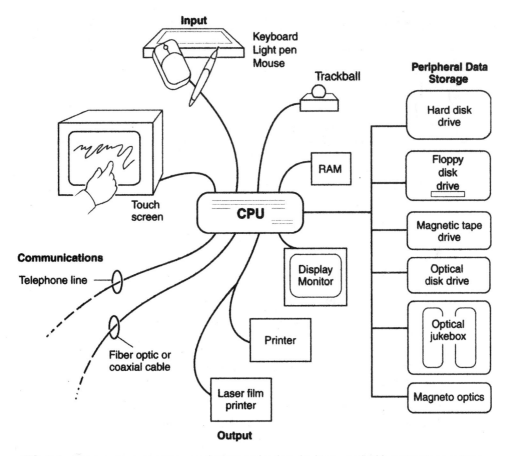

FIG. 6.1. Input, output, memory, and communication devices used with computer systems.

–Modern computers are linked using networks such as **Ethernet,** which can be used to transmit images to remote locations.

–**Baud rate** describes the rate of information transfer in bits per second.

–A baud rate of 56,000 corresponds to 56,000 bits/second or 7,000 bytes/second.

–**Table 6.2** lists network options for transmitting images and the typical transmission times for a standard digitized chest x-ray.

TABLE 6.2. *Types of local area networks and typical time required to transfer a digital chest x-ray**

Mode	Nominal speed (Mbit/sec)	Chest x-ray transfer time
Modem (telephone)	0.056	~45
Ethernet	10	~1 min
Token ring	4–6	~1 min
Fiber distributed data interface	125	<10 sec
Asynchronous transfer mode (ATM)	600	<1 sec

* Approximately 8 MB of information.

TABLE 6.3. *Typical matrix sizes and bytes per pixel in radiology*

Modality	Matrix size	Bytes per pixel
Nuclear medicine	128 × 128	1
Magnetic resonance	256 × 256	2
Computed tomography	512 × 512	2
Ultrasound	512 × 512	1
Digital photospot/DSA	1024 × 1024	2
CR, DR, and film digitizers	2560 × 2048	2
Mammography	4096 × 6144	2

* DSA, digital subtraction angiography; CR, computed radiography; DR, digital radiography.

E. Image information

–**Pixels** are individual picture elements in a two-dimensional image.

–In digital images, each **pixel** intensity is normally coded using either 1 or 2 bytes.

–The total number of pixels in an image is the product of the number of pixels assigned to the horizontal and vertical dimensions.

–The number of pixels in each dimension is called **matrix size.**

–If there are 1,024 (1 k) pixels in both the horizontal and vertical dimensions, then the image contains 1 k × 1 k = 1 M, or $1,024^2$ pixels.

–**Table 6.3** lists typical matrix sizes used in diagnostic radiology.

–The **information content** of images is the product of the number of pixels and the number of bytes per pixel.

–An image with a 512 × 512 pixel matrix and 1 byte coding of each pixel requires 0.25 MB of memory (512 × 512 × 1).

–The same image obtained using 2 byte coding of each pixel requires 0.5 MB of memory (512 × 512 × 2).

–A chest x-ray digitized to a 2 × 2 k matrix using 2 byte coding of each pixel (2,048 × 2,048 × 2) requires 8 MB of memory.

–Modern digital mammography systems are designed with matrix sizes between 4 × 4 k and 4 × 6 k pixels.

–With 2 byte coding of each pixel, a single mammography image would require 32 to 48 MB of memory.

II. Detectors in Digital Imaging

A. Gas and solid state detectors

–Gases may be used to detect x-ray photons by applying a high voltage across a gas chamber and measuring the flow of free electrons produced by ionization of the gas.

–Xenon is a high-atomic number gas (Z = 54; K-edge energy = 35 keV), which is an efficient x-ray detector at high pressure.

–Incident x-rays transfer energy to energetic electrons in Compton and photoelectric interactions.

–Energetic electrons lose energy by undergoing collisions with atoms and thereby producing many ionizations.

–The signal produced by absorption of x-rays is the total electron charge liberated in the gas, which is collected by the positive anode.

–In solid crystals (e.g., NaCl), atoms are arranged in a regular three-dimensional structure.

–Whereas electrons in atoms are arranged in shells, electrons in crystals are arranged in **bands.**

–In solid-state crystals, only the two outer bands of electrons are important. ' are called the (inner) **valence** and (outer) **conduction** band.

–When x-rays interact with a solid-state material, energy is transferred to electrons in the Compton and photoelectric processes.

  –In **photostimulable phosphors,** some of this energy is stored in "electron traps," and can be released at a later time when the phosphor is stimulated with light.

  –In **scintillators,** some of the deposited energy is converted into light which can be detected by a light detector.

  –In **photoconductors,** this charge is collected and measured directly.

B. Photostimulable phosphors

–Computed radiography (CR) uses photostimulable phosphor plates made of europium-activated barium fluorohalide (BaFBr).

–X-ray photons interact with the electrons in the phosphor, creating a latent image.

–After exposure, the plates are read out using a low-energy laser light (red) to stimulate and empty the electron traps.

–High-energy light (blue) is emitted, which can be measured using a light detector (photomultiplier tube).

  –The amount of light detected is proportional to the incident x-ray exposure.

  –The intensity of the detected light signal is stored as a number in a computer.

–Photostimulable phosphor plates can be erased using white light and reused.

–Photostimulable phosphors have a wide dynamic range.

  –Photostimulable phosphors detect x-ray exposures 100 times lower, and 100 times higher, than the 5 μGy (500 μR) required for screen/film.

C. Scintillators

–**Scintillators** or **phosphors** are materials that emit light when exposed to radiation.

–The **conversion efficiency** of a phosphor is the percentage of absorbed energy that is converted into light.

  –Only 2% to 20% of the absorbed energy is converted to light.

–Radiographic screens are examples of scintillators in which the light output is detected by a film.

  –Gadolinium oxysulfide (Gd_2O_2S) is a common radiographic screen.

–Image intensifier input phosphors are scintillators, typically cesium iodide (CsI).

–Scintillators are also being used in digital x-ray detector systems.

  –Digital x-ray detectors based on scintillators are commonly known as "indirect" x-ray detectors **(Fig. 6.2A).**

  –Indirect detectors produce light that is subsequently detected by a two-dimensional array of light detectors.

–CsI is the most commonly used phosphor material in indirect detectors because it has excellent x-ray absorption properties.

  –The conversion efficiency of CsI is 10%, so that 10% of the absorbed x-ray energy is emitted in the form of light energy.

  –CsI in flat-panel detectors is normally manufactured in columns to minimize light diffusion and maintain a high spatial resolution.

D. Photoconductors

–A **photoconductor** is a solid-state device that detects x-rays directly.

–**Selenium** ($Z = 34$; K-edge energy $= 13$ keV) is the most common photoconductor in use in digital radiography.

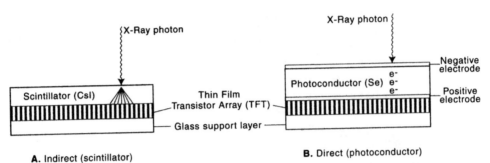

FIG. 6.2. Indirect (scintillator; **A**) and direct (photoconductor; **B**) flat-panel detector systems. Both use a thin film transistor array for signal detection and localization. The indirect detector is based on light production in a scintillating material such as cesium iodide. The direct detector is based on the production and detection of electrons in a photoconductor like selenium. The dispersion of light photons in the scintillator increases blur for indirect systems.

–A typical x-ray detector has a thickness of about 0.5 mm and has a voltage across the device.

–Electrons produced by the deposition of x-ray energy are stored and directly read out.

–The electronic signal in a given region is directly proportional to the amount of x-ray energy deposited in the region.

–Digital x-ray detectors based on photoconductors are known as "direct" x-ray detectors because the deposited x-ray energy in the form of liberated charge is measured directly **(Fig. 6.2B).**

–The charge collection process does not introduce "diffusion," as occurs with light spreading in scintillators.

–Resolution properties of photoconductors are therefore generally excellent.

–Photoconductors based on selenium have poor x-ray absorption properties at higher photon energies because of the relatively low K-shell binding energy.

–Alternatives to selenium include lead iodide (PbI) and mercury iodide (HgI).

–X-ray absorption characteristics of PbI and HgI are expected to be excellent for x-ray imaging applications.

III. Digital X-Ray Imaging

A. Digital systems

–Digital radiography (DR) includes CR and flat-panel detectors that use direct (photoconductors) and indirect (scintillator) detection processes.

–**CR** uses photostimulable phosphors to capture x-ray exposure patterns that are subsequently "read out" using lasers.

–Acquired CR data are stored in a computer and can be processed in a variety of ways before being printed on film or displayed on a monitor.

–CR is based on cassettes and is compatible with analog screen/film imaging systems.

–A single CR reader can process CR cassettes from several radiographic rooms.

–CR systems are ideal for performing portable x-ray examinations when photo-timing cannot be used.

–**Flat-panel detectors** include both direct (photoconductor) and indirect (scintillators) systems.

–Flat-panels comprise a two-dimensional array of elements, each of which can store charge in response to x-ray exposure (light for indirect; charge for direct).

–After exposure, the stored charge is read out electronically.

–Flat-panel detectors are very fast and permit the review of an acquired image within seconds of the exposure.

–Flat-panel detectors are dedicated to a given radiographic room.

–Flat-panel detectors are very expensive.

–Use of flat-panel technology has the potential to significantly improve technologist operational efficiency.

–It is sometimes desirable to convert a conventional analog film print into a digital image for electronic transfer (teleradiology) or processing.

–Commercially available **film digitizers** read the analog image by passing a narrow beam of laser light across the film and converting the transmitted intensity to a digital signal.

–A typical chest x-ray would have 2,000 measurements along one line and 2,500 lines to cover the film.

–Output from a film digitizer has about 5 million pixels (2,500 × 2,000).

B. Image processing

–DR separates image capture, image storage, and image display functions that are all performed by film in screen/film imaging.

–In digital imaging, individual picture elements (pixels) are assigned a location and grayscale value or intensity by groups of bits.

–The full collection of pixels (termed a matrix) can represent an image that can be electronically manipulated (processed) to alter the appearance.

–**Look-up tables** are a method of altering the tonal qualities of an image by mapping intensity values to a desired brightness level **(Fig. 6.3).**

–This is similar to an H and D curve, which maps x-ray intensity values to film optical density.

–**Histogram equalization** eliminates white and black pixels that contribute little diagnostic information and expands the remaining data to use the full dynamic range.

–**Low-pass spatial filtering** is a method of noise reduction in which a portion of the averaged value of the surrounding pixels is added to each pixel.

–Noise is reduced by smoothing the image at the expense of spatial resolution.

–**Unsharp masking** is a method of edge enhancement that involves subtraction of a smoothed version from the original, which is then added to a replicate original.

–Fine details are enhanced at the expense of increased noise and artifacts.

–**Background subtraction** digitally reduces the effect of x-ray scatter to increase image contrast.

–**Energy subtraction** techniques are based on subtracting projection radiographs obtained at two photon energies (i.e., 60 and 110 kVp).

–Chest radiographs obtained at high and low kilovolt peaks can be subtracted to diminish the contribution of bone to the image, thus providing a better depiction of lung and soft tissue.

C. Digital image display

–**Hard-copy** display refers to printing images onto film using a laser camera.

–The film is exposed in a raster fashion by a laser that projects a beam of varying-intensity light across the film.

–The brightness of the beam at each position depends on the (digital) image intensity value at this location.

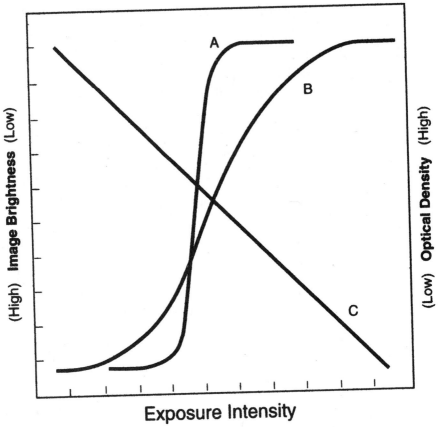

FIG. 6.3. Look-up tables for image processing. The curve shape defines the relationship be-tween the exposure intensity and image density (or brightness). **(A)** High-contrast curve. **(B)** Wide-latitude (low-contrast) curve. **(C)**. Linear response curve with a reversed grayscale.

–A matrix of about 3,500 × 4,300 can be written to a 35 × 43 cm film, with a lim-iting resolution of approximately 5 lp/mm.

–Soft-copy display refers to presenting images on cathode ray tube monitors and flat-panel monitors.

–A monitor where the horizontal dimension is longer is called a landscape display, whereas a longer vertical dimension is a portrait display.

–The luminance of video monitors (80 to 300 cd/m^2) is much lower than that of con-ventional radiographic view boxes (1,500 to 3,500 cd/m^2).

–Image displays used for diagnostic interpretation have a matrix size of 2 × 2.5 k.

–Image displays can also use 1 × 1 k monitor, with only half the resolution.

–**Interpolation** refers to the mapping of an image of one matrix size to a display of another size.

–For example, a 2 × 2 k image displayed on a 1 k monitor requires that 4 pixels from the image be mapped to each pixel on the monitor.

–Video displays use 8 bit images, which register 256 brightness intensity levels.

–Digital images permit the display window width and window level settings to be ad-justed by the operator to modify the image brightness and contrast.

–Image **window width** refers to the range of grayscale values displayed.

  −All pixels with values below the range register as black and all those above as white, and the contrast within the range is increased.
  −**Window level** defines the center value of the window width and, therefore, overall image brightness.

D. Digital image quality

  −Image quality in digital radiology relates to contrast, noise, resolution, and artifacts.
  −Digital and analog image quality are conceptually very similar.
  −Digital image quality is also affected by the discrete nature of the image data.
  −**Image contrast** in a displayed digital image is the difference in monitor intensity of the lesion and that of the surrounding background.
  −A powerful feature of digital images is that their displayed appearance can be easily changed by modifying the display window and level settings.
  −In principle, digital images should never be contrast limited.
  −**Noise** refers to the random fluctuation of pixel values in a region that receives the same radiation exposure.
  −As in screen/film imaging, the dominant source of noise in most digital imaging systems is quantum mottle.
  −Increasing the radiation exposure by a factor of two will reduce quantum mottle fluctuations about the mean value by 41%.
  −Mottle will limit the visibility of low contrast lesions.
  −For digital displays with adjustable contrast, it is the **contrast-to-noise ratio** that will limit the visibility of low-contrast lesions (Chapter 5, Section III.E).
  −The detector size (aperture) and sampling pitch of digital arrays both affect spatial resolution.
  −For example, if there are 2,000 detectors on a line that is 35 cm long, the sampling pitch is 175 μm (35 divided by 2,000).
  −The sampling pitch determines the limiting spatial resolution that is achievable by the digital imaging modality.
  −The limiting spatial resolution, also known as the **Nyquist frequency,** is given by the reciprocal of twice the sampling pitch, or 1/(2 × sampling pitch).
  −If the sampling pitch is 175 μm, the limiting (Nyquist) frequency is 2.9 lp/mm (i.e., 1/[2 × 0.175 mm]).
  −The Nyquist frequency defines the highest spatial frequency that can be faithfully reproduced.
  −Presence of higher spatial frequencies in images result in **aliasing artifacts.**
  −The finite size of each detector element introduces **aperture blurring.**
  −Each detector element produces an average pixel intensity of the x-ray intensity variations within the detector element.

E. Radiation doses in digital radiography

  −In screen/film radiography, the amount of radiation required to generate a satisfactory radiograph is fixed.
  −For a 200 speed screen/film system, for example, a detector exposure of about 500 μR is required.
  −DR systems do not have a specified speed per se and can be used at a range of exposure levels.
  −Virtually any radiation exposure in DR can be used to generate an image with satisfactory intensities by modification of the display settings.

–Comparing radiation doses between DR and screen/film is very tricky and depends on how the question is framed.

–DR is very tolerant of overexposure and underexposure and will reduce the number of repeat examinations because of technical problems (dark and light films).

–Flat-panel detectors are more efficient x-ray absorbers than are radiographic screens, and require less radiation to achieve the same image quality.

–CR uses thinner phosphors than screens, which makes them less-efficient x-ray absorbers; CR would thus require more radiation to achieve the same image quality.

–With all types of flat-panel detectors, patient doses should be lower than screen/film, but the opposite is generally true for CR.

–Of greater importance is the fact that both CR and flat-panel detectors permit the operator to change the radiation exposure for different diagnostic imaging tasks.

–For scoliosis examinations, it may be possible to reduce the doses by an order of magnitude and still produce digital images that answer the clinical question.

IV. Digital Dynamic Imaging

A. Digitizing TV images

–The analog voltage signal from a TV camera must be converted to a digital bit sequence (analog to digital) before it can be processed.

–An **analog-to-digital converter** changes varying voltage levels to the closest binary equivalent.

–The TV output video signal of a fluoroscopy unit may be digitized and stored in a computer for further processing or subsequent display.

–If the TV is a nominal 525 line system, one frame generally consists of 525^2 (250,000) **pixels.**

–Each pixel needs either 1 byte (8 bits) or 2 bytes (16 bits) of space to record the signal level.

–Modern TV cameras may be operated in 1,000 line mode, resulting in a single frame having $1,000^2$ (1 million) pixels, and an information content of 1 or 2 MB.

–Images may be acquired at up to 30 frames/second (525 line systems) or 7.5 frames/second (1,000 line systems).

–TV cameras used in digital systems are selected to have low noise levels and high stability and may also be operated in progressive scan mode.

–The TV camera may be replaced by a **charged coupled device (CCD),** which records the light output from the image intensifier.

–Charged coupled device and TV cameras produce similar fluoroscopy image quality.

–TV resolution is determined by the number of TV/charged coupled device lines.

–Fluoroscopy images are generally quantum noise limited.

B. Digital fluoroscopy

–**Digital fluoroscopy** is a fluoroscopy system, the TV camera output of which is digitized.

–The image data can be passed through a computer to process the images before being displayed on a monitor.

–Image processing in digital fluoroscopy occurs in real time.

–Because the images are acquired by a computer, **last frame–hold** software permits the visualization of the last image when the x-ray beam is switched off.

–**Road mapping** permits an image to be captured and displayed on a monitor, while a second monitor shows live images.

–**Road mapping** can also be used to capture images with contrast material that can be overlaid onto a live fluoroscopy image.

–**Road mapping** is particularly useful for advancing catheters through tortuous vessels.

–**Digital temporal filtering** (frame averaging) is a technique of adding together and then averaging the pixel values in successive images.

–Temporal filtering reduces the effect of random noise.

–Appreciable temporal filtering causes noticeable lag but much lower noise levels.

–Temporal filtering has the potential to reduce patient doses by permitting the use of lower radiation levels while reducing image noise.

–In the future, flat-panel detectors will replace image intensifiers for digital fluoroscopy.

C. Digital photospot imaging

–**Digital photospot imaging** is an alternative to spot film imaging and photospot imaging.

–A short exposure with a high tube current (mA) is made while the real-time video is inactivated.

–The camera scans the image and writes it to the computer memory for later retrieval and processing.

–Digital photospot imaging is widely used for obtaining diagnostic quality images during fluoroscopy examinations.

–Digital photospot images are mainly $1,024^2$, although higher matrix sizes ($2,048^2$) have also been used.

–Digital photospot cameras permit the immediate viewing of radiographic quality images on a monitor.

–A series of digital images demonstrating anatomy and pathology can be rapidly acquired and reviewed.

–Digital photospot images are also normally printed to a laser camera.

–Digital photospot images can be conveniently processed, transmitted, and stored.

–Digital photospot is rapidly replacing spot/photospot imaging in clinical practice.

–**Fig. 6.4** shows the components of a digital imaging system.

D. Digital subtraction angiography

–In **digital subtraction angiography (DSA),** a fluoroscopically acquired digital **"mask" image,** obtained without vascular contrast, is subtracted from subsequent frames obtained following contrast administration.

–DSA images show only the contrast-filled vessels.

–**Table 6.4** shows the typical exposure factors used in DSA imaging.

–DSA can detect low-contrast objects, so less **contrast material** is needed.

–DSA can be used to visualize contrast differences of less than 1% in x-ray transmission.

–Differences of 2% to 3% may often be missed with conventional screen/film combinations.

–Venous (rather than arterial) contrast administration is not used because the reduced concentration of iodine contrast reaching the arteries produces images of poor quality.

–DSA data are stored in a computer so that the image appearance can be modified by changing displayed window settings or enhanced.

–Digital data permit quantitative data to be obtained.

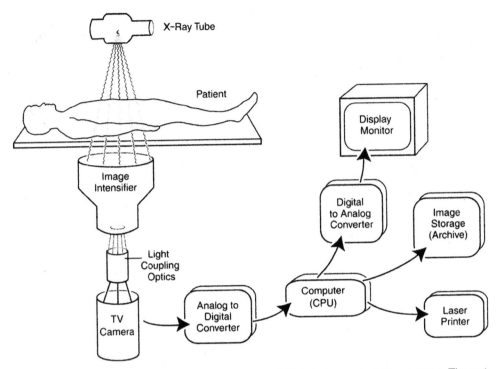

FIG. 6.4. Components of a digital fluoroscopy and digital photospot imaging system. The output signal from the TV camera is digitized by the analog-to-digital converter, allowing the image to be processed in real time. The digital images can be processed to improve contrast and viewed on a display monitor, printed to a laser camera, and stored in an archive.

–The mean rate of flow of iodine contrast through a vessel, or the degree of vessel stenosis, can be determined.

–DSA and temporal subtraction techniques in general are quite susceptible to patient motion, including breathing, cardiac motion, and vascular pulsation.

E. Dose and image quality

–The matrix size in digital fluoroscopy and DSA is usually 1,024 × 1,024.

–The resolution achieved is determined by the camera resolution and is typically 2 lp/mm (1,000 line TV system).

–Spatial resolution can be improved, however, by reducing the field of view.

–Because noise is randomly distributed in each image, the **noise level** in the final subtracted image **is higher** than that in either individual image.

TABLE 6.4. *Typical radiographic techniques used in a 23 cm image intensifier for neuro-digital subtraction angiography*

Parameter	Typical values
Voltage	70–80 kVp
Current	100–250 mA
Pulse duration	30–100 msec
Acquisition rate	2–8 frames/sec
Image matrix size	$1,024^2$

–DSA images, however, benefit from the removal of "anatomical background."

–DSA image quality may be degraded if the patient moves between acquisition of the mask frame and subsequent frames containing the contrast material.

–Corrections for patient motion may be made by computer manipulation of the digital images stored in memory.

–One method of **motion correction** is to incorporate spatial displacement of the mask frame.

–Another correction is to select a later frame for use as the mask (remasking).

–Doses in real time digital fluoroscopy are comparable to those of conventional fluoroscopy, with a typical image intensifier input dose of 0.01 to 0.02 μGy (1 to 2 μR) for each frame.

–Digital photospot and DSA imaging are both digital and do not have an intrinsic speed per se but rather permit a wide range of exposures to create the image.

–Digital photospot and DSA have doses that are about a hundred times higher per frame than in digital flouroscopy.

–Image exposures in digital photospot and DSA imaging should be set by the requirements of the diagnostic task at hand.

–Digital photospot and DSA exposures are generally set to be lower than those used with screen/film imaging.

–A single digital photospot or DSA image generally uses 1 to 2 μGy (100 to 200 μR), which is much lower than the 5 μGy (500 μR) used with screen/film.

V. Picture Archiving and Communications Systems

A. Networks

–**Computer networks allow two or more computers to exchange information.**

–**Network protocols** are the codes and conventions under which a network operates.

–**Bandwidth** defines the maximum amount of information that can be transferred over a data channel per unit of time.

–Bandwidth is measured in megabits per second or gigabits per second.

–**Topology** refers to the network layout and connection of the various components.

–**Token ring** topology is a closed loop of point-to-point connections.

–**Ethernet** is a standard often used for local area networks.

–**Backbone** refers to a large network that connects smaller networks.

–A **bridge** connects network segments.

–Local area networks (**LANs**) are devices connected by cable or optical fiber.

–Wide area networks (**WANs**), such as the Internet, use remote telecommunication devices.

–A **router** is a computer system that connects and directs information from one network to another by selecting the best available pathway.

B. Image transmission

–**Client** refers to a computer requesting information from another computer (**server**).

–**Push** technology refers to an opposite scenario in which a passive client receives information broadcast from a server.

–**Domain** refers to the name identification for a particular machine. E-mail addresses contain various levels of domain names (local name@domain.top-level domain).

–Internet protocol (**IP**) is a low-level protocol for assigning addresses to information packets.

–The **Internet** uses high-level transmission control protocol (**TCP**) and Internet protocol.

–TPC breaks down information into pieces of manageable size called **packets** for movement on the internet.

–The **World Wide Web** (WWW) is the collection of computers that exchange information over the internet using the hypertext transfer protocol (HTTP).

–Image data sets are large and benefit from image **compression,** which reduces the size of data files by removing or encoding redundant information.

–**Lossless** compression is completely reversible and levels of data compression up to 1:5 can be achieved.

–Lossy compression achieves higher savings but introduces some degree of irreversible data loss.

–JPEG (Joint Photographic Expert Group) is a widely available lossy image compression standard.

C. Clinical implementation

–**DICOM** (Digital Imaging and Communications in Medicine) is an image-based medical protocol that specifies image formats.

  –ACR-NEMA is a joint committee of the American College of Radiology and the National Electrical Manufacturers Association that developed DICOM.

–**Picture archiving and communications systems (PACSs)** are digital radiology systems that have the potential to eliminate the use of film.

–**Fig. 6.5** shows the components of a PACS.

–The first "filmless" radiology departments appeared in the 1990s.

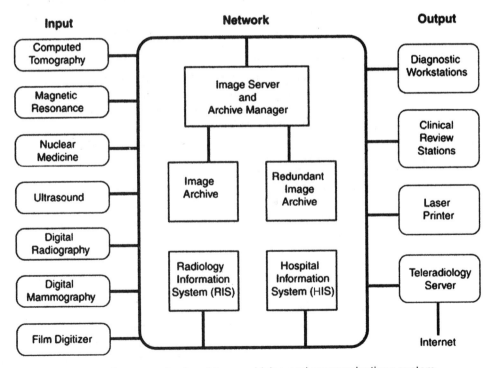

FIG. 6.5. Components of a picture archiving and communications system.

–The Baltimore Veterans Affairs Medical Center in Maryland and the U.S. Army Hospital in Madigan, Washington, were the first PACS sites in the United States.

–The OMSZ hospital in Vienna and the Hammersmith Hospital in London were the first all-digital radiology departments in Europe.

–PACS offers health care information **integration,** including radiology records and reports, medical records, and laboratory information.

–PACSs need to be integrated to Radiology Information System (RIS) and Hospital Information Systems (HIS).

–Networks make image data widely available to multiple users at the same time.

–Networks also permit instantaneous access to users in multiple locations.

–Radiographic images can be transmitted around the world in seconds.

–**PACS** are part of the imaging chain and require quality control monitoring.

–Display monitors need regular checks to ensure that image brightness and contrast are satisfactory.

–Test patterns used to evaluate monitor performance have been developed by the Society of Motion Picture and Television Engineers (SMPTE).

D. Benefits and limitations

–PACSs are expected to reduce the time and financial cost associated with film and paper storage and transfer.

–One benefit of PACSs is the ability to manipulate data and the use of computer-aided detection/diagnosis.

–PACS permit rapid image retrieval, and simultaneous and remote viewing.

–The use of PACS also compacts storage, reducing archival space (file rooms) and requiring fewer personnel (file room clerks).

–Problems of lost, misplaced, and sequestered films are potentially eliminated.

–PACS promises to improve operational efficiency, reduce costs, and provide a much faster service in terms of report time to referring physicians.

–One major limitation to the widespread introduction of PACSs is the high capital costs involved.

–Technical personnel required to support PACS are expensive.

–Other difficulties associated with PACS include security and reliability.

–The amount of image data generated by a radiology department performing 100,000 exams per year is very large (i.e., several terabytes).

–Maintaining access to prior images after the installation of a new archive is a major concern for all radiology departments.

Review Test

1. How many bits are required to store 512 shades of gray?

(A) 6
(B) 8
(C) 9
(D) 10
(E) 12

2. If all 8 bits in a byte are set to one, then the decimal number is:

(A) 8
(B) 255
(C) 311
(D) 511
(E) 1,023

3. How many 512^2 images (16 bit pixel) can be stored on a 2 GB disk?

(A) 500
(B) 1,000
(C) 4,000
(D) 10,000
(E) 50,000

4. How much memory is needed to store a 1 k^2 radiograph with 256 shades of gray?

(A) 0.1 MB
(B) 1.0 MB
(C) 10 MB
(D) 100 MB
(E) More than 100 MB

5. Which is *not* true concerning digital computers?

(A) ROM is read only memory.
(B) RAM is random access memory.
(C) Word is a set of consecutive bits treated as an entity.
(D) Byte is a binary digit used to represent one or zero.
(E) A file is a collection of interrelated records treated as a unit.

6. Parallel processing:

(A) Involves running several tasks simultaneously
(B) Requires an array processor
(C) Cannot be performed in machine code
(D) Requires the sharing of peripheral devices
(E) Can be performed on a single CPU.

7. Input devices for a computer do not include:

(A) Keyboard
(B) Trackball
(C) Touch screen
(D) Light pen
(E) Array processor

8. Which of the following definitions regarding digital computers is *false*?

(A) A byte consists of 8 bits.
(B) File is a collection of data treated as a unit.
(C) Microprocessor is a single integrated circuit.
(D) Modem maintains the power supply to computers.
(E) PACS stands for "picture archiving and communications system."

9. Computers can communicate using all the following communication channels *except:*

(A) Coaxial cables
(B) Telephone lines
(C) Fiber optic cables
(D) Microwave links
(E) High-frequency generators

10. Going from a 256^2 to a 512^2 image will double the image's:

(A) Spatial resolution
(B) Pixels
(C) Gray levels
(D) Transmission time
(E) Storage requirements

11. Which of the following x-ray detector materials emits light?

(A) Xenon
(B) CsI
(C) Selenium
(D) PbI
(E) HgI

12. Photostimulable phosphors do *not* include:

(A) Barium fluorohalide
(B) Red light lasers
(C) Light detectors (blue)
(D) Analog-to-digital converters
(E) TV cameras

13. Photoconductors convert x-ray energy directly into:

(A) Light
(B) Charge
(C) Heat
(D) Current
(E) RF energy

14. Processing a digital x-ray image by unsharp mask enhancement would increase the:

(A) Limiting spatial resolution
(B) Visibility of edges
(C) Patient dose
(D) Matrix size
(E) Bit depth per pixel

15. Which of the following does *not* involve image processing?

(A) Histogram equalization
(B) Low-pass filtering
(C) Background subtraction
(D) K-edge filtering
(E) Energy subtraction

16. Digital image displays in radiology cannot:

(A) Display 2×2.5 k images
(B) Show 256 shades of gray
(C) Have a brightness of 1,500 cd/m^2
(D) Resolve 2 lp/mm
(E) Use flat-panel monitors

17. The Nyquist frequency for a 1 k digital photospot image (25 cm image intensifier size) is:

(A) 1 lp/mm
(B) 2 lp/mm
(C) 4 p/mm
(D) 8 lp/mm
(E) 10 lp/mm

18. For comparable image mottle, which has the highest patient dose?

(A) Screen/film
(B) Photostimulable phosphor
(C) Direct flat-panel detector
(D) Indirect flat-panel detector
(E) Digital photospot

19. Digital fluoroscopy does not permit:

(A) Real-time imaging
(B) Last frame hold
(C) Temporal filtering
(D) Road mapping
(E) Elimination of dose rate limits

20. Image noise in digital fluoroscopy cannot be reduced by:

(A) Increasing tube voltage
(B) Increasing tube current
(C) Reducing the matrix size
(D) Temporal filtering
(E) Increasing fluoroscopy examination time

21. Digital photospot imaging does not generally require:

(A) Exposure time less than 0.1 s
(B) Tube current above 100 mA
(C) Voltage over 120 kV
(D) 1,000 line TV camera
(E) Detector dose of 1 μGy/frame (100 μR/frame)

22. The matrix size in a DSA image is typically:

(A) 128×128
(B) 256×256
(C) 512×512
(D) $1,024 \times 1,024$
(E) $2,048 \times 2,048$

23. DSA image acquisitions normally do not make use of:

(A) High voltages (over 120 kV)
(B) Low-noise TV systems
(C) 2 lp/mm resolution
(D) Up to eight frames/second
(E) 2 μGy/frame (200 μR/frame)

24. The most important component affecting spatial resolution in DSA is the:

(A) Focal spot size
(B) Image intensifier input phosphor thickness
(C) Image intensifier output phosphor thickness
(D) Digitization matrix
(E) Computer CPU

25. Changing DSA matrix from $1,024^2$ to $2,048^2$ would not increase the:

(A) Pixel size
(B) Data digitization rate
(C) Spatial resolution
(D) Data storage requirement
(E) Image processing time

26. Which of the following results in the highest patient dose per acquired frame?

(A) Digital fluoroscopy
(B) Cine
(C) Photospot
(D) Digital photospot
(E) Spot film

27. Which of the following does *not* relate to computer networks?

(A) Token ring
(B) Ethernet
(C) Backbone
(D) JPEG
(E) Bridge

28. The DICOM standard does *not* specify the image's:

(A) Type
(B) Matrix size
(C) Bit depth
(D) Display settings
(E) Reimbursement rate

29. Benefits of digital (PACS) images do *not* generally include:

(A) Improved spatial resolution
(B) Image processing
(C) Computer-aided detection
(D) Convenient storage
(E) Image transmission

30. Limitations of PACS could include all the following except:

(A) High capital costs
(B) Reliability
(C) Access to "old" images
(D) Security
(E) Teleradiology

Answers and Explanations

1–C. Nine bits can store 512 shades of gray ($2^9 = 512$).

2–B. When all bits are set to zero, the number is zero. Because there are 2^8 or 256 levels, the maximum level is 255.

3–C. Four thousand; as each image needs 0.5 MB of information, and 2,000 MB (2 GB) divided by 0.5 MB per image, is 4,000 images.

4–B. One megabyte as there are 1 M pixels, and each needs 1 B (8 bit) to code for 256 gray levels.

5–D. One byte is 8 bits; whereas 1 bit is a binary number representing zero or one.

6–A. Serial processing performs tasks sequentially, whereas parallel processing has tasks running at the same time.

7–E. An array process is a hardware component used by the CPU to perform specific calculations as in computed tomography image reconstruction.

8–D. A modem is used to transmit information on telephone lines.

9–E. High-frequency generators are used to produce high voltages across x-ray tubes.

10–A. Resolution will double, data pixels/storage/transmission time will quadruple, and the number of gray levels will not change.

11–B. Xenon is a gas detector, and selenium/PbI/HgI are photoconductors.

12–E. TV cameras are used in fluoroscopy.

13–B. Absorbed x-ray photon energy is directly converted into charge which is stored and subsequently read out; the amount of charge is proportional to the absorbed x-ray energy.

14–B. Unsharp mask enhancement is an image processing algorithm that enhances the visibility of any edge in the image (e.g., tube or catheter placement).

15–D. A K-edge filter is a material placed into the x-ray beam to preferential transmit x-ray photons just below the K-shell binding energy (e.g., molybdenum in mammography).

16–C. The brightness of a radiology display system is typically below 300 cd/m^2, whereas view boxes are typically 1,500 cd/m^2.

17–B. A 1 k matrix size permits 500 line pairs, which can be allocated to 250 mm; the best possible resolution is thus (500 line pairs)/(250 mm) or 2 lp/mm.

18–B. Photostimulable phosphors are normally thinner than other detectors and are less efficient x-ray detectors; accordingly, they require more radiation exposure to achieve a given level of image quality (mottle).

19–E. The entrance exposure limit remains 100 mGy/min (10 R/min).

20–E. Image noise in fluoroscopy has no relation to total examination time.

21–C. Tube voltages in digital photospot imaging would be between 70 and 120 kVp; high voltages would not be required.

22–D. DSA matrix sizes are 1,024 × 1,024, achieved by the use of a 1,000 line TV system.

23–A. DSA uses normal voltages, and 80 kVp would be ideal for maximizing absorption by iodine contrast.

24–D. The digitization matrix ($1,024^2$) is the primary determinant of DSA spatial resolution.

25–A. A doubling of the matrix size will *halve* the pixel dimension.

26–E. The spot film will deliver the highest dose per frame.

27–D. JPEG is an image compression standard.

28–E. The DICOM standard specifies technical information about medical images but not the reimbursement rates.

29–A. In general, digital devices for DR have inferior spatial resolution of screen/film radiography.

30–E. Moving images to remote sites is a major benefit of PACS.

7

Mammography

I. Diagnosing Breast Cancer

A. Breast cancer

–Breast cancer accounts for 32% of cancer incidence and 18% of cancer deaths in women in the United States.

–The National Cancer Institute estimated that there were approximately 192,200 new cases of breast cancer in the United States in 2001.

–The number of annual breast cancer deaths was once 40,200 and has declined because of early detection and improved treatment.

–Breast cancer ultimately develops in one in eight women in the United States.

–**Fig. 7.1** shows breast cancer incidence and mortality rates.

–Early detection with screening mammography significantly reduces breast cancer mortality rates for women over 50 years of age.

–Screening asymptomatic women between the ages of 40 and 50 is controversial.

–The American Medical Association, American Cancer Society, and American College of Radiology (ACR) all recommend screening of asymptomatic women.

–The ACR recommends a baseline mammogram by age 40, biannual examinations between ages 40 and 50, and yearly examinations after age 50.

B. Cancer detection task

–Detection of breast cancer requires specialized imaging equipment and diagnostic expertise.

–Recognition of breast cancer depends on detection of subtle architectural distortion, masses near normal breast tissue density, skin thickening, and microcalcifications.

–**Microcalcifications** are specks of calcium hydroxyapatite ($Ca_5[PO_4]_3OH$), which may have diameters as small as 0.1 mm (100 μm).

–The small differences in attenuation of x-rays between normal and malignant tissue result in low subject contrast and make cancer detection difficult.

–Detection of microcalcifications is difficult because their small dimensions also result in low subject contrast.

–**Table 7.1** summarizes the key physical properties of the major breast tissues and pathologic conditions.

C. Modern mammography

–Mammography is a low-cost and low-dose procedure that can detect early stage breast cancer.

–Screen/film mammography is technically demanding and requires radiographs with excellent resolution and contrast.

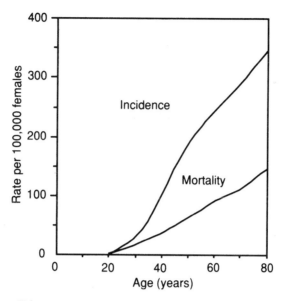

FIG. 7.1. Breast cancer incidence and mortality.

–This imaging equipment must be shown to be functioning properly by means of a comprehensive quality control (QC) program.

–Dedicated mammography equipment is essential for quality and low-dose screen/film imaging.

–Modern mammography equipment uses small focal spots, low tube voltages techniques, low-ratio grids, and phototiming.

   –Low tube voltages are used to maximize the relative contribution of the photoelectric effect, thereby increasing subject contrast and minimizing scatter.

–Special screens, films, and dedicated film processing are also important in mammography.

–Breast compression devices are used, and the imaging chain is configured for optimal patient positioning.

–Typical x-ray imaging specifications for dedicated mammography equipment are given in **Table 7.2.**

–Screening mammography normally includes a **craniocaudal** and a **mediolateral oblique** view of each breast.

   –Diagnostic mammographic examinations may include additional views and magnification to resolve ambiguous findings.

TABLE 7.1. *Properties of breast tissue*

Tissue type	Density (g/cm^3)	Linear attenuation coefficient at 20 keV (cm^{-1})
Adipose	0.93	0.45
Fibroglandular	1.035	0.8
Carcinoma	1.045	0.85
Skin	1.09	0.8
Calcification	2.2	12.5

TABLE 7.2. *Typical specifications for a dedicated mammography unit*

Parameter	Specification
Generator power rating	3 kW
X-ray tube voltage	24–35 kVp (1 kVp steps)
Tube current	100 mA
Target material	Molybdenum ($Z = 42$)
Window material	Beryllium ($Z = 4$)
Added filtration	30 μm molybdenum
Half-value layer	0.30–0.37 mm aluminum at 28 kVp
Nominal focal spot sizes	0.3 mm/0.1 mm

Z, atomic no.

II. Mammography Imaging Chain

A. X-ray spectra

–In visualizing breast tissue, the x-ray energy level that optimizes subject contrast is approximately **20 keV.**

–Higher energy photons decrease subject contrast.

–Lower-energy photons have inadequate breast penetration and substantially increase the patient radiation dose.

–Both **molybdenum** and **rhodium** are used as target materials in the anode because they produce characteristic radiation at optimal energy levels.

–**Molybdenum** has characteristic x-rays of 17.9 and 19.5 keV.

–**Rhodium** has characteristic x-rays of 20.2 and 22.7 keV.

–For these characteristic x-rays to be produced, the x-ray tube peak voltage must be higher than these values, that is, typically 25 to 34 kVp.

–Molybdenum filters (30 μm thick) remove most bremsstrahlung radiation above the molybdenum K-edge energy of 20 keV, because the photoelectric absorption is high.

–Removal of this high-energy bremsstrahlung radiation improves subject contrast.

–The molybdenum also filters out the very low energy x-rays that would only contribute to patient dose.

–**Fig. 7.2** shows the x-ray spectra from a molybdenum target.

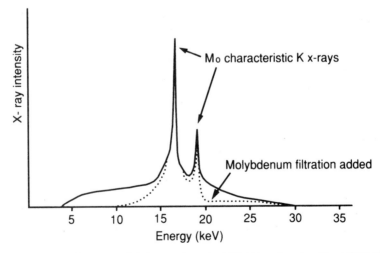

FIG. 7.2. X-ray spectra from a molybdenum target at 30 kVp, showing the effect of adding a molybdenum filter.

–For rhodium anodes ($Z = 45$; K-edge $= 23.2$ keV), a rhodium filter is used to remove the high-energy bremsstrahlung radiation.

–The slightly higher energy x-rays from rhodium provide better penetration of thick or dense breasts.

B. X-ray tubes

–Three-phase or high-frequency generators are used to minimize voltage fluctuations and reduce exposure times.

–Typical x-ray tube currents are 80 to 200 mA.

–Exposure times are usually about 1 second but can be as long as 4 seconds for dense thick breasts.

–The x-ray tube is tilted by about 25 degrees to minimize the effective focal spot size.

–The normal focal spot is only 0.3 mm and is kept small to minimize focal spot blur.

–The small focal spot (0.1 mm) is used for magnification mammography.

–The small focal spot can only tolerate low currents (25 mA), which can result in very long exposure times of several seconds.

–A beryllium ($Z = 4$) x-ray tube window is used to minimize x-ray beam attenuation.

–The **heel effect** (higher x-ray intensity on the cathode side) is used to increase the intensity of radiation near the chest wall, where greater penetration is needed.

–This is accomplished by placing the cathode side of the tube toward the patient.

–For a normal compressed breast (4.5 cm), a typical x-ray tube voltage is 25 kVp, and tube current exposure time product is 120 mAs on a screen/film system.

C. Grids

–Scatter to primary ratios in mammography range from 0.6 to 1.0.

–Although these ratios are low compared with those of general radiology, they can noticeably reduce image contrast.

–Grids are commonly used to **maximize image quality** by reducing scatter.

–Scatter increases with breast thickness and peak voltage.

–Mammography is normally performed using a moving grid.

–Carbon fiber is the preferred interspace material, because aluminum would attenuate too many of the low-energy x-rays used in mammography.

–A high transmission cellular (HTC) grid has been developed for use in mammography, which has a focused cellular pattern that reduces scatter in *both* directions.

–The HTC grid has a self-supporting structure, which eliminates the need for interspace material, and thus allows more primary radiation to reach the detector.

–Typical values for gridline densities range from 30 to 60 lines/cm, and typical grid ratios are 4:1 or 5:1.

–Grids decrease scatter but increase patient dose up to three-fold.

–Grids are sometimes not used if the compressed breast is very thin.

D. Screen/films

–Rare earth intensifying screens, such as terbium-activated gadolinium oxysulfide (Gd_2O_2S:Tb), are used in mammography.

–**Single screens** are used, which may incorporate light absorbers to limit screen diffusion and improve resolution.

–The photon absorption efficiency in mammography screens can be as high as 70% because of the use of low-energy x-ray photons.

–**Single emulsion films** are normally used to reduce receptor blur by eliminating crossover and parallax effects.

–The film is placed between the x-ray source and screen to reduce blur.

–X-rays are mainly absorbed at the front of the screen and should be closest to the film to minimize blur.

–A typical screen/film combination in mammography requires 0.05 to 0.2 mGy (5 to 20 mR) at the screen to generate a satisfactory film density.

–Mammography films generally have **high gradients** (over three) and a low film latitude.

–Limited latitude, however, is normally not a problem when there is adequate breast compression.

–The high-contrast film/screen with a narrow exposure latitude requires very good automatic exposure control (AEC) to ensure consistent film quality (density).

E. Film processors

–Mammography films have relatively thick single emulsions, which makes them much more sensitive to **processor artifacts.**

–Optimal film processing is critical to ensure high image quality, and dedicated mammography processors are recommended.

–**Optimal film densities** in mammography are **between 1.5 and 2.0,** which is higher than that of conventional radiography.

–Higher film densities are needed in mammography because this results in the best film contrast.

–Special processors with extended cycle times of 3 minutes and higher developer temperatures can be used.

–The extended development time optimizes development of the latent image, resulting in increased film speed and contrast.

–Optimal film processing requires careful QC, which results in improved image quality and reduced patient dose.

III. Clinical Imaging

A. Compression

–Optimal mammography requires the use of breast compression.

–Compression results in **greater sharpness, less scatter,** and **reduced patient dose.**

–Compression reduces the thickness of the breast and allows low voltages to be used, thereby improving subject contrast.

–Compressed breasts are normally 3 to 8 cm thick.

–Compression immobilizes the breast and minimizes any motion.

–Compression spreads the breast tissue, making lesions easier to detect.

–Compression brings the breast closer to the image plane (object to film distance), minimizes image magnification, and reduces focal spot blur (geometric unsharpness).

–Compression also reduces exposure times, minimizing patient motion blur associated with long exposure times.

–Spot compression may be used to achieve maximum compression in a limited region of interest.

–Compression is achieved using radio translucent paddles that have an x-ray transmission of about 80% at 30 kVp.

–Compression force is normally between 111 and 200 N (25 and 45 lb).

–The principal drawback of compression is patient discomfort.

B. Magnification mammography

–Magnification mammography improves visualization of mass margins and fine calcifications.

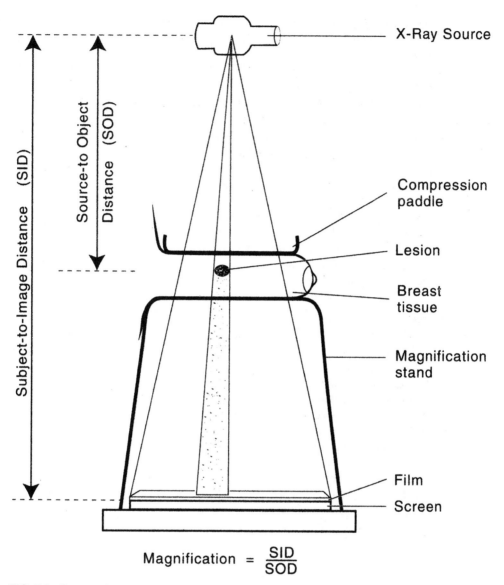

Magnification = $\dfrac{\text{SID}}{\text{SOD}}$

FIG. 7.3. Geometric principles of magnification. A radiolucent magnification stand is placed between the compressed breast tissue and image receptor. The air gap reduces scatter, and a grid is not used. In this example, the source-to-image receptor distance is twice the source-to-object distance, resulting in a 2× magnification.

–Magnification is achieved by moving the breast away from the film using a 15 to 30 cm standoff, and by keeping the source to image receptor distance constant.
–The geometric principles of magnification are illustrated in **Fig. 7.3.**
–The magnification is the ratio of the source-to-image receptor distance (SID) to the source-to-object distance (SOD); magnification is given as SID/SOD.
  –A typical SID is 65 cm, and SOD in magnification is 35 cm, so that magnification is normally 1.85.
–The presence of an air gap reduces the amount of scatter reaching the film and eliminates the need for a grid.

–The amount of breast coverage in a single magnification radiograph is reduced.

–**Small focal spots** (0.1 mm in diameter) are essential to minimize geometric unsharpness.

  –Use of a small focal spot requires longer exposure times, which may result in increased patient motion and blur.

  –Magnification generally improves image quality.

C. Viewing mammograms

–**Film viewing conditions** are very important in mammography.

–High-luminance viewboxes, low ambient light, and complete film masking should be implemented in both the radiologists and technologist's area.

–For optimal viewing of the images, bright viewboxes with luminance values of approximately 3,000 candelas per square meter (cd/m^2) should be used.

–Conventional viewboxes in radiology are approximately 1,500 cd/m^2.

–Viewing rooms should be darkened (below 50 lux), and hot lights should be available.

–Extraneous light decreases contrast perception.

  –Regions beyond the mammogram border should be covered to reduce glare and thereby improve visibility of low-contrast lesions.

–A magnifying glass should be used to view microcalcifications.

D. Stereotaxic localization

–Stereotaxic localization has been developed to perform **core needle biopsies.**

–Stereotaxic localizations are best achieved using digital imaging systems, which eliminate time-consuming film processing.

  –The field of view of digital systems range from 50 × 50 mm to 50 × 80 mm, with a pixel size as small as 25 μm.

  –Digital systems use a charged coupled device to capture the light from the screen, via optical lenses or fiberoptic tapers.

  –The resultant limiting spatial resolution in the imaging plane is 8 to 15 lp/mm.

–Two views of the breast are normally acquired (within 15 degrees of normal).

  –Images of the lesion will shift by an amount that depends on the lesion depth, which permits a three-dimensional localization of the lesion.

–A biopsy needle gun is positioned and fired to capture the required tissue sample.

–Benefits of core needle over open biopsies are a short procedure time, minimal local anesthetic, reduced risk, and no residual scarring of breast tissue.

–The limitations of core needle biopsy devices include their high cost and the limited field of view of real-time images.

E. Digital mammography

–**Computed radiography** has been used for screening mammography, but the low resolution (5 lp/mm) can limit visualization of microcalcifications.

–Full field of view digital systems have recently been introduced into clinical practice.

–A typical matrix size in digital mammography is 4 × 6 k, with a pixel size of 40 to 50 μm.

–The limiting spatial resolution of digital mammography is about 10 lp/mm.

–This is inferior to screen/film, which can reach 20 lp/mm.

–A major benefit of digital mammography is the ability of image processing to improve lesion visibility in underexposed or overexposed regions.

–Current clinical trials of digital mammography have shown this modality to be at least as good as screen/film mammography.

–Digital mammography is very expensive, which is a major inhibitor to rapid diffusion of this technology.

–A digital screening examination and prior examination contain 400 MB of data, which is difficult to view and manipulate using current displays.

–Digital mammograms can be processed using **computer-aided diagnosis** (CAD) software, which can identify malignant lesions and microcalcification clusters.

–CAD systems can assign a "probability of malignancy" for each identified lesion.

–Mammography CAD software has been shown to have sensitivities as high as 90% and can identify lesions missed by mammographers.

  –CAD software has also been shown to improve the performance of mammographers when used as a "second reader."

–Although CAD systems can have a high false-positive rate of up to one or two false-positives per image, these systems continue to improve and have a promising future.

IV. Image Quality and Dose

A. Image quality

–The limiting spatial resolution of state-of-the-art mammographic screen/film combinations is 15 to 20 lp/mm.

–Magnification imaging with a small focal spot can improve the achievable spatial resolution.

–**Quantum mottle** is the major sources of noise in screen/film mammography.

  –**Film granularity** is a secondary source of image noise in screen/film mammography.

–Increasing voltages reduces exposure time and patient dose when film density is kept constant.

–Low–voltage techniques increase contrast but also increase patient dose **(Fig. 7.4).**

–Grids may improve the contrast by a factor of two, but also increase the radiation dose by a factor of two to three.

–The screen/film cassettes must be meticulously cleaned and carefully handled to minimize artifacts and maintain high image quality.

B. Breast dose

–The glandular tissue in the breast is sensitive to cancer induction by radiation.

–The **average glandular dose (AGD)** is the preferred measure of dose in mammography and is determined using a special phantom.

–The AGD depends on x-ray beam techniques (kV and mAs), breast thickness, and composition **(Fig. 7.4).**

  –A composition of 50% glandular tissue and 50% adipose tissue is generally assumed for dosimetry purposes.

  –An average-sized (compressed) breast is taken to be 4.2 cm thick.

–Doses should be determined annually by a certified medical physicist.

  –The AGD is obtained using the measured entrance skin exposure when imaging an ACR phantom that simulates a 4.2 cm breast with 50% glandularity.

  –The x-ray beam voltage and the half-value layer also influence the AGD in mammography.

–The ACR recommends that the **AGD** for a 4.2-cm thick breast should be **less than 3 mGy (300 mrad) per film for screen/film with a grid.**

  –If no grid is used, the AGD should be less than 1 mGy per film (100 mrad).

–Typical AGD values are between 1.5 and 2 mGy per film (150 to 200 mrad) for mammography with a grid.

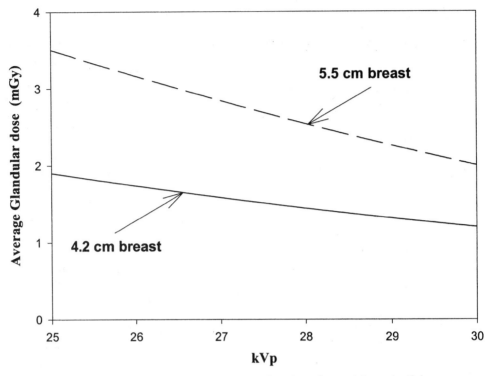

FIG. 7.4. Average glandular dose as a function of x-ray tube potential.

C. Radiation risks

–The principal risk after radiation exposure is the induction of breast cancer in the glandular tissue.

–Epidemiological studies of high-dose radiation-induced breast cancer include studies of atomic bomb survivors, tuberculosis patients who underwent extended fluoroscopy, and radiation therapy patients.

–Most radiation-induced breast cancers result from an AGD in the range of 1 to 20 Gy (100 to 2,000 rad) with little data from doses below 0.5 Gy (50 rad).

–Radiation risks for women undergoing mammography are based on extrapolations of risk estimates made at high doses.

–Based on current risk estimates, exposing 1 million 45-year-old women to an AGD of 1 mGy (100 mrad) may result in two excess breast cancer deaths.

–Although increasing the voltage reduces the AGD in mammography **(Fig. 7.4)**, it also reduces image contrast and is generally not recommended.

D. Risk versus benefits

–For a two-view screening examination, with a total AGD of 3 mGy (300 mrad), the (theoretical) radiation risk in 1 million examined women is about six.

  –This mammogram radiation risk is equivalent to the risk of dying in an accident when traveling 5,000 miles by airplane or 450 miles by car.

–Screening 1 million women is expected to identify 3,000 cases of breast cancer.

–Without a screening program, the breast cancer fatality rate is about 50%.

–Screening programs are expected to reduce the fatality rate by about 40%, or to save about 600 lives.

–The benefit to risk associated with mammography screening is therefore high.

  –It is also important to note that the benefits of screening have been demonstrated in epidemiological studies.

  –The radiation risks at low doses of the order of a few mGy are theoretical and mainly based on extrapolations of observed effects at doses of the order of 1 Gy.

–Radiation doses in mammography are very low and should not deter any women from having a screening examination.

V. Mammography Quality Standards Act

A. Mammography accreditation

–Successful breast cancer detection requires high-quality images that optimize contrast and resolution with minimal radiation dose.

–A comprehensive mammography program requires the combined efforts of physician, technologists, and physicist.

–Factors effecting image quality include proper patient positioning, compression, image interpretation conditions, and exposure conditions.

–The U.S. Food and Drug Administration (FDA) developed the Mammography Quality Standards Act (MQSA), which requires all 10,000 mammography facilities in the United States to be certified.

–MQSA was passed in 1994, and the final rules became effective in April 1999.

–It is against federal law to practice mammography without certification by the FDA.

–To obtain certification, the facility must receive accreditation by an approved body such as the ACR.

–The ACR developed an accreditation program in 1990 to improve the quality of screen/film mammography.

–Accreditation is currently based on the five steps listed in **Table 7.3.**

–Mammography facilities meeting the ACR standards receive a certificate of accreditation in mammography.

–Some states (Ark., Calif., Iowa, and Tex.) have introduced their own mammography accreditation programs, which are generally very similar to that of the ACR.

B. Mammographer requirements

–The **mammographer** is ultimately responsible for ensuring that QC requirements are met.

–The **MQSA** requires that a lead physician takes responsibility for meeting QC requirements.

–All interpreting physicians participate in the facility medical outcomes audit.

–Mammographers must follow facility procedures for corrective action when poor quality images are encountered.

–Accredited physicians are required to have interpreted at least 200 mammograms in the previous 24 months.

TABLE 7.3. *American College of Radiology accreditation requirements*

Site survey questionnaire completed	Assessment of clinical images by independent
Assessment of image quality using a phantom	radiologists
Dosimeter assessment of mean glandular dose	Assessment of quality control program

–The **mammographer** is responsible for ensuring technologists have adequate training and identifying a single technologist to oversee the QC program.
–Technologists must have the time and equipment necessary to perform QC tests.
–The **mammographer** is responsible for selecting a medical physicist to perform the annual testing.
–A qualified individual must be designated to oversee the radiation protection program.
–All records on qualifications, techniques, procedures, and so forth, must be properly maintained and updated in a mammography QC procedures manual.

C. Technologists requirements

–**Technologists** have well-defined QC responsibilities in all mammography facilities.
–MQSA requirements include processor QC on a daily basis.
  –Processor QC is performed by exposing and developing sensitometry strips and by measuring speed, contrast, and base plus fog levels.
  –All major processor problems must be corrected before clinical work begins.
–Screens and darkrooms must be cleaned every day.
–Weekly tests include obtaining an image of the ACR phantom and assessment of viewbox and reading conditions.
–The x-ray imaging equipment should be inspected every month.
–Quarterly tests include a repeat analysis and analysis of fixer retention on film.
  –Repeat rates are expected to be between 2% and 5%, and caused by positioning, patient motion, and overexposure or underexposure.
–Darkroom fog, screen/film contact, and compression testing is performed on a semiannual basis.
–The technologists QC program is reviewed annually by a qualified medical physicist.
–It is estimated that these activities require approximately 160 hours per year.

D. Physicist requirements

–The **responsibilities** of the **medical physicist** include assessing image quality and evaluating patient dose.
–Medical physicists must be adequately trained in mammography, perform at least 6 annual tests every 2 years, and receive the required continuing medical education credits.
–Imaging tests performed annually by the medical physicist are shown in **Table 7.4.**
–Medical physics tests must be performed when an x-ray unit or processor is installed or reassembled.
  –Equipment evaluation is required after replacement of the x-ray tube, filter, collimator, or AEC.
–**Phantom images** are used to assess film optical density, contrast, uniformity, and image quality produced by the imaging system and film processing.

TABLE 7.4. *Mammography quality control tests to be performed annually by a certified medical physicist*

Unit assembly and cassette performance	Uniformity of screen speeds
Collimation	Radiation output
System resolution	Entrance skin exposure and mean glandular dose
Peak voltage accuracy and reproducibility	Image quality (mammography phantom)
Beam quality (half-value layer)	Artifact evaluation
Automatic exposure control performance	

–Phantoms are equivalent to a compressed breast (4.2 cm) with equal glandular and adipose components.
  –The ACR phantom contains various sized fibers (six), speck groups (five), and masses (five).
  –To pass, the phantom image must show a minimum of four fibers, three speck groups, and three masses.
–The MQSA requires more stringent equipment performance as of October 2002.
  –X-ray tube output must be greater than 7 mGy/s, averaged over 3 seconds.
  –Spatial resolution from focal spot blur must be no worse than 11 lp/mm parallel to the anode-cathode axis and 13 lp/mm perpendicular.
  –The AEC shall maintain film optical density within 0.15 of the mean density.

VI. Alternative Breast Imaging

A. Ultrasound breast imaging

–High-resolution and high-frequency transducers (7.5 or 10 MHz) are used for ultrasound imaging of the breast.
–Ultrasound can improve diagnostic accuracy and decrease the need for surgical biopsy in women who have suspicious findings at screen/film mammography.
–The main clinical role of ultrasound is to **differentiate cysts from solid masses.**
–Ultrasound may also be used to evaluate palpable masses not seen on mammograms and for biopsy guidance.
–Ultrasound is ineffective for routine screening of asymptomatic patients.

B. Magnetic resonance breast imaging

–Magnetic resonance imaging (MR) may supplement conventional imaging methods in the diagnosis of breast disease.
  –MR is mainly used when a mammogram results in a problematic diagnosis of breast cancer.
–MR can also be used to assess the integrity of breast implants.
–Special breast coils are used to perform three-dimensional imaging of the breast with a typical volume matrix of $128 \times 256 \times 256$ pixels.
–Fat-suppression techniques may be used to generate T1-weighted images.
–Breast MR normally uses gadolinium–diethylenetriaminepentaacetic acid contrast (0.1 mmol/kg).
  –Contrast-enhanced MR has a high sensitivity and is better able to identify tumor margins.
–The improved sensitivity of MR may be used to determine whether patients with presumed solitary nodules actually have multifocal disease.
–Lack of contrast enhancement from fat and scar tissue may also be used to evaluate mammographically suspicious lesions.
  –Benign lesions such as fibroadenomas are often difficult to distinguish from malignancies.
–MR can distinguish silicone from enhancing tumor.
–MR-guided biopsies cannot be performed with current commercial scanners.

C. Nuclear medicine

–Nuclear medicine breast imaging is normally requested when the conventional mammogram is difficult to interpret (e.g., dense breast or fibrosis).

–**Scintimammography** uses technetium 99m-labeled sestamibi, which is administered intravenously.

–Imaging is performed early (immediately after injection) and later (60 to 90 minutes after injection).

  –Malignant lesions enhance early, whereas benign lesions enhance only on later images.

–Data acquisition is usually in planar mode (128 × 128).

  –Standard single-proton emission tomography (SPECT) imaging is difficult to perform because of activity in the heart and liver.

–**Positron emission tomography (PET)** imaging uses fluorine-18–labeled deoxyglucose (FDG) and the level of uptake is a direct measure of metabolic activity.

–Malignant tumors have high avidity for FDG; benign lesions have low avidity and fibrotic processes show no uptake.

–PET is used for staging, restaging, and monitoring of effectiveness of treatment for patients with breast cancer.

–PET is the nuclear medicine modality of choice.

D. Miscellaneous

–**Light diaphanography** involves shining light through the breast and detecting its transmission using special cameras.

  –Clinical diaphanography screening results have been poor.

  –A major problem of diaphanography is the significant amount of scatter compared with light absorption.

  –Differential absorption effects appear to be caused by increases in vascularity, which results in nonspecific findings.

–**Thermography** involves imaging the infrared radiation emitted by tissues; the amount emitted depends on body temperature.

  –Carcinomas near the breast surface may thus show up as hot spots when compared with the contralateral breast.

  –The ACR deems thermography to be ineffective for detecting breast cancer, and its use for this purpose is not recommended.

Review Test

1. Which is *not* used for a well-designed screen/film mammography unit?

(A) Low x-ray tube voltage
(B) Aluminum filtration
(C) Compression
(D) Phototiming
(E) Small focal spots

2. The low voltage used in screen/film mammography reduces:

(A) Subject contrast
(B) Dose
(C) Microcalcification visibility
(D) Scatter
(E) Film processing time

3. Dedicated film screen mammography equipments uses all of the following except:

(A) Tungsten targets
(B) SID of 65 cm
(C) 0.3 mm focal spot
(D) Molybdenum filters
(E) Long exposure times (1 to 2 seconds)

4. Filters in mammography do *not:*

(A) Use molybdenum or rhodium
(B) Preferentially attenuate x-ray energies over 20 keV
(C) Absorb low energy x-rays
(D) Have K-edges of approximately 33 keV
(E) Reduce x-ray tube output

5. Modern mammography equipment does not use:

(A) 100 kW generators
(B) Small focal spots (0.1 to 0.3 mm)
(C) Automatic exposure control
(D) Built-in compression paddles
(E) Grids

6. Differences between screen/film radiography and mammography may *not* include:

(A) Tube voltage
(B) Tube current
(C) Exposure time
(D) Film processor
(E) View box luminance

7. In mammography, a fiber interspaced grid is preferred over aluminum because it:

(A) Reduces the dose
(B) Improves resolution
(C) Removes more scatter
(D) Reduces image mottle
(E) Improves contrast

8. Mammography screen/film cassettes are *unlikely* to have:

(A) Carbon fiber cassette fronts
(B) Single emulsion film
(C) High-gradient films
(D) Single intensifying screen
(E) 300 μm thick screen

9. The optimal film density in mammography will *not:*

(A) Be between 1.5 and 2.0
(B) Need a developer temperature of 55°C
(C) Require a viewbox luminance greater than 3,000 cd/m^2
(D) Maximize image contrast
(E) Require a screen/film dose of 0.05 to 0.2 mGy (5 to 20 mR)

10. Contrast in screen/film mammography is best improved by using:

(A) Tungsten targets
(B) Latitude film
(C) A high kilovolt peak
(D) A grid
(E) Aluminum filters

11. All the following can degrade mammography image quality *except:*

(A) Lack of compression
(B) Long exposure times
(C) Poor screen/film contact
(D) Single-screen cassettes
(E) Low processor temperatures

12. Breast compression in mammography:

(A) Improves image contrast
(B) Eliminates the need for a grid
(C) Requires the use of a wide-latitude film
(D) Increases radiation dose
(E) Permits the use of higher tube voltages

13. Mammography compression will achieve all of the following except:

(A) Reduce geometric blur
(B) Improve contrast
(C) Reduce radiation dose
(D) Diminish motion blur
(E) Reduced x-ray transmission

14. Magnification radiography using current imaging equipment:

(A) Reduces the entrance skin exposure
(B) Improves definition of fine detail
(C) Requires large focal spots larger than 0.3 mm
(D) Reduces film density
(E) Requires moving the film further from the tube

15. Geometric unsharpness in mammography is:

(A) Unimportant
(B) Minimized with a large focal spot
(C) Reduced by a small SID
(D) Increased with magnification
(E) Reduced with a large air gap

16. Optimal viewing of screen/film mammograms requires all of the following except:

(A) A bright viewbox (3,000 cd/m^2)
(B) Availability of a hotlight
(C) Use of a magnifying glass
(D) Masking around the films
(E) Overhead lighting (200 lux)

17. Benefits of stereotaxic localization for core biopsies include all the following *except:*

(A) Short procedure time (30 minutes)
(B) Absence of ionizing radiation
(C) Minimal local anesthetic
(D) Reduced risk
(E) Reduced scarring

18. A limitation of CR for breast imaging is its inferior:

(A) X-ray detection efficiency
(B) Display contrast
(C) Noise characteristic
(D) Dose performance
(E) Limiting spatial resolution

19. The small focal spot in mammography is generally *not:*

(A) 0.1 to 0.15 mm
(B) Limited to about 25 mA tube current
(C) Able to resolve more than 11 lp/mm
(D) Used for magnification imaging
(E) Able to reduce exposure times

20. Mammography image mottle is determined primarily by:

(A) Quantum mottle
(B) Film grain size
(C) Grid ratio
(D) Viewbox luminance
(E) Variations in screen thickness

21. Breast doses in mammography are most likely to be reduced by *increasing* the:

(A) X-ray tube voltage
(B) X-ray tube current
(C) Focal spot size
(D) Grid ratio
(E) Number of views taken

22. The ACR does *not* recommend that the mammography AGD should be:

(A) For a 4.2 cm-thick breast
(B) For a 50% glandularity breast
(C) Below 1 mGy (less than 100 mrad) with no grid
(D) Below 3 mGy (less than 300 mrad) film with a grid
(E) Below 1 mGy (less than 100 mrad) for magnification views

23. The AGD per film in screening mammography with a grid is likely to be:

(A) Below 1 mGy (less than 100 mrad)
(B) 1 mGy (100 mrad)
(C) 2 mGy (200 mrad)
(D) 3 mGy (300 mrad)
(E) Above 3 mGy (more than 300 mrad)

24. The radiation risk of a screening mammogram for a 45-year-old woman is all of the following except:

(A) About 1 in 200,000
(B) From the induction of breast cancer
(C) Much lower than the potential benefit
(D) Associated with a long latent period
(E) Proven in epidemiological studies

25. The MQSA does *not* require facilities to have:

(A) Annual physics testing
(B) Daily processor sensitometry
(C) Minimum image quality standards
(D) ACR accreditation
(E) FDA certification

26. To pass ACR accreditation, a phantom image must show all of the following except:

(A) Four fibers
(B) Three groups of microcalcifications
(C) Three masses
(D) Minimal artifacts
(E) Film density between 1.0 and 1.2

27. The primary use of ultrasound in breast imaging is:

(A) Routine screening of asymptomatic women
(B) Visualization of microcalcifications
(C) Differentiation of benign from malignant masses

(D) Staging of malignant disease
(E) Identifying fluid filled cysts

28. Breast imaging using MRI would *not* use:

(A) Fat-suppression techniques
(B) Special breast coils
(C) Iodine contrast
(D) Gadolinium-diethylenetriaminepentaacetic acid contrast
(E) Three-dimensional imaging techniques

29. Which radionuclide does PET breast imaging use?

(A) Fluorine 18
(B) Technetium 99m
(C) Iodine 123
(D) Iodine 131
(E) Thallium 201

30. The use of thermography to detect breast cancer:

(A) Involves ionizing radiation
(B) Uses thermoluminescent dosimeters
(C) Is most effective near the chest wall
(D) Is deemed by the ACR to be ineffective
(E) Has high specificity

Answers and Explanations

1–B. Screen/film mammography uses molybdenum or rhodium filtration, not aluminum filtration

2–D. As the photon energy is reduced, the photoelectric effect becomes more important, and Compton scatter is reduced.

3–A. Molybdenum targets are normally used in a mammography x-ray tube, not tungsten.

4–D. Iodine has a k-edge energy of 33 keV, whereas filters used in mammography (Mo and Rh) have k-edges at approximately 20 keV.

5–A. A typical technique in mammography is 25 kV and 100 mA, which corresponds to a power rating of only 2.5 kW.

6–D. The same film processor *may* be used for both mammography and conventional radiography.

7–A. Aluminum attenuates more of the primary rays than fiber, leading to higher patient doses.

8–E. The blur introduced by a 300 μm thick screen would be unacceptable and limit microcalcification visibility (mammography detects objects as small as 150 μm).

9–B. Developer temperature is typically 33°C, not 55°C.

10–E. Grids will improve contrast.

11–D. Single screens improves spatial resolution relative to conventional cassettes with two screens.

12–A. Compression generally improves image contrast.

13–E. X-ray transmission will (obviously) be increased if the breast is compressed (i.e. thinner).

14–B. Magnification improves detail visibility and is achieved by moving the breast closer to the x-ray tube.

15–D. Geometric blur increases with magnification; small focal spots are used in magnification mammography.

16–E. Darkened rooms are preferred; an illuminance of 200 lux would reduce the ability to detect low contrast lesions.

17–B. Radiographs are obtained to correctly localize the needle.

18–E. The limiting spatial resolution of CR is 5 lp/mm, which is much worse than that of screen/film (15 to 20 lp/mm).

19–E. A small focal spot limits the tube current to 25 mA and therefore results in much longer exposure times.

20–A. Quantum mottle is the dominant source of noise in mammography and is determined by the radiation exposure at the screen/film (0.05 to 0.2 mGy; 5 to 20 mR).

21–A. Increasing the tube voltage will make the beam more penetrating, thereby reducing the radiation dose. High voltages also reduce the resultant image contrast, which in turn may reduce the benefit of the examination.

22–E. The ACR does not specify "magnification" doses per se.

23–C. 2 mGy (200 mrad) is a typical value likely to be encountered in clinical practice; 3 mGy is the ACR maximum, and 1 mGy would be too low for the US.

24–E. Radiation breast cancer risks are all theoretical at doses encountered in mammography (3 mGy).

25–D. Facilities need to be accredited, but the accreditation offered by states such as Arkansas, California, Iowa, or Texas would be just as good as that offered by the ACR to obtain FDA certification.

26–E. A phantom image with a film density of 1.0–1.2 would be far too low; one normally obtains phantom images with densities in the range 1.5–2.0.

27–E. The primary role of ultrasound in breast imaging is the differentiation of cysts from solid masses.

28–C. Iodine contrast is used in x-ray imaging not MR.

29–A. PET breast imaging uses fluoro-deoxyglucose labeled with fluorine 18.

30–D. Thermography, the imaging of infrared radiation that is emitted by all bodies, is ineffective for detecting breast cancer.

8

Computed Tomography

I. Basic Physics

A. Hounsfield units

–**Computed tomography (CT)** is a **tomographic** imaging technique introduced in the early 1970s that generates cross-sectional images in the axial plane.

–**CT images** are maps of the relative linear attenuation values of tissues.

–The **relative attenuation coefficient** (μ) is normally expressed in **Hounsfield units (HU),** which are also known as CT numbers.

–The HU of material x is $HU_x = 1,000 \times (\mu_x - \mu_{water})/\mu_{water}$, where μ_x is the attenuation coefficient of the material x, and μ_{water} is the attenuation coefficient of water.

–By definition, the HU value for water is always zero.

–HU value for air is $-1,000$ (μ_{air} is negligible compared with μ_{water}).

–**Table 8.1** lists typical HU values for a range of tissues.

–Because μ_x and μ_{water} are dependent on photon energy (keV), HU values depend on the kilovolt peak and filtration.

  –Therefore, HU values generated by a CT scanner are only approximate and related to the tube voltage used to generate the image.

B. Image acquisition

–For a fixed position of the x-ray tube, a **fan beam** is passed through the patient.

–Measurements of the transmitted x-ray beam intensities are made by an **array** of detectors.

–The total x-ray transmission measured by each detector is the result of the sum of the attenuation by all the tissues the beam has passed through and is called the **ray sum.**

–The collection of ray sums for all the detectors at a given tube position are called **projections.**

–A typical projection will have up to 1,000 individual data points.

–**Projection** data sets are acquired at different angles around the patient.

–A CT image generally requires about 1,000 projections.

–CT images are derived by mathematical analysis of projection data sets.

C. Image reconstruction

–Generating an image from the acquired data involves determining the linear attenuation coefficients of the individual pixels in the image matrix.

–A mathematical **algorithm** takes the multiple projection data **(raw data)** and reconstructs the cross-sectional CT image **(image data).**

TABLE 8.1. *Hounsfield units for representative materials with corresponding values of physical and electron densities*

Material	Density (g/cm^3)	Electron density (e/cm^3) $\times$ 10^{23}	Approximate HU value
Air	<0.01	<0.01	−1000
Lung	0.25	0.83	−300
Fat	0.92	3.07	−90
Water	1.00	3.33	0
White matter	1.03	3.42	30
Gray matter	1.04	3.43	40
Muscle	1.06	3.44	50
Cortical bone	1.8	5.59	1000+

* HU, Hounsfield units.

–Modern scanners use **filtered back projection** (FBP) image reconstruction algorithms.

–Iterative (trial and error) methods such as **algebraic reconstruction techniques** (ART) have been used for image reconstruction.

–Image reconstruction involving millions of data points may be performed in less than a second using **array processors** (number crunchers).

–Different mathematical **filters** may be used in filtered back projection reconstruction, offering tradeoffs between spatial resolution and noise.

–Some filters permit reconstruction of fine detail but with increased noise in the image, such as in bone algorithms.

–Soft tissue filters provide some smoothing, which decreases image noise but also decreases spatial resolution.

–Soft tissue filters improve the contrast to noise ratio and generally improve the visibility of low contrast lesions.

–The choice of the best filter to use with the reconstruction algorithm depends on the clinical task.

D. Image display

–**Field of view (FOV)** is the diameter of the body region area being imaged (e.g., 25 cm for a head or 40 cm for an abdomen).

–CT **pixel size** is determined by dividing the FOV by the matrix size, which is generally 512 × 512 (0.5 k) in CT.

–For example, pixel sizes are 0.5 mm for a 25-cm diameter FOV head scan (25 cm divided by 512) and 0.8 mm for a 40-cm FOV body scan (40 cm divided by 512).

–**Voxel** is a volume element in the patient.

–Voxel volume is the product of the pixel area and slice thickness.

–**Fig. 8.1** shows the relation among FOV, matrix size, voxel, and pixels.

–CT images are viewed on monitors or printed onto film using a laser printer.

–The brightness of each pixel in the image is directly related to the average attenuation coefficient of the tissue in the voxel.

–Each pixel is normally represented by 12 bits, or 4,096 gray levels, which is larger than the display range of monitors or film.

–CT images can be viewed in stack mode on a workstation, where the section viewed can be changed by movement of a mouse.

–Stack mode is ideal for following arteries from image to image.

–**Window width** and **level** optimize the appearance of CT images by determining the contrast and brightness levels assigned to the CT image data **(Fig. 8.2).**

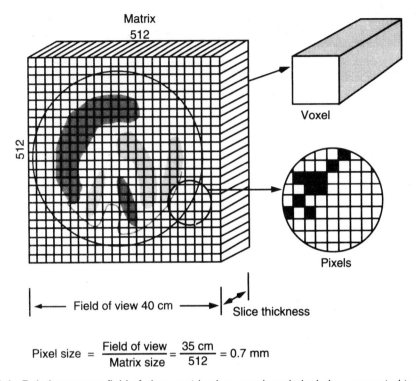

$$\text{Pixel size} \ = \ \frac{\text{Field of view}}{\text{Matrix size}} = \frac{35 \text{ cm}}{512} = 0.7 \text{ mm}$$

FIG. 8.1. Relation among field of view, matrix size, voxel, and pixels in a computed tomography image.

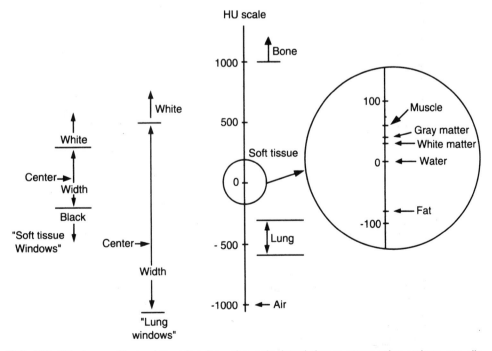

FIG. 8.2. Window settings determine how the calculated tissue attenuation values are displayed. Window width determines the range from white to black. Window center defines the middle value.

TABLE 8.2. *Typical window and level settings used in clinical computed tomography*

Type of examination	Window	Level
Head	80	40
Chest (mediastinum)	450	40
Chest (lung)	1500	−500
Abdomen (liver)	150	60

–Viewing CT images with a window width of 100 HU and a window level (center) of 50 HU results in an image in which HU values of zero or less appear black, HU values of 100 or more appear white, and HU values of 50 appear midgray.

–Window (width and level) settings affect only the displayed image, not the reconstructed image data stored in the computer.

–**Table 8.2** shows typical window and level settings used in clinical CT.

E. Image processing

–**Multiplanar reformatting (MPR)** is a method for generating coronal, sagittal, or oblique images from the original axial image data.

　–Because pixels from adjacent sections are used, the long-axis resolution is generally worse than in plane resolution and determined by collimation thickness (1 to 10 mm).

–Multiplanar reformatting software performs some interpolation, but in most cases, the resulting images have a characteristic "stair-stepping" artifact at tissue interfaces.

–Multiplanar reformatting image quality can be improved by using thin collimation and overlapping intervals for the original axial data reconstruction.

–**Three-dimensional or volume rendering** of CT data requires **segmentation** of the image data to select the tissue or structures of interest.

–**Shaded surface display** is a method for creating surface renderings that simulate a lighted object.

　–A threshold CT number is identified below which no image data are represented.

　–A surface contour is generated so that it encompasses pixels having a CT number above the threshold.

　–An appearance of illumination from a point lightsource is introduced to provide a three-dimensional appearance.

II. Scanner Design

A. X-ray tubes and collimators

–CT x-ray techniques use high x-ray tube voltages, tube currents of hundreds of milliamperes, and scan times between 0.5 and 2 seconds.

–**High-frequency power supplies** are used in CT to provide a very stable tube current and voltage.

–CT large focal spots (1 mm) are used at high power ratings (up to 60 kW).

　–The small focal spot (0.6 mm) is used at low power ratings below about 25 kW.

–**Heat loading** on CT x-ray tubes is generally high, requiring high anode heat capacities.

　–Modern systems have x-ray tube capacities greater than 3 MJ and high heat dissipation rates (10 kW).

(heel) –The x-ray tube axis is positioned perpendicular to the imaging plane to reduce the heal effect.

–Copper or aluminum filters are used to reduce x-ray beam hardening effects.

–The heavy filtration used with CT scanners typically produces a beam with an aluminum half-value layer of up to 10 mm.

–A **bowtie filter** is used to minimize the dynamic range of exposures at the detector.

–**Collimation** defines the section thickness and reduces scatter.

–Collimators are located at the x-ray tube as well as the x-ray detectors.

–Adjustable collimators allow section thickness to range between 1 and 10 mm.

B. Computed tomography radiation detectors

–Detectors measure the intensity of radiation transmitted through the patient.

–CT detectors should have a high x-ray detection efficiency, a fast response, and should operate over a wide dynamic range.

–In CT detectors, an electric signal that is proportional to the incident radiation intensity, is digitized and stored in a computer.

–**Xenon gas** ionization detectors consist of a gas-filled chamber with anodes and cathodes maintained at a potential difference.

–Incident x-ray photons ionize the gas, producing electron-ion pairs.

–Gas detectors are usually relatively deep and maintained at a high pressure (25 atm) to increase x-ray detection efficiency, and are used in third-generation scanners.

–Gas detectors are more stable than are solid-state detectors and have a wide linear response with no lag.

–**Scintillation** crystals produce light when x-ray photons are absorbed, and are coupled to a light detector (photomultiplier tube or photodiode).

–The most common material used in solid-state detectors is **cadmium tungstate** ($CdWO_4$), which is an efficient x-ray detector.

–Cesium iodide, calcium fluoride, and bismuth germanate may also be used.

–Only solid-state detectors are used for fourth-generation scanners, which require thin detectors because of the detection geometry.

C. First- and second-generation scanners

–In 1972, the **EMI scanner** was the first CT scanner introduced into clinical practice.

–EMI scanners used a pencil beam and two sodium iodide (NaI) detectors that moved across the patient (i.e., translated).

–The EMI scanner generated approximately 160 data points per projection on a point-by-point basis.

–The x-ray tube and detector were rotated 1 degree, and another projection was obtained.

–180 projections were obtained over a 180-degree rotation, taking approximately 5 minutes to generate a pair of images.

–This initial EMI design is called a **first-generation system.**

–**Second-generation scanners** also use translate-rotate technology but have multiple detectors and a fan-shaped beam.

–Second-generation scanners allowed larger rotational increments and faster scans, with a single image being generated in approximately 1 minute.

D. Third- and fourth-generation scanners

–**Third-generation scanners** use a wide rotating fan beam coupled with a large array of detectors (rotate-rotate system).

–The geometric relationship between the tube and detectors does not change as it rotates 360 degrees around the patient.

–**Fourth-generation scanners** have a rotating tube and fixed ring of detectors (up to 4,800) in the gantry (rotate-fixed system).

–Third- and fourth-generation scanners acquire a single section in 0.5 to 2 seconds.

–The imaging performance of third- and fourth-generation CT scanners is approximately equal.

–**Multislice CT** has resulted in the demise of fourth-generation CT systems, which are cost-prohibitive for more than one slice thickness.

E. Electron-beam computed tomography

–**Electron-beam CT,** also known as **fifth-generation CT,** uses an electron gun that deflects and focuses a fast-moving electron beam along a 210 degree arc of a large diameter tungsten target ring in the gantry.

–The x-ray beam produced is collimated to traverse the patient and strike a detector ring.

–Two detector rings permit the simultaneous acquisition of two image sections.

–There is no motion by the x-ray tube or detector array, which allows images to be obtained in as little as 50 milliseconds with minimum motion artifacts.

–The major advantage of electron-beam CT is the speed of data acquisition, which can freeze cardiac motion.

–The whole heart can be acquired in approximately 0.2 second (8 images).

–Serial images of a given section can be acquired every 50 milliseconds (cine mode).

–Electron-beam CT may also be useful in patients unable to cooperate for routine studies that require breath holding (e.g., pediatric and trauma patients).

–Electron-beam CT scanners can also operate as a conventional CT system by averaging multiple images acquired by repeat scans of a given section.

III. Modern Scanners

A. Axial computed tomography scanning

–All CT examinations begin with acquisition of a topographic or scout image.

–The scout image is obtained by advancing the patient couch through the gantry with the tube in a fixed position.

–Axial CT parameters to be selected include scan time (0.5 to 2 seconds), tube current (50 to 400 mA), voltage (120 to 140 kVp), and section thickness (1 to 10 mm).

–A FOV and image reconstruction filter are also selected.

–Use of cables to supply high voltage to the CT x-ray tube limit rotation to one revolution.

–Most modern CT scanners make use of **slip ring** technology in which high voltage is supplied to the tube through contact rings in the gantry.

–Slip ring scanners are fast and can scan several sections in a single breath-hold.

–X-ray tube currents should be reduced for small patients, who transmit much more radiation than adults.

–Section thickness is reduced for small patients to reduce partial volume effects.

–**Table 8.3** shows typical CT technique factors for adults and young children.

TABLE 8.3. *Typical computed tomographic technique protocols**

Type of examination	mAs		Section thickness (mm)	
	Adult	5-year-old	Adult	5-year-old
Head	300	240	7	5
Chest	180	60	7	5
Abdomen	240	80	7	5

* All scans performed at 120 kVp.

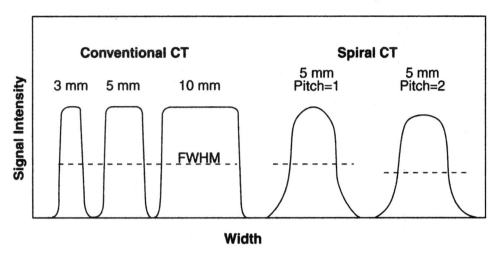

FIG. 8.3. Computed tomography (CT) slice-sensitivity profile. For axial scanning, the full-width half maximum of the slice-sensitivity profile is slightly greater than the nominal slice thickness. Slice-sensitivity profiles are broader for helical CT and increase with increasing pitch.

B. Helical (spiral) computed tomography

–Helical scanners may be either third or fourth generation designs.

–In helical CT acquisitions, the patient is moved along the horizontal axis as the x-ray tube rotates around the patient.

–The x-ray beam central ray follows a helical path during the CT scan.

–The relation between patient and tube motion is called **pitch,** defined as the table movement during each revolution of the x-ray tube divided by the collimation width.

–For a 5 mm section, if the patient moves 10 mm during the time it takes for the x-ray tube to rotate through 360 degrees, the pitch is two.

–Increasing pitch reduces the scan time and patient dose.

–Increasing pitch increases the **slice-sensitivity profile** and effective slice width **(Fig. 8.3).**

–Image reconstruction is obtained by interpolating projection data obtained at selected locations along the patient axis.

–Images can be reconstructed at any level and in any increment but must have a thickness equal to the collimation used.

–The ability to rapidly cover a large volume in a single breath-hold eliminates respiratory misregistration and reduces the volume of intravenous contrast required.

–Image reformatting into the coronal, sagittal, or oblique plane is improved.

–Continuous scanning limits either the tube current that can be used, or the length of the acquisition.

C. Multislice computed tomography

–Multislice CT makes use of multiple detector arrays to make use of a wider portion of the x-ray fan beam during data acquisition.

–Section thickness in multislice CT is determined by detector width rather than by collimation thickness, as in conventional CT.

–For example, four parallel rows of detectors, each 2.5 mm wide, can be used to simultaneously record four adjacent image sections in a single rotation of the x-ray tube.

–Data for four 2.5 mm sections can be combined to produce two 5 mm sections or a single 10 mm section.

–This technology makes better use of the x-ray tube output and decreases heat loading for a given coverage range.

–Current CT scanners offer up to eight or 16 sections in a single 360 degree rotation of the x-ray tube.

–The number of sections acquired in a single x-ray tube rotation will continue to increase, culminating in area detectors being used for CT.

D. Computed tomography fluoroscopy

–CT images can be reconstructed in nearly real time during continuous rotation of the tube.

–In CT fluoroscopy, the CT image is constantly updated to include the latest projection data (e.g., 60 degree increments).

–Images are typically updated at the rate of six per second, which provides excellent temporal resolution.

–Any motion at the image level can then be followed in nearly real time by observing the updated reconstruction.

–This facilitates advancement of a needle for biopsies or drainage procedures.

–Low tube currents (20 to 50 mA) are used to minimize radiation doses.

IV. Image Quality

A. Spatial resolution

–**Spatial resolution** is the ability to discriminate between adjacent objects and is a function of pixel size.

–Additional factors that affect CT spacial resolution include the focal spot size, detector size, and choice of image reconstruction filter.

–If the CT FOV is d and the matrix size is M, the pixel size is d/M.

–For a typical head scan with an FOV of 25 cm and a matrix of 512 pixels, the pixel size is 0.5 mm.

–Because two pixels are required to define a line pair (lp), the best achievable spatial resolution is 1 lp/mm at this FOV.

–In practice, the pixel size is smaller than the limiting resolution imposed by the finite sizes of the focal spot and x-ray detectors.

–**Axial resolution** within the scan plane can be improved by operating in a **high-resolution mode** using a smaller FOV or a larger matrix size.

–CT spatial resolution may also be improved by using a smaller focal spot and by designing systems with smaller detectors.

–Typical resolution in CT scanning ranges from 0.5 to 1.5 lp/mm.

–Detail (bone) reconstruction filters must be used to achieve the best spatial resolution.

–Section thickness (collimation) effects resolution in the longitudinal plane and is important in sagittal and coronal reconstructions.

–The **slice-sensitivity profile (Fig. 8.3)** is a measure of the effective section thickness.

–The pitch ratio is the most important factor that affects the slice-sensitivity profile.

B. Noise

–Image noise is an important determinant of CT image quality and limits the visibility of low-contrast structures.

–CT image noise is determined primarily by the number of photons used to make an image (**quantum mottle**).
  –When a detector receives a total count of 100 photons, the standard deviation is $\sqrt{100}$, or 10 (i.e., 10% of the mean).
  –A total of 68% of repeat measurements are within one standard deviation of the mean (i.e., between 90 and 110 counts).
–Quantum mottle decreases as the number of photons increases.
  –If the count is increased to 1,000, the standard deviation is 32 ($\sqrt{1,000}$), or 3.2% of the mean; if the count is 10,000, the standard deviation is 100 ($\sqrt{10,000}$), or 1% of the mean.
–CT noise is generally reduced by increasing the tube voltage, current, or scan time, if all other parameters are constant.
–CT noise is also reduced by increasing voxel size (i.e., by decreasing matrix size, increasing FOV, or increasing section thickness).
–Noise does not change with pitch in helical CT scanning.
–The typical noise with a modern CT system is approximately 3 HU (i.e., 0.3% difference in attenuation coefficient).
–At a fixed technique, small patients transmit more radiation and thus noise will be reduced; this permits a reduction of techniques in small patients (**Table 8.3**).
–Noise in reconstructed images is also affected by the back projection filter used, with detail filters increasing noise, and soft-tissue filters reducing noise.
–Image noise becomes more conspicuous as the window width is reduced.

C. Contrast

–CT is far superior to projection radiography in detecting low-contrast differences.
–**CT contrast** is the difference in the HU values between tissues.
–CT contrast generally increases as tube voltage decreases but is not affected by tube current or scan times.
–CT contrast can be artificially increased by adding a contrast medium such as iodine.
–**Table 8.4** shows how lesion contrast is reduced as the photon energy increases.
  –Increasing photon energy reduces contrast much more for high–atomic number lesions, which contain iodine, than for soft-tissue lesions.
–Image noise can prevent detection of low-contrast objects, such as tumors, with a density close to the adjacent tissue.
–Under ideal circumstances, a lesion that differs by about 5 HU from its surroundings, corresponding to a 0.5% difference in attenuation, can be detected.
–Screen/film radiography requires the lesion to differ by 3% to 5% for detection.

TABLE 8.4. *Relative computed tomographic image contrast as a function of photon energy*

Effective photon energy (keV)	Relative image contrast	
	Soft tissue ($Z = 7.6$)	Iodine ($Z = 53$)
50	1.0	1.0
60	0.93	0.68
70	0.88	0.48
80	0.84	0.37

Z, atomic no.

–The **displayed image contrast** is determined primarily by the CT window (width and level) settings, with narrow windows offering high contrast.

–Window (level and width) settings allow the operator to emphasize the subtle density differences detected by CT.

D. Artifacts

–CT images may have **artifacts** that degrade diagnostic quality.

–**Partial volume artifact** is the result of averaging the linear attenuation coefficient in a voxel that is heterogenous in composition.

–Partial volume artifact increases with increasing pixel size and section thickness.

–**Motion artifacts** are the result of the 0.5 to 2 second scan times, which allow both involuntary (cardiac) and voluntary patient motion.

–Structures therefore move from one voxel to another during data acquisition, introducing errors in the reconstruction.

–Random or unpredictable motion (e.g., a patient's sneeze) produces **streak artifacts** in the direction of motion.

–In high-density structures, such as metal implants, the detector may record no transmission, complicating the filtered back projection and resulting in **star artifacts.**

–In these cases, the reconstruction algorithm generates streaks adjacent to the high-density structures.

–**Beam-hardening artifacts,** or "cupping" artifacts, are caused by the polychromatic nature of the x-ray beam (beam hardening).

–As the lower-energy photons are preferentially absorbed, the beam becomes more penetrating, causing underestimation of the attenuation coefficient (HU).

–Software algorithms have been developed to reduce beam-hardening artifacts.

–Beam-hardening artifacts are most marked at high-contrast interfaces, such as between dense bone in the skull and the brain.

–**Ring artifacts** may arise in third-generation systems if one or more detectors are faulty or miscalibrated.

–Artifacts caused by equipment defects are rare on modern CT systems.

V. Doses

A. Dose distributions

–The dose profile in a CT scanner is not uniform along the patient axis.

–Doses at the patient surface may be higher than the dose at the center of the patient.

–In head scans, the surface-to-center ratio is approximately 1:1.

–In body scans, the surface-to-center ratio is approximately 2:1.

–Because of scattered x-rays, the **CT section dose profile** is not perfectly square but has tails that extend beyond the section edges.

–The radiation dose profile is analogous to the slice-sensitivity profile.

–Tissues beyond the section are exposed to radiation, thus increasing dose as the number of slices increases.

–Manufacturers specify CT doses by the **CT dose index (CTDI),** which is the integral of the axial dose profile for a single CT slice divided by the slice thickness.

–The CTDI can be measured using a pencil-type ionization chamber in phantoms that simulate heads (16 cm diameter acrylic) and bodies (32 cm diameter acrylic).

–CTDI measurements are made at the surface ($CTDI_{peripheral}$) and at the center ($CTDI_{center}$) of the phantom.

–**Fig. 8.4** shows how average CTDI values vary with x-ray tube potential (kVp).

–CTDI increases with tube voltage at a rate that is greater than linear.

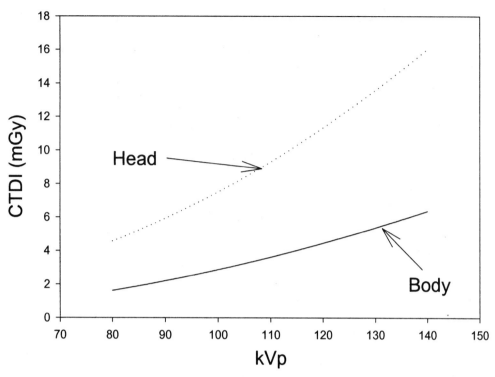

FIG. 8.4. Average value of the computed tomography dose index (CTDI) per 100 mAs versus x-ray tube potential (kVp).

–CTDI values for body scans are lower than those for head scans because of the greater attenuation of x-rays in the body.
–A weighted CTDI, expressed as $CTDI_w$, can be generated using the formula $CTDI_w$ = [⅔($CTDI_{peripheral}$) + ⅓($CTDI_{center}$)].
–CTDI doses do not quantify the patient risk because they take no account of section thickness, the number of sections scanned, or the radiosensitivity of irradiated organs.

B. Organ doses

–The highest dose to any part of the patient in a typical head CT examination performed at 120 kVp/300 mAs is about 40 mGy (4 rad).
–The highest dose to any part of the patient in a body CT examination performed at 120 kVp/250 mAs is about 20 mGy (2 rad).
–The dose to the eye lens is about 40 mGy (4 rad), which is well below the threshold for inducing eye cataracts 2 Gy (200 rad).
–Patient skin doses are typically between 20 and 40 mGy (2 to 4 rad), well below the threshold dose for the induction of erythema.
–In **CT fluoroscopy,** higher skin doses are possible and are proportional to the fluoroscopy time and the selected technique.
  –By minimizing the total patient exposure in CT fluoroscopy, it should be possible to prevent the induction of deterministic (skin) effects.
–If the embryo/fetus is directly exposed in CT, the embryo dose will be about 15 mGy (1.5 rad) at 120 kVp/250 mAs.

TABLE 8.5. *Typical effective doses in computed tomography*

Type of examination	Effective dose
Head	1–2 mSv (100–200 mrem)
Chest	6 mSv (600 mrem)
Abdomen	4 mSv (400 mrem)
Lower extremities	<1 mSv (<100 mrem)

–If the embryo is 8 cm from the directly irradiated region, the mean dose will be no more than 10% of the dose in the directly irradiated region.

C. Effective doses

–Because deterministic effects do not occur in CT, the major patient radiation risk is the induction of cancer.
  –The patient cancer risk depends on the dose and radiosensitivity of all exposed organs and tissues, and is best quantified by the effective dose parameter.
–**Effective doses** in CT are much higher than those in conventional radiography **(Table 8.5).**
–The effective dose for head CT examinations in infants and young children can be up to four times higher than that for adults when performed using the same techniques.
–Body CT examinations in infants and young children can be double those of adults when performed using the same techniques.
–Effective doses in children are higher than in those in adults because of the much smaller organ sizes (dose is energy deposited divided by mass)
–It is estimated that CT scans account for about 10% of all examinations performed in the United States but contribute 65% of the total patient dose from x-rays.
–The high doses associated with CT examinations prompted the U.S. Food and Drug Administration to issue an advisory in 2001 to reduce radiation doses to pediatric and small adult patients.

D. Patient doses

–Patient effective dose (and risk) is directly proportional to the total energy imparted (deposited) in the patient.
–The **effective dose** is directly proportional to the tube current and the scan time.
–Increasing the x-ray tube potential from 80 to 140 kVp increases the patient dose by a factor of five.
–The effective dose is directly proportional to the product of the slice thickness and the total number of slices in the CT examination.
–In helical CT at a pitch of 1.0, radiation doses are the same as in conventional CT using contiguous slices.
–Patient doses are inversely proportional to the selected pitch; a pitch of 1.5 will reduce doses to 67% of those for a pitch of 1.0 and a pitch of 2.0 will halve the patient dose.
–For multislice CT, radiation doses should be similar to those of helical CT for the same techniques (kVp/mAs) and scan length (slice thickness × number of slices).
–Performing pre- and postcontrast CT scans of the abdomen generally doubles the patient dose.
–Performing multiphase studies also increases the patient dose according to the number of series that are performed.
–Some manufacturers multiply the weighted CTDI by the total scan length (slice thickness × number of slices) to generate a **dose length product**.
–The dose length product is proportional to the total dose (energy) imparted to the patient and can be used as an indicator of the relative risk in CT.

Review Test

1. The fundamental measurement made by a CT scanner is the:

(A) Sorting of CT numbers
(B) Determination of gray scale
(C) Pixel density
(D) Relative x-ray attenuation
(E) Voxel atomic number

2. Which of the following has a Hounsfield unit value of approximately −90?

(A) Fat
(B) Gray matter
(C) Water
(D) Bone
(E) Lung

3. Tissue characterization is difficult because the value of a CT number may change because of:

(A) Window level
(B) Window width
(C) Tube current
(D) Scan time
(E) Volume averaging

4. The measured x-ray transmissions from a single CT fan beam through a patient is called a:

(A) Filter
(B) Back-projection algorithm
(C) Tomographic slice
(D) Primary beam
(E) Projection

5. Which image reconstruction algorithm is used in current commercial CT scanners?

(A) Two-dimensional Fourier transform
(B) Three-dimensional Fourier transform
(C) Back projection
(D) Filtered back projection
(E) Algebraic reconstruction algorithm

6. If a CT display is set at a window width of 100 and a window center of 50, the:

(A) HU value of water changes to 50
(B) White matter will look gray
(C) Gray matter will look white
(D) Bone will look black
(E) Lung will look white

7. The CT image display contrast:

(A) Must be selected prior to the x-ray exposures
(B) May be altered after the CT scan

(C) Does not modify the appearance of the CT image
(D) Can be used to change the Hounsfield unit values of image data
(E) Uses an array processor

8. Which of the following *cannot* be used to process CT images?

(A) Window/level adjustment
(B) Multiplanar reformatting
(C) Phase encoding
(D) Volume rendering
(E) Shaded-surface display

9. CT anode heat loading increases with all of the following *except* an increase in:

(A) Tube voltage
(B) Tube current
(C) Scan time
(D) Section thickness
(E) Number of sections

10. CT collimators are:

(A) Variable for different section thicknesses
(B) Not necessary for helical scans
(C) Usually made out of Plexiglas
(D) Bowtie shaped
(E) Cooled using fans

11. Which would *not* likely be used as detectors in CT scanners?

(A) Bismuth germanate
(B) $CdWO_4$
(C) Xenon gas
(D) NaI
(E) Air ionization chambers

12. Fourth-generation CT detectors are frequently made of:

(A) Low-pressure air ionization chambers
(B) Geiger tubes
(C) $CdWO_4$
(D) High-pressure xenon
(E) Selenium

13. Electron-beam CT can acquire a CT image in:

(A) Less than 1 millisecond
(B) 1 millisecond
(C) 8 milliseconds
(D) 25 milliseconds
(E) 50 milliseconds

14. The main advantage of helical CT over conventional (axial) CT is improved:

(A) Spatial resolution
(B) Low contrast detection
(C) Data acquisition rate
(D) Patient dose
(E) Image reconstruction time

15. Multislice CT improves the utilization of the:

(A) X-ray tube output
(B) Collimators
(C) Bow tie filter
(D) X-ray detectors
(E) Analog-to-digital converters

16. CT fluoroscopy minimizes radiation doses by using lower:

(A) Filtration
(B) Voltage
(C) Current
(D) Collimator thickness
(E) Field of view

17. The theoretically best possible CT resolution for a 512^2 matrix and 25 cm FOV is:

(A) 0.5 lp/mm
(B) 1.0 lp/mm
(C) 2.0 lp/mm
(D) 5.0 lp/mm
(E) 10.0 lp/mm

18. CT scanner spatial resolution could improve with an increase of:

(A) Focal spot size
(B) Detector elements size
(C) Tube voltage
(D) Scan time
(E) Reconstruction matrix

19. Visibility of small high-contrast CT lesions would most likely improve with decreasing:

(A) Patient dose
(B) Scan time
(C) Field of view
(D) Slice thickness
(E) Tube voltage

20. Visibility of large low-contrast CT lesions may improve with increasing:

(A) Filtration
(B) mAs
(C) Matrix size
(D) Display window width
(E) Size of film image

21. Image noise is *not* affected by the:

(A) Section thickness
(B) Reconstruction algorithm
(C) Patient thickness
(D) mAs
(E) Display settings (window/level)

22. The difference in x-ray attenuation between white (40 HU) and gray matter (50 HU):

(A) Is 0.1%
(B) Is 1%
(C) Is 10%
(D) Is 25%
(E) Cannot be determined

23. Partial volume artifacts in CT are generally reduced by reducing the:

(A) Section thickness
(B) Scanning time
(C) Image matrix size
(D) Focal spot size
(E) Tube voltage

24. CT number depends on all the following *except:*

(A) Beam hardening
(B) Tissue heterogeneity
(C) mAs
(D) X-ray attenuation
(E) Tube voltage

25. Ring artifacts in a third-generation CT scanner are caused by:

(A) Kilovolt peak drift
(B) Tube arcing
(C) Faulty detector elements
(D) Patient motion
(E) Poor collimation

26. Which of the following is *least* likely to be a source of CT image artifacts?

(A) Anode wobble
(B) Faulty detectors
(C) Metallic implants in patient
(D) Limited sampling of projection data
(E) Radiofrequency source near CT scanner

27. Which of the following is not a source of CT artifacts?

(A) Patient motion
(B) Metal implants
(C) Beam hardening
(D) Low tube current
(E) Faulty calibration data

28. Representative patient doses in CT are expected to include all the following *except:*

(A) Head skin dose of 40 mGy (4 rad)
(B) Head central axis dose of 40 mGy (4 rad)
(C) Body skin dose of 20 mGy (2 rad)
(D) Body central axis dose of 40 mGy (4 rad)
(E) Embryo dose (abdomen CT) of 15 mGy (1.5 rad)

29. The dose to the fetus during an abdominal CT scan would *not* increase with increasing:

(A) Patient size

(B) Tube voltage
(C) Tube current
(D) Scan time
(E) Number of sections

30. The scattered radiation dose 1 meter from a patient undergoing a head CT scan is:

(A) Less than 0.04 mGy (below 4 mrad)
(B) About 0.04 mGy (4 mrad)
(C) About 0.4 mGy (40 mrad)
(D) About 4 mGy (400 mrad)
(E) More than 4 mGy (over 400 mrad)

Answers and Explanations

1–D. Relative attenuation of x-rays, because the Hounsfield units associated with each pixel are linearly related to the average linear attenuation coefficient of the tissue associated with this pixel.

2–A. Fat is −90 HU.

3–E. Volume averaging, because the CT number is an average of the linear attenuation coefficients of the materials within the voxel.

4–E. A projection is a profile of transmitted x-ray intensities through the patient at any given location of the x-ray tube, with up to 1,000 projections acquired and used to reconstruct the CT image.

5–D. Filtered back projection is currently used on virtually all commercial CT scanners to reconstruct images from projection data.

6–B. White matter will be in the middle of the display range.

7–B. Changing the display contrast (window center and width) alters the *appearance* of the CT image but not the reconstructed image data (HU).

8–C. Phase encoding is used in magnetic resonance imaging and has no connection with CT.

9–D. Section thickness selection does not directly affect x-ray heat loading.

10–A. The collimators are located at the x-ray tube and detectors and have a variable width that defines the CT section thickness.

11–E. Because air (obviously) absorbs a negligible amount of radiation, an air ionization chamber would be a terrible CT x-ray detector.

12–C. Fourth-generation CT systems use solid state detectors such as $CdWO_4$; gas detectors are used *only* in third-generation scanners.

13–E. EBCT can acquire a CT image in a period as short as 50 milliseconds.

14–C. Fast patient data acquisition is the major benefit of helical CT.

15–A. The principle benefit of multislice CT is the improved utilization of the x-ray tube output.

16–C. Low current values are normally used in CT fluoroscopy (20 to 50 mA) to reduce doses to patients and operators.

17–B. 1 lp/mm; a matrix size of 512 can display about 250 lp over a region that is 250 mm (25 cm) and that corresponds to 1 lp/mm.

18–E. Spatial resolution could improve with an increase in reconstruction matrix size *if* resolution was limited by matrix size (not focal spot or detector size).

19–C. Decreasing the FOV would improve spatial resolution.

20–B. Low-contrast objects are difficult to see because of noise, and increasing the mAs increases the number of photons used and hence reduces CT image noise.

21–E. The CT display will not affect the image noise contained in the image data set itself. However, modifying the display settings would affect the *appearance* of any noise.

22–B. By definition 10 HU always corresponds to a difference in attenuation coefficient of 1% relative to water (HU is a relative attenuation scale in which water is equal to 0).

23–A. A lower slice thickness will reduce partial volume effects.

24–C. mAs will have no effect on CT numbers but will affect the precision with which they are measured (noise).

25–C. A faulty detector reading on third-generation scanners gives rise to ring artifacts. The closer the artifact to the image center, the more central the detector element that is faulty in the linear detector array.

26–E. Radiofrequency sources are unlikely to have any effect on the x-ray detection and therefore should produce no artifacts.

27–D. Low tube currents give rise to noticeable quantum mottle effects but not to artifacts per se.

28–D. A body central axis dose would be about 10 mGy (1 rad), which is about half the skin dose.

29–A. Increasing the patient size will always reduce the embryo dose because there is more attenuation of the x-ray beam.

30–B. Skin dose to patient will be about 40 mGy (4 rad), and the scatter will be about 0.1% of this level at a distance of 1 meter.

9

Nuclear Medicine

I. Radiopharmaceuticals

A. Production of radioactivity

–**Radionuclides** may be produced in a nuclear reactor by adding neutrons to nuclides (e.g., ^{59}Co + neutron → ^{60}Co).

–Radionuclides produced in a generator generally decay by a beta-minus process (see Chapter 1, section V.A).

–Radionuclides can be produced in **cyclotrons,** where protons or deuterons are added to stable nuclides (e.g., ^{201}Hg + deuteron → ^{201}Tl + 2 neutrons).

–Cyclotron-produced radionuclides generally decay by either a beta-plus process (^{15}O) or electron capture (^{123}I) (see Chapter 1, sections V.B and V.C).

–Radionuclides may also be produced as **fission products** of heavy nuclides.

–In nuclear medicine (NM), **generators** are used to produce radionuclides.

–Technetium (^{99m}Tc) is obtained from the parent ^{99}Mo in a generator, and ^{113m}In is obtained from a ^{113}Sn generator.

–Both ^{99m}Tc and ^{113m}In decay by isomeric transition.

–**Table 9.1** lists the characteristics of radionuclides used in NM.

B. Radiopharmaceutical characteristics

–**Radiopharmaceuticals** are designed to mimic a natural physiologic process.

–The evaluation of function rather than anatomy sets NM studies apart from other imaging studies.

–NM diagnostic studies use **gamma rays** produced in the nucleus of an atom.

–To minimize the patient radiation dose, radiopharmaceuticals should do the following:

–Have a short half-life that is compatible with the duration and objectives of the NM study.

–Produce monochromatic gamma rays with energies between 100 and 300 keV.

–Minimize production of particulate radiation, such as beta particles, internal conversion electrons, and Auger electrons.

–Radiopharmaceuticals should localize in the organ or tissue of interest, be nontoxic, and contain no chemical or radionuclide contaminants.

–Ideally, radionuclides should be readily and economically available.

–Technetium fulfills these requirements and is the most commonly used radionuclide.

C. Radiopharmaceutical localization

–Radiopharmaceutical **localization mechanisms** include the following:

–**Active transport** such as thyroid uptake scanning with iodine.

TABLE 9.1. *Characteristics of common radionuclides*

Nuclide	Photons (keV)	Production mode	Decay mode	Half-life ($T_{1/2}$)
^{67}Ga	93, 185, 296, 388	Cyclotron	EC	78 hr
^{99m}Tc	140	Generator	IT	6 hr
^{111}In	173, 247	Cyclotron	EC	68 hr
^{123}I	159	Cyclotron	EC	13 hr
^{125}I	27, 36	Reactor	EC	60 d
^{131}I	364	Fission product	β	8 d
^{133}Xe	80	Fission product	β	5.3 d
^{201}Tl	70, 167	Cyclotron	EC	73 hr

β, beta decay; EC, electron capture; IT, isomeric transition.

–**Compartmental** localization such as blood pool scanning with human serum albumin, plasma, or red blood cells.

–**Simple exchange** or **diffusion** such as bone scanning with pyrophosphates.

–**Phagocytosis** such as liver, spleen, and bone marrow scanning with radiocolloids.

–**Capillary blockade** such as lung scanning with macroaggregate (8 to 75 μm) or organ perfusion studies with intraarterial injection of macroaggregates.

–**Cell sequestration** such as spleen scanning with damaged red blood cells.

D. Technetium generator

–The ideal gamma energy of 140 keV, convenient half-life of 6 hours, and ready availability from a generator make ^{99m}Tc the most popular radionuclide.

–^{99m}Tc is used in approximately 80% of all NM examinations.

–Pertechnetate (^{99m}TcO$_4$) is produced directly from ^{99}Mo using a saline eluant.

–The technetium generator is shielded with lead and consists of an alumina column loaded with ^{99}Mo.

–^{99}Mo decays to ^{99m}Tc, and saline is added to the generator when ^{99m}Tc is needed.

–Saline passes through the column to elute (wash off) the ^{99m}Tc in the form of sodium pertechnetate.

–The ^{99}Mo is not soluble in saline and therefore remains in the column.

–^{99m}Tc decays by isomeric transition with 88% nuclear transformations, resulting in the emission of a 140 keV gamma rays.

  –The remainder of energy is emitted as internal conversion electrons, characteristic x-rays, and Auger electrons.

–The half-life of ^{99}Mo is 67 hours, which allows the generator to remain useful for approximately 1 week (about 2.5 half-lives).

–A ^{99m}Tc generator is eluted daily over the course of a week and then replaced.

–**Transient equilibrium,** in which the activity between the parent (^{99}Mo) and daughter (^{99m}Tc) are equal, is reached in approximately four half-lives (24 hours).

  –In transient equilibrium, parent and daughter decay together, with the half-life of the parent.

–**Secular equilibrium** occurs after approximately four half-lives in generator systems in which the half-life of the parent is much greater (100 times) than that of the daughter.

E. Imaging radiopharmaceuticals

–Radiopharmaceuticals are designed to concentrate in a particular organ or tissue.

–Oral or intravenous administration of pertechnetate results in uptake in the thyroid, salivary glands, and stomach as a result of its similarity to iodide and chloride ions.

–^{99m}Tc can be used to label a wide range of biological entities, including diethylen-etriaminepentaacetic acid (DTPA), dimercaptosuccinic acid (DMSA), iminodi-acetic acid (HIDA), iron complexes, macroaggregated albumin (MAA), polyphos-phate, red blood cells, and sulfur colloid.

  –As an example, sulfur colloid is available as a commercial kit containing 0.3 mm particles.

  –After sulfur colloid is injected, approximately 70% localizes in the liver within 10 to 20 minutes; the remainder is distributed in the spleen and bone marrow.

–Radioiodine is used for thyroid imaging and to evaluate thyroid function (uptake), and ^{123}I- or ^{131}I-labeled hippuran is used to evaluate kidney function.

–^{99m}Tc-MAG3 is replacing hippuran for kidney function studies.

–Radioactive gases (e.g., ^{133}Xe) may be used in lung ventilation imaging.

–Other radiopharmaceuticals used in nuclear medicine include thallium for cardiac imaging, ^{51}Cr-labeled red blood cells, ^{67}Ga-labeled citrate to detect tumor and in-fection, and ^{111}In-labeled leukocytes to detect acute infections.

–Images of the radioisotope distribution are acquired using gamma cameras.

II. Planar Imaging

A. Gamma ray detection

–Sodium iodide (NaI) scintillation crystals are used to detect gamma rays emerging from patients.

  –The **photopeak** is produced when an incident gamma ray is completely absorbed in the crystal (photoelectric effect).

  –An **iodine escape peak** occurs at approximately 30 keV below the photopeak and is the result of characteristic K-shell x-rays from iodine that escape the crystal.

–**Scatter events** in the NaI crystals occur when the energy of the scattered electron is absorbed in the crystal but the scattered photon escapes.

–The **Compton edge** represents the maximum energy transferred to a scattered elec-tron in the Compton process.

–Compton scattering of gamma rays in tissue produces low-energy photons that can be subsequently absorbed by the NaI crystal.

–**Pulse pile-up** events occur when the energy of two photons is registered simultane-ously.

–**Fig. 9.1** shows the detection of the three gamma rays emitted by ^{67}Ga using a NaI scintillation crystal.

  –The photopeak for each gamma ray occurs at an energy proportional to the photon energy.

  –Pulse height analysis permits the identification of photopeak events.

–Photoelectric absorption events in the crystal, from gamma rays that have not un-dergone Compton scatter in the patient, should be used for nuclear imaging.

B. Gamma cameras

–**Gamma cameras** (also known as **Anger cameras**) are the most common imaging devices used in NM **(Fig. 9.2).**

–**Scintillation crystals** absorb incident gamma photons by the photoelectric process and produce many light photons.

  –Most crystals are made of NaI, activated with a trace of thallium, and are about 10 mm thick.

  –NaI crystals are fragile and easily damaged.

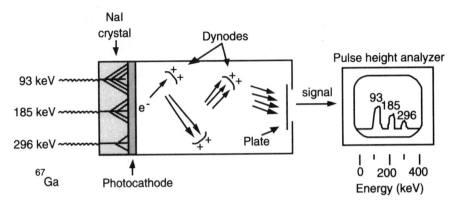

FIG. 9.1. Incident photons are absorbed by the sodium iodide crystal, producing scintillations (light), which are converted to photoelectrons in the photocathode. These are accelerated and multiplied as they move between the charged dynodes toward the plate, where they are detected. The pulse height analyzer determines signal strength as a function of energy.

–Light output can be detected by **photomultiplier tubes (PMTs).**
–The output voltage from PMTs is directly proportional to the amount of energy absorbed by the scintillating material.
–**Table 9.2** summarizes how photopeak detection efficiency increases with increasing detector thickness and decreases with increasing photon energy.
–As crystal thickness increases, sensitivity improves but resolution gets worse.
–Light output from the NaI crystal is detected by an array of PMTs.
–Gamma cameras typically use 37, 61, or 91 PMTs.
–Signals from PMTs generate data about the location of each photon interaction **(spatial data).**
–The position and energy of the gamma ray is determined by **pulse arithmetic circuit** based on the relative strength of the signal received by several PMTs.

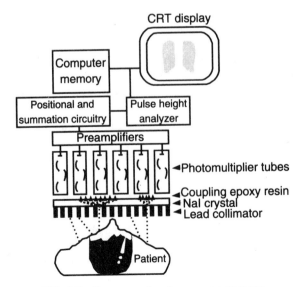

FIG. 9.2. Components of a gamma camera.

TABLE 9.2. *Sodium iodide crystal photopeak detection efficiency*

Photon energy (keV)	Photons (%) detected by sodium iodide crystal with detector thickness of:		
	5 mm	10 mm	25 mm
100	94	100	100
140*	72	92	100
200	32	54	85
300	12	22	46
500	3	6	15

* ^{99m}Tc.

–The term **counts** refers to the registration of gamma rays by the detector.

–The **intrinsic sensitivity** or **efficiency** of a crystal is the percentage of incident gamma rays detected.

–Images are built up count-by-count, with between 500,000 and 1 million data points per image.

–Modern gamma cameras are all digital and use computers to store image data.

  –Gamma cameras also have spatial uniformity corrections made to the acquired image data that correct for system spatial nonlinearity.

–Gamma cameras have lead shielding to prevent unwanted background radiation from the room or other areas of the patient from contributing to the image information.

C. **Pulse height analysis**

  –A **pulse height analyzer (PHA)** is an electronic device used to determine which portion of the detected spectrum is used to create images **(Fig. 9.3).**

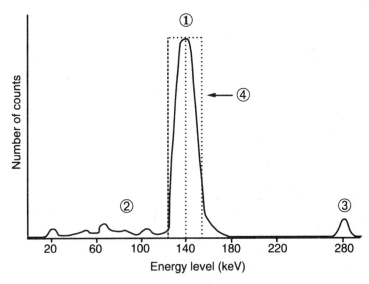

FIG. 9.3. Technetium spectrum and photopeak window settings. The photopeak *(1)* is the result of complete absorption of ^{99m}Tc gamma rays in the crystal. The iodine escape peak, Compton scatter events, and secondary x-rays from lead occur below this *(2)*. The sum peak *(3)* is the result of two photons being simultaneously absorbed in the crystal and counted as one. The area within the dashed line *(4)* shows the acceptance range of a pulse height analyzer (PHA) set at 140 keV with a 20% window.

–The PHA is placed between the detector and counting portion of the camera system **(Fig. 9.2).**

–The PHA can be set to allow only certain photon energy levels to be counted, thus decreasing the Compton scatter and pulse pile-up in the resultant image.

–The PHA allows the operator either to set the upper and lower energy limits or to set a peak energy level and associated window.

–The **window,** measured as a percentage, determines the acceptable range of energy levels around the peak for subsequent counting.

  –For example, a peak of 140 keV with a 20% window ($\pm 10\%$) accepts photon energy levels ranging from 126 to 154 keV **(Fig. 9.3).**

–A wide window accepts more photons and produces an image more quickly, but it includes more scatter photons, which degrade image quality.

–Some radionuclides, such as ^{67}Ga, require that multiple windows be set because there are several gamma ray energy levels **(Fig. 9.1).**

D. Collimators

–Collimators are used to provide spatial information by allowing photons arriving only from certain directions to reach the crystal.

–Collimators are typically made of lead and contain multiple holes **(Fig. 9.4).** The lead strips between the holes are called **septa.**

–**Parallel hole** collimators project the same object size onto the camera, and the field of view (FOV) does not change with distance **(Fig. 9.4A).**

–**Converging collimators** produce a magnified image, and FOV decreases with distance **(Fig. 9.4B).**

–**Diverging collimators** project an image size that is smaller than the object size, and FOV increases with distance from the collimator **(Fig. 9.4C).**

–**Pinhole** collimators are cone-shaped with a single hole at the apex, and generate a minified or magnified image depending on the object-to-collimator distance.

  –The image is inverted and the FOV increases rapidly as the observer moves away from the pinhole **(Fig. 9.4D).**

E. Collimator performance

–Collimators are the major factors in determining the spatial resolution performance, and system sensitivity.

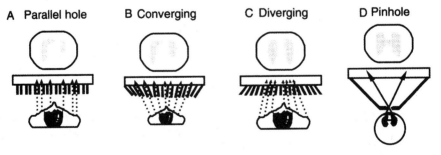

| A Parallel hole | B Converging | C Diverging | D Pinhole |

Liver / spleen scan   Liver /spleen scan in child   Lung scan   Thyroid scan

FIG. 9.4. Collimators used in nuclear medicine. **(A)** Parallel hole collimator is used for routine imaging. **(B)** Converging hole collimator magnifies the image. **(C)** Diverging hole collimator reduces image size. **(D)** Pinhole collimator.

TABLE 9.3. *Typical full-width half maximum resolution values for different types of clinical collimators*

Distance from collimator (cm)	Spatial resolution at FWHM (mm)		
	High resolution	All-purpose collimator	High sensitivity
0	2	3	5
5	5	7	10
10	8	10	15
15	12	14	20

FWHM, full-width half maximum.

–The resolution of a collimator is expressed as the **full-width half maximum (FWHM)** of a line source.

–Collimator **sensitivity** is the fraction of gamma rays reaching it from all directions that pass through the holes.

–Collimator sensitivity is low, with approximately 10^{-4} (or only 0.01%) of the emitted photons being detected.

–Collimators generally involve a tradeoff between spatial resolution and sensitivity.

  –Resolution is increased if the size of the holes is reduced (thicker septa) or if the collimator is made thicker.

  –These same changes decrease the number of photons reaching the crystal, thus reducing system sensitivity.

–Parallel-hole collimators are classified for high-sensitivity (i.e., low-resolution), general-purpose, and high-resolution (i.e., low-sensitivity) uses.

–**High-sensitivity** collimators are thinner and have larger and, therefore, fewer holes and lower resolution.

–**High-resolution** collimators have smaller and, therefore, more holes and lower sensitivity; these can transmit half as many photons as the general-purpose collimator.

–**Low-energy** collimators, for use with ^{99m}Tc and ^{201}Tl, have thin septa.

–**Medium-energy** collimators, used with ^{67}Ga, ^{131}I, and ^{111}In, have thicker septa and, therefore, fewer holes and lower sensitivity.

–**High-energy** collimators are used for ^{131}I and ^{18}F, and have even thicker septa.

–**Table 9.3** summarizes the variation of resolution as a function of distance from the source to the collimator; resolution decreases with increasing distance from the collimator.

F. Nuclear Medicine (NM) Images

–NM images can be viewed in real time on a display monitor during the acquisition.

  –A "persistence screen," in which each count remains on the screen for a prolonged period, can be used to help patient positioning.

–Analog-to-digital converters are used to generate the digital information.

  –A typical NM matrix size is 128×128, with a bit depth of 8 (256 gray levels).

–Images can be acquired for a set number of counts (usually 500,000 to 1 million) or for a set time period (usually several minutes).

–Some studies require the collection of a series of images or frames to record a dynamic process such as cardiac motion or renal function.

–Image processing includes calculating plots of counts in select regions of interest and background subtraction.

–First pass cardiac studies are usually recorded in a series of short acquisitions lasting only a few dozen milliseconds and triggered by the patient's electrocardiogram.

–In these gated cardiac studies, the information from several hundred frames is added to generate a composite cine loop, which has an adequate number of total counts.

III. Tomography

A. Single photon emission computed tomography

–Single photon emission computed tomography (SPECT) provides computed tomographic views of the three-dimensional distribution of radioisotopes in the body.

–Parallel-hole collimators are commonly used for SPECT imaging.

  –Hybrid converging and parallel-hole collimators offer superior resolution and sensitivity performance and are sometimes used for brain SPECT.

–In SPECT, the gamma camera rotates 180 or 360 degrees around the patient, acquiring data that allow tomographic images to be generated.

  –Typically, 64 or 128 projections are taken.

  –SPECT images are typically reconstructed using a 128 × 128 matrix.

–Scan profiles from these projections are used as inputs for filtered-back projection reconstruction algorithms to compute tomographic images.

  –Transverse, sagittal, and coronal views can be generated.

  –Rotating three-dimensional representations can also be created and displayed.

–Iterative reconstruction algorithms can be more accurate and can be used with fast computers.

–Problems in SPECT relate to obtaining quantitative information and long acquisition times.

–To obtain quantitative information, corrections need to be made for scatter and attenuation.

B. Clinical single photon emission computed tomography

–**Multiheaded cameras** are used to increase system sensitivity and reduce scan times.

–The use of **elliptical orbits** (i.e., body contouring) for gamma camera travel around the patient allows the distance to the patient to be minimized, thus improving sensitivity and resolution.

–The spatial resolution of SPECT is generally poorer than that of planar imaging.

  –SPECT needs to use high-sensitivity collimators to obtain an adequate number of counts in each projection image.

–In addition, noise is a major factor in SPECT because of the low number of photons used to create data for each voxel.

–Most SPECT equipment uses two gamma camera heads, but sometimes three or even four heads are incorporated to reduce data acquisition time.

–The major benefit of SPECT is the improved contrast that results from the elimination of overlapping structures.

–SPECT studies are susceptible to image artifacts caused by nonuniformities and by axis of rotation misalignment.

  –The image reconstruction algorithm amplifies the detrimental effects of image noise and nonuniformities.

–Common clinical SPECT applications include myocardial ischemia or infarctions, evaluation of abnormalities seen on planar bone scans, and cerebral blood flow.

C. Positron emission tomography physics

–**Positron emission tomography (PET)** makes use of short-lived positron emitters such as ^{11}C ($T_{1/2} = 20$ minutes), ^{13}N ($T_{1/2} = 10$ minutes), ^{15}O ($T_{1/2} = 2$ minutes), and ^{18}F ($T_{1/2} = 110$ minutes).

–Most short-lived radioisotopes require a cyclotron for production.

–^{18}F in the form of fluorodeoxyglucose is the most commonly used agent.

–Rubidium (^{82}Rb, $T_{1/2} = 75$ seconds) and gallium (^{68}Ga, $T_{1/2} = 68$ minutes) can be obtained from a generator.

–PET is based on the simultaneous detection of the two 511 keV annihilation photons produced when a positron loses its kinetic energy and combines with an electron **(Fig. 9.5).**

–**Annihilation coincident detection,** or simultaneous detection using coincident circuitry, allows extrapolation to locate the emission site.

–Collimators are used to define planes and limit the number of coincidence counts but are not needed for localization of photons.

–The PET scanner consists of a ring of **bismuth germanate (BGO)** detectors, coupled to photomultiplier tubes.

  –Lutetium oxyorthosilicate (LSO) and gadolinium oxyorthosilicate (GSO) are promising inorganic scintillators that may replace BGO.

–The spatial resolution of commercial PET systems (FWHM) can approach 5 mm.

–Images are generated using filtered-back projection algorithms.

–Recent developments include the development of hybrid PET/CT scanners, which permit PET and CT images to be fused together.

  –CT images also provide accurate patient attenuation data, which is useful for performing attenuation corrections in PET reconstruction algorithms.

D. Positron emission tomography imaging

–Radiopharmaceuticals that can be used for PET imaging include fluorodeoxyglucose (^{18}F-FDG), used to study metabolism, and ammonia (^{13}N), used to study perfusion.

–PET studies can produce absolute quantitative information on processes such as perfusion and metabolism.

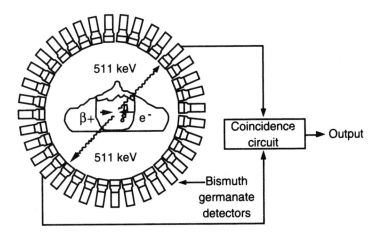

FIG. 9.5. Positron emission tomography.

–Because a collimator is not required, PET images normally have a large number of counts (and low noise).

–Serial studies can be performed because of the short half-life of PET radionuclides.

–The major limitation of PET is the large cost of building a PET imaging center with an on-site cyclotron and radiopharmaceutical production facilities.

–Until recently, most facilities used PET as a research tool.

–Reimbursement for PET studies has recently improved, and PET is rapidly becoming a widely available and important clinical tool.

–PET is proving to be a valuable diagnostic and staging tool in oncology imaging.

–PET is also very useful in cardiac and neurological imaging.

IV. Quality Control

A. Generator quality control

–If the technetium generator is damaged, ^{99}Mo or alumina can break into the saline elute.

–Alumina interferes with the proper formation of ^{99m}Tc radiopharmaceutical kits.

–Color indicator paper is used to test for alumina breakthrough.

–^{99}Mo has gamma ray energy levels of 740 and 780 keV, and breakthrough results in an unnecessary and high radiation dose to the patient.

–A **dose calibrator** is used to determine the content of ^{99}Mo each time the generator is eluted.

–A lead shield blocks the ^{99m}Tc gamma rays, allowing ^{99}Mo gamma rays to be counted.

–The legal limit for molybdenum breakthrough is 5.5 kBq (0.15 μCi) of ^{99}Mo per 37 MBq (1.0 mCi) of ^{99m}Tc.

B. Radiopharmaceutical quality control

–**Radionuclide purity** is the presence of unwanted radionuclides in the sample and is checked using a well counter to search for unwanted energy levels.

–For example, ^{99}Mo in ^{99m}Tc, ^{123}I may contain ^{124}I, and ^{201}Tl may contain ^{202}Tl.

–**Radiochemical purity** is the chemical purity of the isotope and is checked by thin-layer chromatography.

–For example, there may be free pertechnetate in ^{99m}Tc-labeled DTPA.

–**Chromatography** separates compounds that are soluble in saline.

–For example, free pertechnetate is soluble in saline, but sulfur colloid is not.

–**Chemical purity** refers to the amount of unwanted chemical contaminants in the agent.

–**Sterility** means that the radiopharmaceutical is free of any microbial contamination.

–Even if a preparation is sterile, it may still contain **pyrogens,** which can cause a reaction if administered to a patient.

–All sterility and pyrogenicity tests should be performed before the agent is administered to patients.

–Sterility and pyrogenicity tests are not feasible with each dose for short-lived radionuclides (e.g., ^{99m}Tc), but they should be performed periodically.

C. Gamma camera quality control

–The photopeak window of the PHA is checked daily by placing a small amount of a known radioisotope in front of the camera.

–**Field uniformity** is the ability of the gamma camera to reproduce a uniform distribution of activity.

–Differences in the PMT response and transmission of light in the crystal contribute to nonuniformity.

–Nonuniformities of greater than 10% are unacceptable for clinical imaging.

–Modern cameras have a uniformity of better than 2% between adjacent areas.

–Field uniformity is checked daily by placing a uniform flood source in front of the camera and generating a histogram of pixel activity.

–The flood source is usually a sealed dish of ^{99m}Tc or ^{57}Co.

–**Extrinsic floods** are obtained with the collimator in place.

–**Intrinsic floods** are performed without the collimator.

–An **uncorrected flood** is obtained with the computer correction circuitry turned off.

–**Resolution** (i.e., the ability to separate two points) and **linearity** (i.e., the ability to accurately image a straight line) are checked using a parallel-bar phantom.

D. Dose calibrator quality control

–A **dose calibrator** is an ionization chamber used to measure the activity of a radioisotope dose in megabecquerels (megacuries).

–Each dose is measured in a dose calibrator before injection into the patient.

–**Constancy** (i.e., precision) is checked daily by measuring two standardized long half-life sources (e.g., ^{57}Co, ^{137}Cs).

–Day to day measurements should vary by less than 5%.

–**Accuracy** is checked at installation and annually using calibrated sources.

–**Linearity** is checked quarterly by measuring the decay of ^{99m}Tc over 72 hours or more, or by using calibrated shields.

V. Image Quality

A. Spatial resolution

–**Resolution** is the ability to distinguish two adjacent radioactive sources.

–An image of a line source of activity is known as the **line spread function.**

–Measurement of the FWHM of the line spread function is a common measure of resolution in NM.

–**Intrinsic resolution** refers to the camera, including crystal, PMTs, and electronics.

–Intrinsic resolution is degraded with increased detector thickness because of increased light diffusion in the NaI crystal.

–Intrinsic resolution is typically between 3 and 5 mm.

–**System resolution (R)** depends on the intrinsic resolution of the gamma camera (R_i) and resolution of the collimator (R_c).

–System resolution is $R = \sqrt{Ri^2 + Rc^2}$.

–System resolution decreases with distance from the collimator.

–FWHM values in NM are approximately 10 mm with an all-purpose collimator and 7.5 mm with a high-resolution collimator.

–Resolution is degraded if the PMTs separate from the crystal.

B. Image contrast

–Contrast in NM images is generally high because radiopharmaceuticals localize well in the organ of interest.

–Some radioactivity is always found in other tissues, and photons from this activity generate undesirable **background counts.**

–**Background counts** degrade image contrast.

–The ratio of organ-specific uptake to unwanted uptake in other tissues is called the **target-to-background ratio.**

–Contrast is also affected by **septal penetration** and **scatter.**

–When images are printed on film or displayed on a monitor, image contrast is also affected by the characteristic curve of the film or monitor.

C. Image noise

–Noise degrades image quality and is classified as **random** or **structured.**

–Random noise, or **quantum mottle,** results from statistical variation in pixel counts.

–Because of the low number of photons used to create a typical NM image, quantum mottle is a major factor in image quality.

–Noise is the primary factor determining the quality of NM images.

–If too few counts are recorded, the high quantum mottle can reduce lesion detectability.

–Noise can be quantified by the standard deviation about the mean pixel value in a nominally uniform region of interest.

–The noise can be reduced by increasing the administered activity, increasing the imaging time, or increasing the sensitivity of the collimator.

–Section III.B in Chapter 5 discusses the relationship between Poisson statistics and quantum mottle.

–**Structured noise** includes nonuniformities in the gamma camera and is a minor contributor to overall noise.

–Most modern gamma cameras use computers to perform corrections for nonuniformities, thereby reducing the significance of structured noise.

–Overlying objects in the patient (e.g., uptake in the gastrointestinal tract when imaging the kidneys) can also result in structured noise.

D. Artifacts

–Gamma camera artifacts are caused by many different sources.

–Damaged collimators can cause significant uniformity problems.

–Patient motion is a common source of artifacts.

–Metal objects worn by the patient produce photopenic areas that can mimic pathologic cold lesions.

–**PMT failure** can also produce a cold defect and shows up well on a flood image.

–**Off-peak images** contain excessive Compton scatter and occur when the PHA window is outside the main photopeak.

–**Edge packing** refers to the increased brightness at the edge of the crystal.

–Edge packing is caused by internal reflection of light at the edge of the crystal and absence of PMTs beyond the crystal edge.

–**Cracked crystals** produce linear defects in the image.

VI. Dosimetry

A. Half-lives

–**Physical half-life ($T_{1/2}$)** is the time required for a radionuclide to decay to half its original activity **(Fig. 9.6).**

–The **decay rate,** or activity, of a source is the number of disintegrations occurring each second.

–Lambda (λ) is the **decay constant,** and activity equals $N \times \lambda$, where N is the number of atoms in the sample.

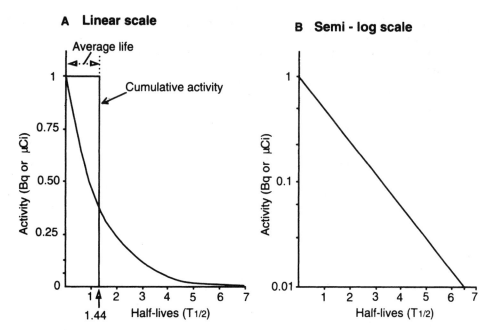

FIG. 9.6. (A) Physical half-life ($T_{1/2}$) is the decay of radioactive substances. The cumulative activity of a radiopharmaceutical is equal to the area under the curve, which is also the product of the average life (1.44 times the half-life) and the initial activity, as shown by the shaded box. **(B)** Radioactive decay is exponential and can be plotted as a straight line on a semi-log scale.

–The activity of a source decays exponentially as $e^{-\lambda xt}$, where t is time expressed in the same units as λ: $T_{1/2} = 0.693/\lambda$.

–The **biological half-life (T_b)** is determined by the clearance of the radionuclide from the organ, tissue, or body.

–The **effective half-life (T_e)** of a radionuclide in any organ encompasses both radioactive decay and biological clearance and is shorter than the physical or biological half-life.

–The relation between $T_{1/2}$, T_b, and T_e is $1/T_e = 1/T_b + 1/T_{1/2}$.

–If a radionuclide has a physical half-life of 6 hours and a biological half-life of 3 hours, then $1/T_e = 1/6 + 1/3$, and $T_e = 2$ hours.

–The effective half-life is always less than the physical or biological half-life.

–If either the biological or physical half-life is much longer than the other, the effective half-life approximates to the shorter of the two.

B. Cumulative activity

–The total number of nuclear transformations in an organ or tissue is called **cumulative activity ($\tilde{A}$).**

–Cumulative activity is the area under a curve of activity in an organ or tissue plotted as a function of time.

–The **average life** of a radioactive nucleus is **1.44 × $T_{1/2}$,** or $1/\lambda$.

–In the SI system, the number of transformations is expressed in becquerel-seconds (Bq-s) as 1.44 × initial activity in organ (Bq) × $T_{1/2}$ (seconds).

–In non-SI units, the number of transformations is expressed in microcurie-hours (μCi-hours) and is calculated as 1.44 × initial activity (μCi) in organ × $T_{1/2}$ (hours).

–In general, Ã = 1.44 × A_o × T_e, where A_o is the initial activity in the organ, and T_e is the effective half-life.

–Cumulative activity data are obtained empirically for each radiopharmaceutical by monitoring the time course of activity.

–Cumulative activity values are often different for normal patients and patients with certain diseases.

C. S factor

–The radiation dose *(D)* to any organ or tissue is obtained by dividing the total energy absorbed *(E)* in the organ by the organ mass *(M)*.

–Absorbed dose is $D = E/M$ and is measured in grays (Gy).

–The energy absorbed in a target organ per nuclear emission in the source organ is the product of [(average number of emissions per transformation) × (average energy associated for each emission) × (fraction of emitted energy deposited in the target organ)].

–The total energy deposited in the target organ is then obtained by summing over all the radiations emitted by the nuclide.

–Dividing the absorbed energy by the target organ mass gives the **S factor,** which is the absorbed dose in a target organ per unit of cumulative activity in a source organ.

–The S factor is dependent on organ shape, size, and the location of the radioactivity.

–S factor units are Gy/Bq-s (rad/μCi-hr).

–Calculated S factors for radionuclides used in NM for numerous source and target organs and tissues are available in the scientific literature.

D. Patient doses

–The dose to a target organ, from activity in one source organ, is obtained by multiplying the source organ cumulative (Ã) and the corresponding source target S factor.

–In general, organ dose D = Ã × S.

–The total dose to an organ is obtained by summing the doses from all source organs that contain radioactivity.

–The maximum organ doses from diagnostic NM procedures are approximately 50 mGy (5 rad).

–Normally, more than one organ or tissue receives a significant radiation dose in NM studies.

–The **effective dose, E,** combines all organ doses and their relative radiosensitivity, and is the best indicator of patient risk in NM.

–Effective doses are typically 5 mSv (500 mrem) for most common NM examinations **(Table 9.4).**

–Effective doses in PET imaging are similar to those in NM, and 4 mSv (400 mrem) is a representative value.

–Although PET radionuclides are very short-lived, the energy emitted per transformation is relatively high.

–Organ doses in ^{131}I therapy application can be as high as hundreds of Gy (tens of thousands of RAD).

–The amount of ^{131}I administered for therapy can be as high as 10 GBq (hundreds of millicuries).

E. Operator doses

–NM technologists receive much higher occupational doses than do x-ray technologists.

TABLE 9.4. *Effective doses in nuclear medicine*

Procedure	Radiopharmaceutical	Administered activity	Effective dose per procedure
Brain	^{99m}Tc gluconate	750 MBq (20 mCi)	7.5 mSv (750 mrem)
Bone	^{99m}Tc pyrophosphate	750 MBq (20 mCi)	6.0 mSv (600 mrem)
Liver/spleen	^{99m}Tc sulphur colloid	200 MBq (5 mCi)	2.0 mSv (200 mrem)
Biliary	^{99m}Tc HIDA	200 MBq (5 mCi)	4.5 mSv (450 mrem)
Cardiac (MUGA)	^{99m}Tc red blood cells	750 MBq (20 mCi)	5.5 mSv (550 mrem)
Cardiac	^{99m}Tc pyrophosphate	600 MBq (15 mCi)	3.5 mSv (350 mrem)
Cardiac	^{201}Tl thallus chloride	75 MBq (2 mCi)	7.0 mSv (700 mrem)
Lung	^{99m}Tc MAA	150 MBq (4 mCi)	2.5 mSv (250 mrem)
Renal	^{99m}Tc DTPA	600 MBq (15 mCi)	6.0 mSv (600 mrem)
Inflammation	^{67}Ga gallium citrate	200 MBq (5 mCi)	20.0 mSv (2000 mrem)
Thyroid uptake	^{131}I sodium iodide	0.2 MBq (0.05 mCi)	1.2 mSv (120 mrem)
Thyroid scan	^{99m}Tc pertechnetate	200 MBq (5 mCi)	2.5 mSv (250 mrem)
Thyroid uptake	^{123}I sodium iodide	7.5 MBq (0.2 mCi)	0.55 mSv (55 mrem)
Infection	^{111}In leukocytes	2 MBq (0.05 mCi)	1.2 mSv (120 mrem)

HIDA, hepato-iminodiacetic acid; MUGA, multiple gated acquisition; MAA, macroaggregated albumin; DTPA, diethylenetriaminepentaacetic acid.

–NM technologists are surrounded by patients full of radioactivity.

–The gamma ray energies in NM are much higher than in diagnostic radiology and therefore much more difficult to shield.

  –The average gamma ray in NM is 140 keV (^{99m}Tc), which is higher than photon energies in x-ray imaging (about 40 keV).

–The average annual exposure for NM technologists in a year is between 1 and 5 mSv (100 to 500 mrem).

  –Ninety-five percent of x-ray technologists receive no measurable occupational exposure.

–Handling of radionuclides requires the use of leaded syringes to minimize extremity doses.

  –Extremity doses need to be monitored using ring dosimeters, which are worn on a finger.

–NM operators also run the risk of the intake of radionuclides such as ^{131}I.

  –Technologists who handle volatile radionuclides such as ^{131}I need to have their thyroids monitored on a regular basis.

Review Test

1. An ideal radiopharmaceutical would have all the following *except:*

(A) Long half-life
(B) No particulate emissions
(C) Target specificity
(D) 150 to 250 keV photons
(E) Rapid biological distribution

2. Which of the following is *not* a radiopharmaceutical localization mechanism?

(A) Diffusion
(B) Phagocytosis.
(C) Capillary blockage
(D) Elution
(E) Cell sequestration

3. What determines the residual activity of a 1-week-old ^{99}Mo/^{99m}Tc generator?

(A) Initial activity of molybdenum
(B) Number of times the generator was milked
(C) Half-life of ^{99m}Tc
(D) Half-life of ^{99}Tc
(E) Thickness of PB shielding

4. ^{99m}Tc generators *cannot* be:

(A) Produced in a cyclotron
(B) Used to dispense more than 1 Ci
(C) Shipped by air
(D) Purchased by licensed users
(E) Used for more than 67 hours

5. For ^{99m}Tc, which of the following *cannot* contribute to the patient dose?

(A) Auger electrons
(B) Beta particles
(C) Internal conversion electrons
(D) Gamma rays
(E) Characteristic x-rays

6. A long-lived radionuclide with a daughter ($T_{1/2} = 10$ hours) reaches equilibrium in:

(A) About 3 hours
(B) About 10 hours
(C) About 40 hours
(D) About 200 hours
(E) More than 200 hours

7. A pulse height analyzer window width of 20% detects ^{99m}Tc gamma rays with energies of:

(A) 140 keV only
(B) Between 135 and 145 keV

(C) Between 120 and 140 keV
(D) Between 126 and 154 keV
(E) Between 118 and 168 keV

8. Gamma camera crystals:

(A) Are made of cesium iodide
(B) Convert about 95% of gamma ray energy to light
(C) Are generally 100 μm thick
(D) Have lead backing
(E) Absorbs more than 90% of 140 keV photons

9. NM images acquired using a computer will typically have all of the following except:

(A) 500,000 to 1 million counts
(B) Matrix sizes of 128^2
(C) 256 grayscale levels
(D) Approximately 10 MB of data
(E) Uniformity corrections

10. The pulse height analyzer in NM imaging increases:

(A) Detector efficiency
(B) Scattered photons
(C) Contrast-to-noise ratio
(D) Count rate
(E) Image distortion

11. Which does not change as the distance from the face of a parallel-hole collimator is increased?

(A) Resolution
(B) Sensitivity
(C) Energy resolution
(D) Imaging time
(E) Patient dose

12. Imaging of the thyroid yields the highest resolution with a:

(A) High-sensitivity collimator
(B) Diverging collimator
(C) High-energy collimator
(D) Low-energy all-purpose collimator
(E) Pinhole collimator

13. Gamma cameras are normally capable of resolving:

(A) 0.01 lp/mm
(B) 0.06 lp/mm
(C) 0.3 lp/mm
(D) 1.0 lp/mm
(E) More than 1.0 lp/mm

14. SPECT requires all of the following except:

(A) Gamma-emitting radioisotopes
(B) Gamma camera rotation
(C) Coincidence detection
(D) Pulse height analysis
(E) Filtered-back projection reconstruction algorithms

15. PET scanners detect:

(A) Positrons of the same energy in coincidence
(B) Positrons and electrons in coincidence
(C) Photons of different energies in coincidence
(D) Annihilation photons in coincidence
(E) Annihilation photons in anticoincidence

16. PET scanners:

(A) Need high-energy parallel-hole collimators
(B) Cannot handle very high count rates
(C) Suffer from significant attenuation losses
(D) Detect 1.022 MeV photons
(E) Have FWHM of 5 mm

17. The best radionuclide spatial resolution is normally achieved using:

(A) SPECT
(B) Low-energy all-purpose collimator
(C) High-resolution collimator
(D) High-sensitivity collimator
(E) PET

18. Advantage of PET over gamma cameras include all of the following *except:*

(A) More physiological tracer compounds
(B) Better resolution
(C) Less mottle
(D) Rapid radiopharmaceutical decay
(E) Availability of the positron radioisotopes

19. Which of the following is *not* a quality control test performed on a gamma camera?

(A) Field uniformity
(B) ^{99}Mo breakthrough
(C) Extrinsic flood
(D) Spatial resolution
(E) Linearity

20. The intrinsic (R_i) and collimator (R_c) resolution are related to the system resolution R as:

(A) $R = R_i + R_c$
(B) $R = (R_i + R_c)^2$
(C) $R = (R_i + R_c)^{1/2}$
(D) $R = R_i^2 + R_c^2$
(E) $R = (R_i^2 + R_c^2)^{1/2}$

21. The resolution of gamma camera does not depend on:

(A) Photon energy
(B) Septal thickness
(C) NaI crystal thickness
(D) Counting time
(E) Distance from the collimator

22. The variance of a NM image pixel with a 100 count would be:

(A) 10
(B) 20
(C) 30
(D) 50
(E) 100

23. A circular cold spot artifact in a gamma camera image is most likely the result of:

(A) A cracked NaI crystal
(B) Using the incorrect collimator
(C) A defective PMT
(D) A faulty power supply
(E) Incorrectly administered activity

24. A radionuclide with a shorter half-life will generally reduce the:

(A) Count rate
(B) Patient dose
(C) Biological clearance
(D) Scatter
(E) Photopeak energy

25. For ^{99m}Tc decaying to ^{99}Tc, which of the following is *not* true?

(A) The half-life of ^{99m}Tc is 67 hours.
(B) The half-life of ^{99}Tc is 2.1×10^5 years.
(C) Activity is N $\times$ λ, where N is the number of atoms, and λ is decay constant.
(D) $\lambda = 0.693/T_{1/2}$, where $T_{1/2}$ is the half-life.
(E) The half-life of ^{99m}Tc is independent of its activity.

26. The effective half-life is:

(A) Longer than the physical half-life
(B) Equal to the biological half-life
(C) Dependent on the administered activity
(D) Shorter or equal to the physical half-life
(E) Independent of biological clearance

27. Cumulated activity in an organ does *not* depend on:

(A) Administered activity
(B) Fractional uptake in organ
(C) Organ mass

(D) Physical half-life
(E) Biological clearance

28. The S factor does *not* depend on:

(A) Number of emission/transformation
(B) Emission energy
(C) Distance to target organ
(D) Target organ mass
(E) Organ activity

29. Which is *not* true for patient doses in SPECT imaging?

(A) Effective doses are approximately 5 mSv (500 mrem).

(B) Maximum organ doses are about 50 mGy (5 rad).
(C) Doses are much higher than chest x-rays.
(D) Doses are similar to PET doses.
(E) Dose is proportional to imaging time.

30. Following administration of ^{131}I to a patient, the dose rate near the patient does not depend on:

(A) Administered activity
(B) Effective half-life
(C) Patient size
(D) Distance to patient
(E) Patient age

Answers and Explanations

1–A. The ideal radionuclide has a short half-life to reduce the radiation dose to the patient.

2–D. Elution is a process whereby a radionuclide is extracted (washed out) from a generator.

3–A. The original activity of ^{99}Mo and its half-life, which determines the activity of molybdenum (and thus of ^{99m}Tc) at the end of the week.

4–A. ^{99}Mo can be produced in a reactor or from fission products, but it cannot be produced in a cyclotron (^{99}Mo is a beta emitter, requiring the addition of neutrons, not protons).

5–B. There are no beta particles associated with ^{99m}Tc.

6–C. It will take approximately four half-lives (i.e., 40 hours) for the daughter activity to be equal or approximately equal to the parent activity.

7–D. If the window width is 20%, the PHA lower energy level is 140% − 10% (126 keV), and the upper energy level is 140 keV + 10% (156 keV).

8–E. A typical NaI crystal (10 mm) will absorb over 90% of 140 keV photons via the photoelectric effect.

9–D. A typical NM image has about 10 kB of data, not 10 MB.

10–C. The pulse height analyzer window is centered around the pulses of the principal photon energy; some signal (contrast) is lost, but a much larger fraction of the noise is excluded.

11–E. Patient dose depends on administered activity.

12–E. For pinhole collimators, the shorter the distance, the larger the magnification; this characteristic makes the pinhole collimator the most suitable tool for high-resolution imaging of small organs such as the thyroid.

13–B. A typical FWHM value for a NM image of a line source is about 8 mm; the maximum resolvable frequency is thus [1/(2 × 8)] cycles/mm, or 0.06 lp/mm.

14–C. Annihilation radiation in PET, but not in SPECT, is obtained using coincidence detection.

15–D. PET detects and uses annihilation photons (511 keV) detected in coincidence.

16–D. The FWHM (resolution) of a PET scanner is typically 5 mm.

17–E. The spatial resolution achieved using PET is superior to that of any gamma camera or SPECT.

18–E. PET systems generally require a cyclotron, which severely limits the availability of positron-emitting radionuclides.

19–B. ^{99}Mo breakthrough is a quality-control test performed on a technetium generator.

20–E. The system resolution is the square root of the sum of the squares of the resolutions of the individual components.

21–D. The counting time has no direct relationship with the gamma camera resolution.

22–E. The variance is the standard deviation squared (variance is σ^2). For NM images that are governed by Poisson statistics, $\sigma = N^{1/2}$, where N is the mean number of counts in a pixel.

23–C. A defective PMT tube can give rise to a cold spot artifact.

24–D. Patient doses should be lower for short lived radionuclides.

25–A. The half-life of ^{99m}Tc is 6 hours. The parent of ^{99m}Tc, ^{99}Mo, has a half-life of 67 hours.

26–D. The effective half-life must be equal or shorter than the physical half-life, depending on the rate of biological clearance.

27–C. The size of the organ has no effect on the computed value of cumulated activity.

28–E. Organ activity is important for determination of cumulated activity but does not affect the S factor per se.

29–E. Patient dose is determined by the amount of activity administered, and "imaging" time is irrelevant to patient dose.

30–E. Patient age has no direct bearing on the local radiation level.

10

Radiation Protection

I. Biological Basis

A. Introduction
- **Ionizing radiation** can induce detrimental biological effects in organs and tissues by depositing energy that may damage important molecules such as **DNA.**
- **Free radicals** are chemically reactive molecules with unpaired electrons that are produced by ionizing radiation and can damage tissue.
  - Chromosome breaks and aberrations are examples of biological damage caused by radiation.
- This deposited energy can break apart biologically important molecules such as DNA and cause cell function to be modified.
- Cells with higher oxygen content are generally more sensitive to radiation.
- The amount of biological damage produced depends on the total energy deposited in a cell or tissue (dose).
- Data on the detrimental effects of radiation come from studies on atomic bomb survivors, radiation workers, and radiation therapy patients.

B. Cellular radiation effects
- Human cells are either **germ cells,** which are involved in reproduction, or **somatic cells,** which make up the remaining organs and tissues.
  - Metabolic functions of cells occur in the cytoplasm.
  - Genetic information is found in the cell nucleus.
- Cell division of reproductive cells is called **meiosis.**
- **Mitosis** is the process of cell division in somatic cells.
  - The stages of somatic cell division include **prophase; metaphase,** which is the most radiosensitive phase; **anaphase; telophase,** and **interphase,** which is the resting stage.
- The **DNA** molecule carries the code needed for cell metabolism and is exactly duplicated when the cell divides.
- Radiation may induce a break in the DNA molecule, or it may damage a section of the DNA molecule, which could result in genetic or somatic damage.
  - A change in the genetic code (mutation) of a germ cell can affect future generations.
- At high doses, radiation can cause **cell death,** defined as the loss of reproductive capacity.
  - A plot of the surviving fraction of cells versus radiation dose is called a **cell survival curve.**
- The radiobiological **LD$_{50}$** is the lethal dose that will kill 50% of irradiated cells.

–Lymphoid tissue and rapidly proliferating tissues, such as spermatids and bone marrow stem cells, are relatively radiosensitive.

–Nerve cells are the least radiosensitive cells.

C. Linear energy transfer

–Radiation can cause damage to cells directly or, more commonly, indirectly by producing ions.

–**Linear energy transfer (LET)** represents the energy absorbed by the medium per unit length of travel (keV/μm).

–Uncharged radiation (photons and neutrons) **transfers energy** to the medium **via** photoelectrons (photons) and recoil protons (neutrons).

–**Photoelectrons** produced in tissue can produce hundreds of ion pairs.

–For a given medium, LET is proportional to the square of the particle charge and is inversely related to particle kinetic energy.

  –Low speed particles with multiple charges, such as slow-moving alpha particles, have the highest LET values.

–Neutrons, protons, alpha particles, and heavy ions are **high-LET** radiations, with values ranging from 3 to 200 keV/μm.

–Photons, gamma rays, electrons, and positrons are **low-LET** radiations, with values ranging from 0.2 to 3 keV/μm.

–High-LET radiations produce more biological damage than do low-LET radiations.

–When considering the biological effect of radiation, both the total amount of energy absorbed (i.e., dose) and the effectiveness of this radiation at causing biological damage (i.e., LET) must be considered.

–Radiobiologists use the term **relative biological effectiveness** to compare the ability of different types of radiations to cause biological damage.

  –Relative biological effectiveness is close to unity for low-LET radiation (1 keV/μm) and a maximum for radiations with an LET of about 100 keV/μm.

  –High-LET radiations can have relative biological effectiveness values three to eight times higher than that of x-rays.

D. Equivalent dose

–**Equivalent dose *(H)*** attempts to quantify the biological damage arising from the deposition of ionizing radiation in tissues by different types of radiation.

–Equivalent dose may also be referred to as the dose equivalent.

–The equivalent dose is the absorbed dose *(D)* multiplied by the radiation weighting factor (w_R) of the radiation, or $H = D \times w_R$.

–The radiation weighting factor is also referred to as the quality factor.

–The **radiation weighting factor** depends on the radiation LET value.

  –For low-LET radiation sources (e.g., electrons, x-rays, gamma rays), $w_R = 1$.

  –For high-LET radiation sources (e.g., alpha particles), w_R can be as high as 20.

–Equivalent dose is expressed as sieverts (Sv) in the SI system and as rems (*radia*tion *e*quivalent, *m*an) in non-SI units: **1 Sv = 100 rem; 1 rem = 10 mSv.**

–In diagnostic radiology and nuclear medicine, x-rays, gamma rays, and beta particles have low LET values, and the radiation weighting factor (w_R) equals one.

  –In this instance, exposure, absorbed dose, and equivalent dose are all approximately equal when using non-SI units **(1 R ~ 1 rad ~ 1 rem).**

–Although all three terms are often used interchangeably, they are conceptually different, as shown in **Fig. 10.1.**

–Equivalent dose is a parameter that is used primarily for radiation protection purposes.

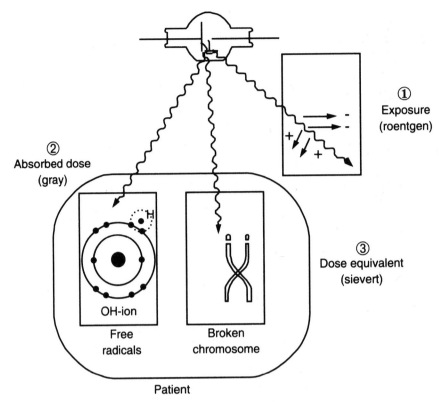

FIG. 10.1. *Exposure* is a source-related term that refers to the ability to ionize air as shown in the ionization chamber *(1)*. *Absorbed dose* refers to the radiation energy absorbed as shown at position *2*, where free radicals are being formed. *Equivalent dose* is used to quantify the biological damage resulting from ionizing radiation as shown at position *3*, where chromosome breaks have occurred.

E. Deterministic effects

–At high doses (i.e., doses above 0.5 Gy [50 rad]), radiation effects are called **deterministic** and are mainly a result of cell killing.

–Lymphocytes are the most radiosensitive cells in the blood, and decreased cell counts have been observed after doses of less than 1 Gy (100 rad).

–Deterministic effects are characterized by a **threshold dose,** below which the effect does not occur **(Fig. 10.2).**

–Deterministic effects include skin erythema (reddening), cataract induction, and induction of sterility.

–The severity of deterministic effects increases with dose.

  –Skin erythema can occur at a skin dose of 5 Gy (500 rad), whereas skin necrosis would be expected to occur at a skin dose of 30 Gy (3,000 rad).

–Cataract formation is dependent on the total dose and on the time over which this dose is delivered.

  –Cataracts can be induced at acute doses as low as 2 Gy (200 rad) and as soon as 6 months after exposure.

  –The threshold dose for chronic cataract induction is about 5 Gy (500 rad).

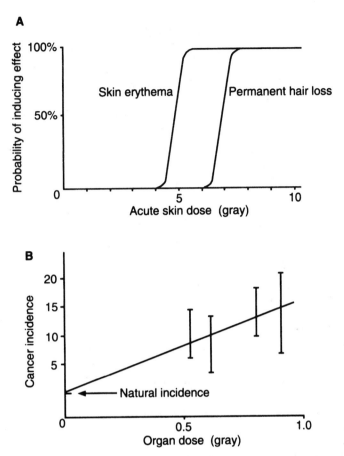

FIG. 10.2. Representative dose response curves for deterministic **(A)** and stochastic **(B)** effects.

–Sperm count can be decreased with 0.15 to 0.3 Gy (15 to 30 rad), but sterility requires 3 to 4 Gy (300 to 400 rad) in women and 5 to 6 Gy (500 to 600 rad) in men.
–**Table 10.1** lists approximate threshold doses for deterministic effects in humans.

F. Stochastic effects

–At low doses (i.e., doses below 0.5 Gy [50 rad]), the **stochastic effects** of **carcinogenesis** and **genetic damage** are of primary importance.
–**Stochastic** means random or probabilistic.

TABLE 10.1. *Threshold doses for deterministic radiation effects (acute exposure)*

Target organ	Dose	Results
Whole body	50–100 Gy (5,000–10,000 rad)	Death from cerebral edema (1–2 d)
Whole body	7–50 Gy (700–5,000 rad)	Death from gastrointestinal failure (3–4 d)
Whole body	2–7 Gy (200–700 rad)	Death from infection due to hematopoietic failure (4–6 wk)
Skin	~5 Gy (500 rad)	Erythema
Sperm cells	5–6 Gy (500–600 rad)	Permanent azospermia
Eye lens	~2 Gy (200 rad)	Cataract induction

–The severity of radiation-induced stochastic effects is *independent* of the radiation dose.

–The radiation dose affects only the *probability* of an occurrence of the stochastic effect.

–As dose increases, the chance of an occurrence of the stochastic effect increases.

–The existence of any threshold doses is controversial, and for radiation protection purposes, stochastic effects are assumed to have **no threshold (Fig. 10.2).**

–Stochastic risks depend on gender and age at exposure.

–Radiation protection is designed to minimize the radiation dose and, therefore, the corresponding stochastic radiation risk.

II. Radiation Risks

A. Radiation-induced cancers

–**Cancer induction** is the main risk of radiation exposure at doses normally encountered in radiology.

–Bone marrow, colon, lung, and stomach are the most susceptible to radiation-induced malignancy.

–The bladder, breast, liver, esophagus, and thyroid are moderately radiosensitive.

–Cancer risks from radiation exposure are generally higher for children than for adults.

–Radiation can induce both benign and malignant tumors.

–Cancer induction has a latency of 5 to 10 years for leukemia but is measured in decades for solid tumors.

–Radiation used to treat acne and tonsillitis has been linked to thyroid cancer.

–Radiation-induced thyroid cancer is more likely in children and women than in men.

–Evidence of the carcinogenic effects of radiation exposure has been observed in radium dial painters, uranium miners, and atomic bomb survivors.

B. Cancer risk estimates

–Radiation risks have been provided by the U.S. National Academy of Sciences Committee on the Biological Effects of Ionizing Radiation (BEIR).

–In 1990, the BEIR V Committee introduced a **linear response** paradigm **(Fig. 10.2).**

–Current radiation risks are based on a **relative risk model** for cancer induction, in which radiation increases the natural incidence of cancer by a constant fraction.

–Previously, an **absolute risk model** was used in which radiation induced a given (absolute) number of cancers in the exposed population.

–International Commission on Radiological Protection (ICRP) currently estimates the fatal cancer radiation risk at 4% per sievert (i.e., 0.04% per rem) for whole-body exposure of a working population.

–The radiation risk factor for the whole population, about 5% per sievert (0.05% per rem), is higher because it includes children, who are more sensitive to radiation.

–Radiation cancer risks are a factor of two higher if the doses are high compared with occupational exposure and are delivered at a high dose rate (acute exposure).

–Quantitative radiation risks from United Nations Scientific Committee on the Effects of Atomic Radiation (UNSCEAR) and BIER are similar to those of the ICRP.

C. Genetic risks

–Before 1950, **genetic effects** were considered the most important risk of radiation exposure.

–Genetic effects (i.e., effects on future generations because of chromosome muta-tions in germ cells) are the result of radiation exposure to the gonads.

–There is virtually no epidemiological evidence of the genetic effects of radiation in humans, and current risk estimates are based on animal experiments.

–Genetic effects depend on the demographics of the exposed populations, with older populations having lower risks than those of younger populations for the same ex-posure.

–For workers, the risk of severe hereditary effects is 0.8% per sievert (i.e., 0.008% per rem) of gonadal radiation according to the ICRP.

–For a whole population, the risk of severe hereditary effects is 1.3% per sievert (0.013% per rem), which is higher because of the inclusion of children.

D. Fetal risks

–The **fetal risk** when exposing pregnant women depends on the gestation period.

–The most likely result of a major radiation exposure during the first 10 days after conception is early intrauterine death.

–The fetus is most vulnerable to radiation-induced congenital abnormalities during the first trimester, specifically, 20 to 40 days after conception.

  –Radiation-induced microcephaly is the most likely abnormality, occurring at 50 to 70 days after conception

  –Growth and mental retardation occur at 70 to 150 days after conception.

  –The greatest effect after 150 days after conception is an increased risk of child-hood malignancies.

–Risks of congenital abnormalities are negligible below 10 mGy (1 rad).

–For doses up to 0.1 Gy (10 rad), any radiation risks are deemed to be low when com-pared with the normal risks of pregnancy.

  –In the United States, a congenital abnormality occurs in approximately 5% of live births, which makes the impact of medical x-rays difficult to evaluate.

–At doses greater than 0.1 Gy (10 rad), the risk of congenital malformation increases.

  –An abortion to avoid the possibility of radiation-induced congenital anomalies is considered only when doses exceed 0.1 Gy (10 rad).

–For a dose of 10 mGy (1 rad) in the second or third trimester of gestation, the risk of childhood leukemia may be increased by as much as 40%.

  –Childhood leukemia is a relatively rare disease, and therefore the absolute risk of radiation induced childhood leukemia is low.

III. Dose Limits

A. Radiation protection organizations

–The **ICRP** was founded in 1928 and issues periodic recommendations on radiation protection.

–**ICRP** Publication 60 (1990) is the latest publication from the ICRP that provides recommendations for radiation workers and members of the public.

–The **International Commission on Radiological Units and Measurements (ICRU)** advises on issues such as measurement units in radiology.

–In the United States, the foremost radiation protection body is the **National Com-mittee on Radiological Protection and Measurements (NCRP).**

–The **NCRP** advises federal and state regulators on radiation protection.

–The **Nuclear Regulatory Commission (NRC)** is responsible for the rules and reg-ulations regarding nuclear materials.

–Some states are known as **agreement states** and arrange with the NRC to self-regulate medically related licensing and inspection requirements for nuclear materials.
–Other states (i.e., nonagreement states) are regulated directly by the NRC.
–Each state is responsible for regulations pertaining to x-ray imaging equipment.
–States coordinate their x-ray protection activities through the **Conference of Radiation Control Program Directors (CRCPD),** which meets annually.

B. Occupational exposure

–Important goals of radiation protection are the prevention of the occurrence of deterministic effects and minimizing stochastic effects of radiation.
–Dose limits can refer to individual organs or to uniform whole-body irradiation.
  –Individual organ dose limits include doses to the eye lens, extremities, and other tissues.
–**Controlled areas** have significant dose equivalent exposure rates and must be supervised by a **radiation safety officer.**
–**Table 10.2** summarizes recommended dose limits for occupational exposure as outlined in ICRP Publication 60 (1990).
–In the United States, the legal (regulatory) **whole-body dose limit for radiation workers** is currently 50 mSv/year **(5 rem/year).**
  –The U.S. dose limit for workers is likely to be reduced in the future to the 20 mSv/year (2 rem/year), as recommended by the ICRP and NCRP.
–**Occupational dose limits** exclude exposures from medical procedures and natural background.
  –People who are occupationally exposed to radiation should be monitored using personnel dosimeters, such as film badges.
–Actual exposures to radiology department staff are relatively low.
  –The typical annual effective dose equivalent exposures are approximately 0.2 mSv (20 mrem) for x-ray technologists.
  –Annual doses to radiation therapy technologists are about 1.5 mSv (150 mrem) and to nuclear medicine technologists are about 2 mSv (200 mrem).
–Doses to the most highly exposed radiation workers (interventional radiologists and nuclear power operators) are unlikely to exceed 5 mSv/year (500 mrem/year).

C. Pregnant workers

–For radiation protection purposes, the fetus is normally considered to be a member of the public by the ICRP.
–In the United States, however, the dose limit for the fetus of a radiation worker (5 mSv) is higher than that of member of the public (1 mSv).
  –This higher fetus legal dose limit permits women of reproductive capacity to seek employment as radiation workers (e.g., nuclear medicine technologists).

TABLE 10.2. *Recommended International Commission on Radiological Protection dose limits for workers (1991)*

Parameter	Dose limit
Whole body	20 mSv/yr (2 rem/yr)
Lens of the eye	150 mSv/yr (15 rem/yr)
Extremities (hands)	500 mSv/yr (50 rem/yr)
Lifetime whole body	<0.8 Sv (<80 rem)
Fetus (9 mo)	1 mSv (100 mrem)

–Setting the fetal dose limit at 1 mSv would have deprived women of reproductive capacity employment as radiation workers.
–The fetus of a radiation worker should not exceed a dose of 0.5 mSv/month (50 mrem/month).
  –The limitation on the rate at which the fetus is exposed helps ensure that any radiation risks to the fetus is kept to a minimum.
–Pregnant radiation workers are monitored by a dosimeter worn on the abdomen to ensure fetal dose limits are not exceeded.
  –The dose to the fetus is normally taken to be half the skin dose to account for attenuation by soft tissues between the fetus and skin surface.

D. Nonoccupational exposure

–Dose limits to members of the public exclude natural background radiation and all medical exposures.
–Dose limits for members of the **public** are generally much lower than those for occupational exposure.
–ICRP Publication 60 (1990) recommends a whole-body dose limit for members of the public of 1 mSv/year (100 mrem/year).
–In the United States, the regulatory dose limit for members of the public is currently 1 mSv/year **(100 mrem/year).**
–X-ray facilities must be designed to ensure that exposure to members of the public does not exceed 1 mSv/year (100 mrem/year).
  –Facilities may be designed to result in even lower doses to members of the public who may be exposed to multiple sources of radiation.
–The public generally receives negligible doses from radiological activities.

IV. Protection Methods

A. Patient protection

–Patient doses should be minimized whenever possible and the **ALARA** (*as low as reasonably achievable*) principle should always be followed.
–Careful attention to close collimation reduces the exposed area, minimizing patient risk.
–Gonadal shielding should be used if the patient is of reproductive age, if the gonads lie in or near the primary beam, and if the shield does not interfere with the examination.
  –For example, a gonadal shield can usually be used for a unilateral hip examination.
–Patient exposure is proportional to mAs and tube voltage squared.
–A short focus-to-skin distance increases the patient entrance skin dose, because the patient exposure is inversely related to the square of the distance from the focal spot.
  –The skin-focus distance should always be greater than 38 cm in fluoroscopy.
–Correct phototiming of exposures prevents overexposure of films and eliminates the need to perform repeated films.
–Interventional neurological and cardiac procedures requiring long fluoroscopy times (hours), and large numbers of film may induce deterministic effects such as epilation.
–In nuclear medicine, it is important that the activity being administered to the patient is verified using a dose calibrator.

B. Operator shielding

–Lead is an effective protective barrier (i.e., it has a high attenuation coefficient) because of its high density and high atomic number.

–Lead aprons used in diagnostic radiology should have 0.25 or 0.5 mm equivalents of lead.

–A 0.5 mm lead apron reduces radiation exposure by at least a factor of 10.

–Individual organs not protected by lead aprons, such as the eye lens or thyroid, can receive much higher doses during fluoroscopy.

–Leaded glass can significantly reduce the dose to the eye.

–Leaded glasses should be used by operators performing interventional radiology.

–A neck shield can significantly reduce the dose to the thyroid.

–Protective gloves should have a lead equivalence of 0.25 mm.

C. Room design

–The design of radiation facilities should always incorporate the **ALARA** principle.

–Design of barriers in radiology departments depends on factors such as **workload** (W), which is how often the machine is in operation (mA-minute/week).

–Room shielding also depends on the **use factor** and **occupancy factor.**

　–The **use factor** (U) is the fraction of time that radiation points in a specified direction).

　–The **occupancy factor** (T) is fraction of time people work on the other side of the barrier.

–The source-to-barrier distance also affects the amount of x-ray shielding required.

–The design of shielding must also take into account the **exposure output** mGy/mAs for primary, scattered, and leakage radiation **(Fig. 10.3).**

–A primary protective barrier absorbs primary radiation.

–A secondary barrier protects workers from scattered radiation.

–For primary barriers, the use factor is one for the floor, $\frac{1}{16}$ for the walls, and zero for the ceiling.

–Occupancy factors are generally one for offices and laboratories, $\frac{1}{4}$ for corridors and restrooms, and $\frac{1}{16}$ for waiting rooms and outside areas used by pedestrians.

–In practice, the shielding used for most x-ray installations is 1.6 mm ($\frac{1}{16}$ inch) of lead in the walls.

–In designing x-ray facilities, there should be no gaps between doors.

–Shielding is normally required to extend at least 2 m from the floor.

D. Protection in radiology

–Methods of controlling radiation exposure are decreasing exposure time, increasing distance from the radiation source, and using appropriate shielding **(Fig. 10.4).**

–Because both primary and scattered radiation fall off as the inverse square of the distance, doubling the distance reduces the exposure level by a factor of four.

–As a general rule, the **scatter dose** level from patients at 1 m is approximately 0.1% of the entrance skin dose.

　–**Table 10.3** illustrates the scatter radiation exposures for common radiological examinations.

　–**Leakage radiation** from the tube housing should be less than 1 mGy/hour (0.1 R/hour) at a distance of 1 m.

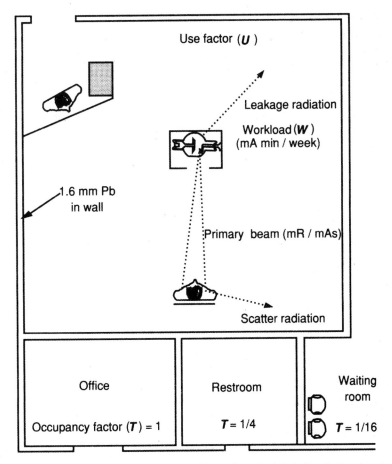

FIG. 10.3. Room shielding needs are calculated based on the intensity of primary, scatter, and leakage radiation.

–During fluoroscopy, workers should not be in the room if not necessary.

–Radiation workers should never hold a patient for a study.

  –A parent or relative should be instructed to position the patient and should be given a lead apron to wear.

–When performing portable examinations, the operator should stand at least 2 m away from the patient.

E. Protection in nuclear medicine

  –Most hospitals have a **radiation safety committee** that is responsible for radiation protection in nuclear medicine departments.

TABLE 10.3. *Representative scatter radiation exposure levels in radiology*

Examination	Exposure (at 1 m)
Posterior-anterior chest x-ray	0.1 μGy (10 μR)
Lateral skull x-ray	1.5 μGy (150 μR)
Anterior-posterior abdominal x-ray	3 μGy (300 μR)
Computed tomography examination	20–40 μGy (2,000–4,000 μR)
Fluoroscopy	10–30 μGy/min (1,000–3,000 μR/min)

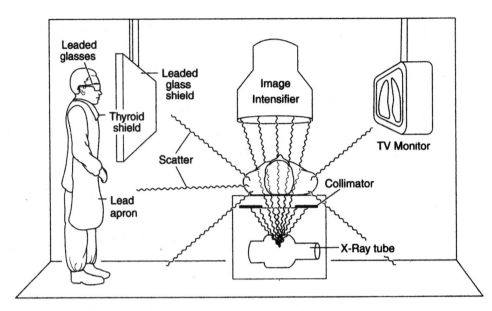

FIG. 10.4. Radiation protection aspects of fluoroscopy. Minimizing the fluoroscopy time, increasing the distance from the patient, and using protective shielding reduce the operator dose.

–**Contamination** is uncontained radioactive material where it is not wanted.

–Protective clothing and handling precautions are required to minimize contamination.

–Volatile radionuclides (^{131}I and ^{133}Xe) should be stored in fume hoods.

–Personnel should wear gloves when handling radionuclides and should dispose of them in radioactive waste receptors after use.

–Effectiveness of contamination control is monitored using Geiger-Mueller survey meters.

–Wipe tests should be performed of radionuclide use areas where a small piece of filter paper is wiped on an area and checked in a NaI gamma well counter.

–In nuclear medicine, patients are "walking sources" of radiation, which result in operator doses that are generally higher than in diagnostic radiology.

–**Table 10.4** shows the exposure rates from commonly used radionuclides.

–Nuclear medicine workers should undergo bioassay, such as thyroid monitoring, for uptakes of iodine radionuclides.

–Disposal of radioactive waste in nuclear medicine is facilitated by the relatively short half-lives of most radionuclides.

–Radioactive waste can be stored for 10 half-lives before being surveyed and disposed of as regular waste.

TABLE 10.4. *Approximate exposure rates from patients administered 370 mBq (10 mCi) of specified radionuclide for a nuclear medicine procedure*

Procedure	Radionuclide	Exposure rate (at 1 m)
Liver spleen (sulfur colloid)	^{99m}Tc	5 μGy/hr (0.5 mR/hr)
Myocardial perfusion	^{201}Tl	3 μGy/hr (0.3 mR/hr)
Infection	^{67}Ga	10 μGy/hr (1 mR/hr)
Tumor staging (FDG)	^{18}F	50 μGy/hr (5 mR/hr)
Thyroid cancer therapy	^{131}I	20 μGy/hr (2 mR/hr)

–Limited amounts of radionuclides can also be disposed of via the sink if the material is water soluble and the amount of radioactivity does not exceed regulatory limits.

V. Population Doses

A. Natural background radiation

–A useful benchmark for comparing radiation exposure is **natural background radiation,** which in the United States is approximately 3 mSv/year (300 mrem/year).

–**Table 10.5** lists the contributions to natural background from cosmic radiation, terrestrial radioactivity, and radionuclides incorporated in the body.

–Cosmic rays are energetic protons and alpha particles (10^{10} to 10^{19} eV), which originate in galaxies.

  –Most cosmic rays interact with the atmosphere, with fewer than 0.05% reaching sea level.

  –Because exposure to cosmic rays increases with elevation, a transcontinental flight in the United States results in a dose of approximately 20 μSv (2 mrem), a transatlantic flight results in 30 to 50 μSv (3 to 5 mrem), and space travel results in approximately 10 μSv/hour (1 mrem/hour).

–Natural background radiation varies with location; in Leadville, Colorado, an additional 0.9 mSv/year (90 mrem/year) is attributed to higher cosmic radiation (3,000 m elevation).

  –Leadville also has elevated levels of terrestrial radioactivity, which results in an additional dose of approximately 0.7 mSv/year (70 mrem/year).

B. Radon

–The biggest contribution to natural background is from domestic **radon.**

–Radon (^{222}Rn) is a radioactive gas formed during the decay of radium.

–Radium (^{226}Ra) is a decay product of uranium found in the soil and has a half-life of 1620 years.

–Radon is an alpha emitter, which has a half-life of approximately 4 days.

–The progeny of radon are also radioactive and include two short-lived beta emitters and two short-lived alpha emitters.

–Radon daughters attach to aerosols and are deposited in the lungs, thereby permitting the bronchial mucosa to be irradiated and inducing **bronchogenic cancer.**

–The average concentration of radon outdoors is 4 to 8 Bq/m^3 (0.1 to 0.2 pCi/L); indoors, the average is 40 Bq/m^3 (1 pCi/L).

–Remedial action is recommended at levels in excess of 160 Bq/m^3 (4 pCi/L).

–Average annual doses from radon are about 2 mSv/year.

C. Population medical doses

–Approximately 300 million diagnostic medical procedures (x-ray, nuclear medicine, and dental) are performed in the United States each year.

TABLE 10.5. *Typical annual background radiation exposure in the United States*

Radiation source	Exposure
Radon	2.0 mSv/yr (200 mrem/yr)
Cosmic rays	0.3 mSv/yr (30 mrem/yr)
External (gamma rays)	0.3 mSv/yr (30 mrem yr)
Internal (e.g., ^{40}K, ^{14}C)	0.4 mSv/yr (40 mrem/yr)

–The effective dose from the x-ray studies averaged over the population (*per caput* dose) each year is approximately 1 mSv (100 mrem).

–The *per caput* dose from nuclear medicine examinations each year is about 0.14 mSv (14 mrem).

–Diagnostic procedures using ionizing radiation are the highest source of manmade radiation exposure.

–The **highest contributor to medical exposure is computed tomography (CT),** which is a relatively high-dose procedure the use of which has grown substantially in the past two decades.

–In the United Kingdom in the 1990s, CT was estimated to account for 4% of all radiological examinations but accounted for 40% of the collective medical dose.

–In U.S. hospitals in 2000, CT was estimated to account for 10% of radiological examinations but accounted for two thirds of the collective medical dose.

–Doses from CT are likely to increase with the advent of multislice CT.

D. Manmade exposure (nonmedical)

–The total annual radiation exposure in North America is about 3.6 mSv, with most of this arising from natural background and medical radiation.

–Public radiation exposure from consumer products accounts for 3% of the total exposure of the North American population to radiation.

–Major sources of exposure from consumer products are building materials and the water supply.

–Other sources of exposure from consumer products include luminous watches, airport inspection systems, and smoke detectors.

–Additional sources of radiation exposure include occupational exposure (0.3%) and fallout from atmospheric weapons testing in the 1950s (less than 0.3%).

–The nuclear fuel cycle contributes about 0.1% of the annual radiation exposure to inhabitants of the United States.

Review Test

1. Radiobiological LD_{50} is the radiation dose that kills:

(A) 50% of exposed cells
(B) 50 exposed cells
(C) All exposed cells within 50 days
(D) e^{-50} of exposed cells
(E) e/50 of exposed cells

2. The cell division stage most sensitive to radiation is:

(A) Prophase
(B) Metaphase
(C) Anaphase
(D) Telophase
(E) Interphase

3. Which cells are considered to be the least radiosensitive?

(A) Bone marrow cells
(B) Neuronal cells
(C) Lymphoid tissues
(D) Spermatids
(E) Skin cells

4. Which is not true of the interaction of ionizing radiation with tissues?

(A) Indirect action causes most of the biological damage.
(B) Ions can dissociate into free radicals.
(C) Cellular DNA is a key target.
(D) It can produce chromosome aberrations.
(E) Direct action is more frequent than indirect action.

5. The LET of x-rays is:

(A) Greater than the LET for alpha particles
(B) Between 0.3 and 3 keV/μm
(C) Independent of relative biological effectiveness
(D) Cannot be defined for energies greater than 2 MeV
(E) Low energy threshold

6. The radiation weighting factor (w_R) is:

(A) Used to convert sievert to gray
(B) Independent of the particle mass
(C) Independent of the particle charge
(D) Increased for high-LET radiation
(E) Increased for sensitive organs

7. Equivalent dose is greater than absorbed dose for:

(A) X-rays
(B) Gamma rays
(C) Electrons
(D) Neutrons
(E) Positrons

8. An x-ray exposure of 1 mGy (100 mR) results in all of the following except:

(A) Absorbed dose of 1 mGy (100 mrad) in tissue
(B) Absorbed dose of 4 mGy (400 mrad) in bone
(C) Equivalent dose of 1 mSv (100 mrem) in tissue
(D) Equivalent dose of 1 mSv (100 mrem) in bone
(E) Negligible cell killing

9. The absorbed radiation dose to induce cataracts is not:

(A) 2 Gy (200 rad) for acute exposure
(B) 5 Gy (500 rad) for chronic exposure
(C) Lower for neutrons than for x-rays
(D) The same for x-rays and gamma rays
(E) Sex dependent

10. Stochastic effects of radiation:

(A) Include carcinogenesis
(B) Have a threshold of 50 mSv/year
(C) Have a dose-dependent severity
(D) Involve cell killing
(E) Can be recognized as caused by radiation

11. Which of the following studies have *not* shown evidence of radiation-induced cancers?

(A) Radiation therapy
(B) Chest fluoroscopy for tuberculosis
(C) Radium dial painters
(D) Diagnostic nuclear medicine scans
(E) Atomic bomb survivors in Hiroshima

12. Radiation-induced thyroid neoplasms include all of the following except:

(A) Can be malignant or benign
(B) Are more common in women
(C) Are more common in children
(D) Have a long latent period
(E) Are generally fatal

13. Which of the following does *not* concern itself with radiation risk estimates?

(A) ICRP
(B) UNSCEAR

(C) BEIR
(D) ICRU
(E) NCRP

14. Which group of irradiated individuals has demonstrated genetic effects of radiation?

(A) Atomic bomb survivors
(B) Cancer radiotherapy patients
(C) Uranium miners
(D) Thyroid treatment (^{131}I) patients
(E) No human group

15. When is gross malformation most likely to occur?

(A) Preimplantation
(B) Early organogenesis
(C) Late organogenesis
(D) Early fetal period
(E) Late fetal period

16. What "threshold" embryo/fetal dose corresponds to a radiation risk smaller than those normally encountered during pregnancy?

(A) Less than 10 mGy (1 rad)
(B) 10 mGy (1 rad)
(C) 30 mGy (3 rad)
(D) 100 mGy (10 rad)
(E) More than 100 mGy (10 rad)

17. An "agreement" state regulates:

(A) Patient CT doses
(B) Leakage radiation
(C) X-ray beam HVL
(D) Nuclear medicine activities
(E) Room shielding

18. NCRP protection standards are based on all the following except that:

(A) The ALARA principle should be used
(B) There are no risks below certain radiation levels
(C) Unnecessary exposures are not permitted
(D) The major health risk is carcinogenesis
(E) Deterministic effects should be prevented

19. By law, the fetus of an x-ray technologist should receive:

(A) No occupational radiation exposure
(B) Less than 50 mSv (5 rem)
(C) Only low-LET radiation exposure
(D) No exposure during weeks 7 to 15
(E) No more than 0.5 mSv (50 mrem) per month

20. The regulatory dose limit for a patient having an x-ray is:

(A) 1 mSv (100 mrem)
(B) 5 mSv (500 mrem)

(C) 20 mSv (2 rem)
(D) 50 mSv (5 rem)
(E) Not limited

21. According to the ALARA concept, annual doses to x-ray technologists should be:

(A) Zero
(B) 1 mSv (100 mrem)
(C) 5 mSv (500 mrem)
(D) 50 mSv (5 rem)
(E) As low as possible

22. One meter away from a CT scanner, the total exposure during a patient examination might be:

(A) 30 μGy (3 mR)
(B) 300 μGy (30 mR)
(C) 3 mGy (300 mR)
(D) 30 mGy (3 R)
(E) Zero

23. A lead apron attenuates 95%; transmission through two lead aprons would be approximately:

(A) 0.25%
(B) 0.5%
(C) 1.0%
(D) 1.25%
(E) 2.5%

24. Which of the following is *not* required to estimate room-shielding needs?

(A) Workload
(B) Use factor
(C) Occupancy factor
(D) Anode angle
(E) X-ray tube output

25. Which would be most effective at reducing the dose level outside an x-ray room?

(A) Adding a HVL of lead
(B) Halving the work load
(C) Doubling the distance to the x-ray source
(D) Halving the use factor
(E) Halving the occupancy factor

26. The radiation shielding of most current x-ray rooms is:

(A) 3 mm Al
(B) 3 mm concrete
(C) 0.3 mm lead
(D) 1.6 mm lead
(E) 5 mm lead

27. The average background annual radiation exposure in the U.S. is:

(A) Less than 1 mSv (100 mrem)
(B) About 1 mSv (100 mrem)

(C) About 3 mSv (300 mrem)
(D) About 5 mSv (500 mrem)
(E) More than 5 mSv (500 mrem)

28. Which of the following contributes the least to annual radiation exposure in the U.S.?

(A) Radon gas
(B) Domestic televisions and computer video display units
(C) Cosmic background
(D) Internal radio nuclides such as ^{40}K
(E) Nuclear weapons testing fallout

29. The largest exposure to the U.S. population is the result of:

(A) Nuclear power production
(B) Test bomb fallout
(C) Diagnostic x-rays
(D) Nuclear medicine
(E) Indoor radon

30. Which imaging modality results in the highest collective medical dose?

(A) Chest x-rays
(B) Fluoroscopy
(C) Interventional radiology
(D) Mammography
(E) CT

Answers and Explanations

1–A. LD$_{50}$ will kill 50% of the exposed cells.

2–B. The metaphase is most radiosensitive.

3–B. Cells that are continually proliferating are the most radiosensitive, so neuronal cells, which do not proliferate, are the least radiosensitive.

4–E. Indirect action is more important, in which deposited energy produces free radicals that go on to produce damaged DNA.

5–B. The LET for x-rays is in the range of 0.3 to 3 keV/μm.

6–D. w_R increases with increasing LET and is used to multiply the absorbed dose to obtain the equivalent dose.

7–D. Neutrons, because they have a w_R of 20.

8–D. For an exposure of 1 mGy (100 mR), the equivalent dose in bone will be 4 mSv (400 mrem) because the absorbed dose in bone will be 4 mGy (f factor for bone is 4).

9–E. Male and female cataract risks are the same.

10–A. Stochastic (random) effects, including carcinogenesis and genetic damage, are the most significant risks encountered in diagnostic radiology.

11–D. There is no evidence that diagnostic tests in nuclear medicine have resulted in higher levels of cancer incidence.

12–E. Only 5% of thyroid cancers are normally fatal.

13–D. The ICRU is primarily concerned with the measurement of radiation.

14–E. There are no human data showing statistically significant genetic effects radiation.

15–B. Early organogenesis is the most sensitive period of embryonic development, when high doses of radiation (i.e., over 100 mGy) could result in gross malformation.

16–D. Note that there is no implication of doses less than 100 mGy being absolutely safe, only that any theoretical risk to the fetus is relatively small. (In practice, for doses below 100 mGy, one would never even consider the issue of any "therapeutic abortion.")

17–D. "Agreement" states have regulations for nuclear materials that are at least as stringent as those of the NRC.

18–B. NCRP assumes a linear dose response curve with no threshold dose for induction of detrimental effects.

19–E. A fetus of a radiation worker is subject to a total dose limit of 5 mSv (500 mrem), with no more than 0.5 mSv (50 mrem) in any month.

20–E. There are no regulatory dose limits for diagnostic radiologic examinations (the benefit to the patient is expected to much greater than any estimated radiation risk, as assessed by the radiologist in charge of the examination).

21–E. The principle is as low as reasonably achievable, which means that doses should be minimized but always below the occupational dose limit.

22–A. 30 μGy (3 mR) because the scattered radiation dose can be taken to be about 0.1% and the typical entrance skin exposure in CT is 30 mGy (3 R).

23–A. Because 5% (one twentieth) gets through the first barrier, and one twentieth of this gets through the second barrier, this corresponds to a transmission fraction of 1/400, or 0.25%.

24–D. The anode angle is irrelevant for estimating room shielding requirements.

25–C. Doubling the distance from a source will reduce the exposure by a factor of four, whereas all the other options would reduce the dose by a factor of two.

26–D. 1.6 mm or $\frac{1}{16}$ mm lead is used in virtually all diagnostic x-ray rooms.

27–C. Annual exposure of North Americans from natural background is 3 mSv, with two thirds from radon.

28–B. Radiation exposure from domestic televisions and computer video display units is negligible.

29–E. Average value of the effective dose from radon is about 2 mSv/year (200 mrem/year).

30–E. CT is by far the largest contributor to the collective dose from medical exposures and will continue to grow in importance for the foreseeable future.

11

Ultrasound

I. Basic Physics

A. Ultrasound waves

–**Sound waves** are a mechanical disturbance that propagate through a medium.
–**Wavelength (λ)** is the distance between successive wave crests.
–**Frequency (f)** is the number of oscillations per second measured in hertz.
 –**Hertz (Hz)** is 1 cycle/second.
–The **period** is the time between oscillations, or $1/f$.
–For sound waves, the relation between velocity *(v)*, measured in m/second, frequency, and wavelength is $v = f \times \lambda$ (m/second).
–Audible sound has frequencies ranging from 15 to 20,000 Hz.
–Ultrasound frequencies are higher than audible sound and are greater than 20 kHz.
–**Diagnostic ultrasound** uses **transducers** with frequencies ranging from 1 to 20 MHz (1 MHz = 10^6 Hz).
–Ultrasound waves are transmitted through tissue as **longitudinal waves** of alternating compression and rarefaction.
–Ultrasound waves may be **reflected, refracted, scattered,** or **absorbed.**
–Reflected ultrasound echoes allow images to be generated.

B. Velocity

–The **velocity** of sound is dependent on the nature of the medium through which it is traveling and is **independent of frequency.**
–Because velocity is constant, increases in frequency result in decreases in wavelength and vice versa $(v = f \times \lambda)$.
–Velocity is inversely proportional to compressibility. The less compressible the medium, the greater the velocity.
 –Sound travels fastest in solids and slowest in gases.
 –The **average velocity** of sound in soft tissue is **1,540 m/second,** with much higher values in bone and metal and much lower values in lung and air.
–**Table 11.1** lists ultrasound velocities for various media.

C. Acoustic impedance

–The **acoustic impedance (Z)** of a material is the product of the density (ρ) and the velocity of sound in the medium: $Z = \rho \times v$.
–The acoustic impedance unit is called the **Rayl,** the units of which are kg/m^2/second.
–Acoustic impedance is independent of frequency in the diagnostic range.
–Air and lung media have low values of acoustic impedance, whereas bone and metal have high values.

TABLE 11.1. *Ultrasound properties*

Material	Velocity (m/sec)	Attenuation coefficient (dB/cm at 1 MHz)	Acoustic impedance $(kg/m^2/sec \times 10^6)$
Air	330	12.0	0.0004
Fat	1,450	0.63	1.38
Blood	1,570	0.18	1.61
Muscle	1,585	3.3	1.70
Bone	3,300	20.0	7.8
Metals	>4,000	<0.02	>30.0

–**Table 11.1** lists acoustic impedance values for various media.
  –Most tissues have acoustic impedance values of about 1.6×10^6 kg/m²/second (Rayl).
–The differences between acoustic impedance values at an interface determines the amount of energy reflected at the interface.

D. Sound intensity

–The **amplitude** of a wave is the **size** of the wave displacement.
–Larger amplitudes of vibration produce denser compression bands and, hence, higher intensities of sound.
–Ultrasound beam **intensity (I)** is a measure of the energy associated with the beam and is proportional to the square of the amplitude.
–Ultrasonic intensities are normally expressed in terms of **milliwatts per square centimeter (mW/cm²).**
–The intensity of a beam may be averaged over the transducer area and over long time periods (many pulses) as a crude measure of ultrasound beam strength.
–The **temporal peak intensity** (I_{TP}) is the highest instantaneous intensity in the beam.
–**Temporal average intensity** (I_{TA}) is the time average intensity.
–I_{TA} is 1,000 times lower than I_{TP} for pulses that are 1,000 times shorter than the repetition frequency.
–The **spatial peak intensity** (I_{SP}) is the highest intensity spatially in the beam.
–**Spatial average intensity** (I_{SA}) is the average intensity over the beam, normally taken to be equal to the transducer area.
–I_{SA} is generally less than I_{SP}.
–The spatial peak and temporal average intensity value (I_{SPTA}) is the highest intensity spatially, and time averaged.
–I_{SPTA} is a good indicator of thermal effects of ultrasound, and is generally less than 100 mW/cm² for ultrasound imaging.
–For some Doppler applications, I_{SPTA} can exceed 1,000 mW/cm².

E. Decibels

–**Relative sound intensity** is measured on a logarithmic scale and may be expressed in bels (B) or **decibels (dB),** where 1 B = 10 dB.
–Relative intensity in decibels is equal to $10 \times \log_{10}(I/I_0)$, where I_0 is the original intensity, and I is the measured intensity.
–Negative decibel values correspond to signal attenuation, and positive values correspond to signal amplification.
–Intensity reduced to 50% is −3 dB; to 10% is −10 dB; to 1% is −20 dB, and to 0.1% is −30 dB.

–A change of $+3$ dB corresponds to a two-fold increase in intensity, $+10$ dB to a 10-fold increase, $+20$ dB to a 100-fold increase, and so on.

II. Interaction with Matter

A. Attenuation

–**Attenuation** is a composite effect of loss by scatter and absorption.

–Attenuation generally **increases with frequency.**

–Because of its high frequency, ultrasound is attenuated more readily than audible sound.

–The attenuation of ultrasound in a homogeneous tissue is exponential.

  –In soft tissues, there is a nearly linear relation between the frequency and attenuation (in dB/cm) of ultrasound.

–At 1 MHz, attenuation in soft tissue is approximately 1 dB/cm.

  –At 5 MHz, attenuation in soft tissue is approximately 5 dB/cm; at 10 MHz, attenuation is approximately 10 dB/cm.

  –For water and bone media, attenuation (in dB/cm) increases approximately as frequency squared.

–The absorbed sound wave energy is converted into **heat.**

–Little absorption and almost no scatter or reflection occur in fluids.

–**Table 11.1** lists ultrasound attenuation coefficients for a range of media.

B. Reflection angle and intensity

–A portion of the ultrasound beam is reflected at tissue interfaces **(Fig. 11.1).**

  –The sound reflected back toward the source is called an **echo** and is used to generate the ultrasound image.

–The percentage of ultrasound intensity reflected depends in part on the **angle of incidence** of the beam.

–Angles of incidence and reflection are equal as shown in **Fig. 11.1,** similar to the reflection of light.

–As the angle of incidence increases, reflected sound is less likely to reach the transducer.

  –No reflection is generally detected by the transducer if the beam strikes the tissue surface at angles greater than about 3 degrees perpendicular to the interface.

–**Specular reflections** occur from large smooth surfaces and are the major contributors to ultrasound images.

–**Nonspecular reflections** are diffuse scatter from "rough" surfaces where the irregular contours are bigger than the ultrasound wavelength.

–The percentage (intensity) of ultrasound reflected also depends on the **acoustic impedance** of the tissues.

–At normal incidence (90 degrees), the fractional amount of ultrasound intensity **reflected** is $[(Z_2 - Z_1)/(Z_2 + Z_1)]^2$ **(Fig. 11.1).**

–Because the amount transmitted and the amount reflected must always equal 1, the amount **transmitted** is $(4Z_1 \times Z_2)/(Z_1 + Z_2)^2$.

  –From chest wall ($Z = 1.7$) to lung ($Z = 0.0004$), the intensity reflected is 99.9% and transmitted is 0.1%.

  –From kidney ($Z = 1.62$) to fat ($Z = 1.38$), the intensity reflected is 0.64% and transmitted is 99.36%.

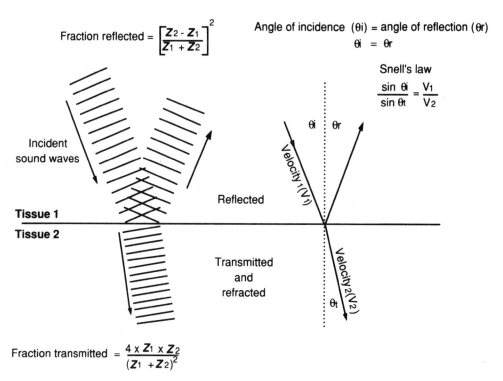

$$\text{Fraction reflected} = \left[\frac{Z_2 - Z_1}{Z_1 + Z_2}\right]^2$$

Angle of incidence (θi) = angle of reflection (θr)

$$\theta i = \theta r$$

Snell's law

$$\frac{\sin \theta i}{\sin \theta t} = \frac{V_1}{V_2}$$

Incident sound waves

Tissue 1

Tissue 2

Reflected

Transmitted and refracted

$$\text{Fraction transmitted} = \frac{4 \times Z_1 \times Z_2}{(Z_1 + Z_2)^2}$$

FIG. 11.1. Reflection and refraction of sound waves.

–**Table 11.2** lists values of reflected intensities for a range of interfaces encountered in diagnostic ultrasound.

C. Tissue reflections

–Air-tissue interfaces reflect virtually the entire incident ultrasound beam.

–Gel is applied between the transducer and skin to displace the air and minimize large reflections that would interfere with ultrasound transmission into the patient.

–Bone-tissue interfaces also reflect substantial fractions of the incident intensity.

–Imaging through air or bone is generally not possible.

–The lack of transmissions beyond these interfaces results in an area void of echoes called **shadowing.**

–In imaging the abdomen, the strongest echoes are likely to arise from gas bubbles.

–Organs such as the kidney, pancreas, spleen, and liver are composed of complex tissue structures that contain many scattering sites.

–Complex tissues result in a speckled texture on ultrasound images.

–Fluids, such as the bladder, blood vessels, and cysts have no internal structure and almost no echoes (i.e., show black).

TABLE 11.2. *Energy reflected from an ultrasound beam perpendicular to tissue interface (%)*

	Muscle	Liver	Bone
Fat	1.1	0.8	49
Muscle	—	0.02	41
Liver	0.02	—	42

–Contrast agents for vascular and perfusion imaging are encapsulated microbubbles (3 to 6 μm) containing air, nitrogen, or insoluble gases (perfluorocarbons).

–The small size of the microbubbles permits perfusion of tissues.

–Ultrasound signals (reflections) are generated by the large difference in acoustic impedance between the gas and surrounding fluids/tissues.

D. Refraction

–**Refraction** is the change in direction of an ultrasound beam when it passes from one medium to another with a different acoustic velocity as shown in **Fig. 11.1.**

–When ultrasound passes from one medium to another, the frequency remains the same but the wavelength changes.

–The change of wavelength occurs to accommodate the new velocity of sound in the second medium and shortens when the velocity is reduced.

–Refraction is described by **Snell's law:** $\sin \theta_i / \sin \theta_t = v_1/v_2$, where θ_i is the angle of incidence, θ_t is the transmitted angle, v_1 is the velocity in medium 1, and v_2 is the velocity in medium 2.

–If the velocity of sound in medium 2 is greater than that of medium 1, the transmission angle is greater than the angle of incidence.

–If the velocity of sound in medium 2 is less than that of medium 1, the transmission angle is less than the angle of incidence.

–Ultrasound machines assume straight line propagation, and refraction effects give rise to artifacts.

–**Total reflection** occurs if the ultrasound velocity in medium 2 is greater than that in medium 1, and the angle of incidence is greater than a critical angle (θ_c).

–At the critical angle, $\sin (\theta_c)$ is equal to v_1/v_2.

III. Transducers

A. Introduction

–A **transducer** is a device that can convert one form of energy into another.

–**Piezoelectric transducers** convert electrical energy into ultrasonic energy, and vice versa.

–*Piezoelectric* means **pressure electricity.**

–High-frequency voltage oscillations are produced by a **pulse generator** and are sent to the ultrasound transducer by a **transmitter.**

–The electrical energy causes the crystal to momentarily change shape (expand and contract depending on the current direction).

–This change in shape of the crystal increases and decreases the pressure in front of the transducer, thus producing ultrasound waves (transmitter).

–When the crystal is subjected to pressure changes by the returning ultrasound echoes, the pressure changes are converted back into electrical energy signals.

–Return voltage signals are transferred from the receiver to a computer to create an ultrasound image.

–Transducer crystals do not conduct electricity but are coated with a thin layer of silver, which acts as an electrode.

–The piezoelectric effect of a transducer is destroyed if heated above its curie temperature limit.

–Transducers are made of a synthetic ceramic (piezoceramic) such as lead-zirconate-titanate (PZT) or plastic polyvinylidene difluoride (PVDF), or a composite.

–A transducer may be used in either pulsed or continuous-wave mode.

B. Transducer characteristics

–The thickness and acoustic velocity of a piezoelectric crystal determine the resonant frequency of the transducer.

–Transducers also emit ultrasound energy at frequencies other than the resonant frequency, but at a lower intensity.

–Transducer crystals are normally manufactured so that their thickness *(t)* is equal to half of the wavelength (λ) (i.e., $t = \lambda/2$).

–Changing the thickness of the crystal changes the frequency but not the ultrasound amplitude or velocity.

–For example, if a crystal has a thickness of 1 mm and the velocity of sound is 4,000 m/second, the resonant frequency is $f = v/\lambda = v/(2 \times t)$, or 2 MHz.

–High-frequency transducers are thin, and low-frequency transducers are thicker.

C. Transducer design

–The **Q factor** is related to the frequency response of the crystal.

–The Q factor determines the purity of sound and the length of time a sound persists, or **ring-down time.**

–**High-Q transducers** produce a relatively pure frequency spectrum; low-Q transducers produce a wider range of frequencies.

–The Q factor is determined by the ratio of the operating frequency to the bandwidth at full-width half maximum.

–Short pulses correspond to reduced Q values and vice versa.

–Most transducers are designed to have short pulses with low Q values.

–Blocks of **damping material,** usually tungsten/rubber in an epoxy resin, are placed behind transducers to reduce vibration (ring-down time) and shorten pulses.

–A **matching layer** of material is placed on the front surface of the transducer to improve the efficiency of energy transmission into the patient.

–The matching layer material has an impedance between those of the transducer and the tissue.

–The matching layer thickness is one fourth the wavelength of sound in that material and is referred to as **quarter-wave matching.**

–**Fig. 11.2** shows the components of a typical piezoelectric transducer.

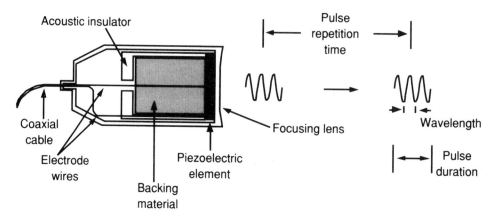

FIG. 11.2. Components of a single element ultrasound transducer and a typical ultrasound pulse.

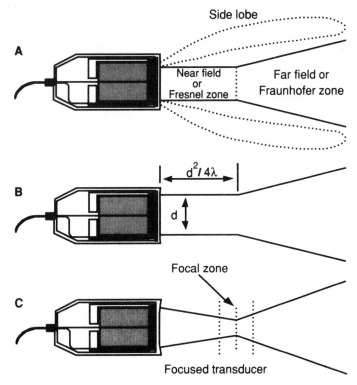

FIG. 11.3. Transducer zones and focus.

D. Ultrasound fields

–The near (parallel) field of the ultrasound beam is known as the **Fresnel zone (Fig. 11.3).**

–The far (diverging) field is known as the **Fraunhofer zone.**

–Beam intensity falls off in both zones because of attenuation, in the far zone because of beam divergence.

–Ultrasound imaging normally uses the Fresnel zone but not the Fraunhofer zone.

–The length of the Fresnel zone is $d^2/4\lambda$, where d is the diameter of the transducer and λ is the wavelength.

–The Fresnel zone increases with increasing transducer size and frequency (lower wavelengths).

–**Table 11.3** lists Fresnel zone dimensions for a 10 mm diameter transducer at different frequencies.

–**Side lobes** are small beams of greatly reduced intensity that are emitted at angles to the primary beam **(Fig. 11.3).**

TABLE 11.3. *Wavelength and Fresnel zone length in soft tissue for 10 mm diameter transducer*

Frequency (MHz)	Wavelength (mm)	Fresnel zone (mm)
1.0	1.5	17
2.0	0.75	33
5.0	0.3	83

E. Focused transducers

–Focused transducers reduce beam width.

–Focused transducers also concentrate beam intensity, thereby increasing penetration and echo intensities and improving image quality **(Fig. 11.3).**

–All diagnostic transducers are focused, which is achieved using a curved piezoelectric crystal or acoustic lens.

–Array transducers also focus by electronic phasing of adjacent crystal elements.

–The **focal zone** is the region over which the beam is focused.

–The **focal length** is the distance from the transducer to the center of the focal zone.

–The **depth of focus** is the distance over which the beam is in reasonable focus.

–A small-diameter transducer has a shorter focal zone and spreads more rapidly in the far zone.

F. Pulse repetition frequency

–**Pulse rate** or **pulse repetition frequency (PRF)** refers to the number of separate packets of sound that are sent out every second.

–Each sonic pulse is short (two to three wavelengths, or a duration of about 1 microseconds); between pulses, the transducer acts as a receiver.

–Common PRFs are approximately 3 kHz, or 3,000 pulses/second.

–High pulse rates limit the penetration depth (range) that may be detected because of the time required for the signal to return.

–A low PRF limits the line density and frame rate, which affects the ability to follow motion.

–For example, a 20 cm deep object requires 260 microseconds for a round trip.

–The maximum number of lines is then $[1/(260 \times 10^{-6})]$, or 3,846, in every second.

–With 3,846 total lines, it is possible to have 113 lines per image and 34 frames/second, or 225 lines per image and 15 frames/second, and so on.

IV. Displays

A. Introduction

–Most ultrasound beams are emitted in brief pulses with a duration of about 1 microsecond.

–The span between emitted pulses allows time for the returning echoes to be received and provides information about the depth of an interface.

–The strength of returning echoes provides information about differences between the two tissues.

–Objects imaged with ultrasound are large in comparison to the wavelength.

–Ultrasound scanners use **time gain compensation (TGC)** to compensate for increased attenuation with tissue depth.

–This is accomplished by increasing the signal gain as the echo return time increases.

–TGC is also known as depth gain compensation, time varied gain, and swept gain.

–Images are normally displayed on a video monitor.

–Images can also be digitized using a frame grabber and stored in a computer.

–Ultrasound images generally have a 512×512 matrix size, with each pixel being 8 bits deep (1 byte), allowing 256 (2^8) gray levels to be displayed.

B. A-mode ultrasound

–**A-mode** (amplitude) displays depth on the horizontal axis, and displays echo intensity (pulse amplitude) on the vertical axis, and can only display the position of a tissue interface.

–For soft tissue ($v = 1{,}540$ m/second), a return time of 13 microseconds corresponds to a depth of 1 cm (round trip of 2 cm).

–A-mode systems have no memory, and a permanent record is obtained by photographing the cathode ray tube (CRT) monitor.

–Little use is made of the spike amplitude.

–A-mode may be used in ophthalmology or when accurate distance measurements are required.

–A-mode provides information only along the line of sight and has been superseded by M-mode (motion) and two-dimensional B-mode (brightness) imaging.

C. M-mode ultrasound

–**M-mode** or **T-M–mode** (time-motion) displays time on the horizontal axis and depth on the vertical axis.

–The spikes of A-mode are converted into dots, and brightness replaces amplitude.

–Sequential ultrasound pulses are displayed adjacent to each other, allowing the change in position of interfaces to be seen.

–M-mode thus displays **time-dependent motion.**

–Longer times are stored digitally.

–M-mode is valuable for studying rapid movement, such as cardiac valve motion.

D. B-mode ultrasound

–**B-mode** displays a static image of a section of tissue.

–The grayscale is used to display the intensity of an echo from a given region.

–The transducer functions as both transmitter and receiver.

–The transducer sweeps the beam back and forth through the patient's body, acquiring single lines of data that display echo intensity as a function of location.

 –Because the sweeping motion covers a sector, this is known as **sector scanning.**

–The sweeping motion can be achieved using different mechanisms.

 –A single transducer can be wobbled back and forth.

 –A stationary transducer can be reflected off an oscillating mirror.

 –A multielement transducer can be continually rotated.

–**Phased arrays** consist of multiple small transducers that are sequentially activated to image a plane **(Fig. 11.4).**

 –Linear arrays have parallel elements.

 –Curvilinear phased arrays diverge and allow a wider field of view (FOV).

 –Linear and curvilinear arrays use a subset of their elements to form each ultrasound beam.

–Phased arrays electronically steer the ultrasound beam to form a sector.

 –Phased arrays use all of their elements to form each ultrasound beam.

–A single image frame is created by adding together individual lines.

–**Line density** is the number of vertical lines per field of view.

–The frame rates for **real time imaging** are 15 to 40 frames/second, which permits motion to be followed.

E. Scan converter

–Scan converters create two-dimensional images from echo data from distinct beam directions.

–Scan converters permit image data to be viewed directly on a video display.

–Scan conversion is required because the formats of image acquisition and display are different.

–Modern scan converters use digital methods for processing and storing data.

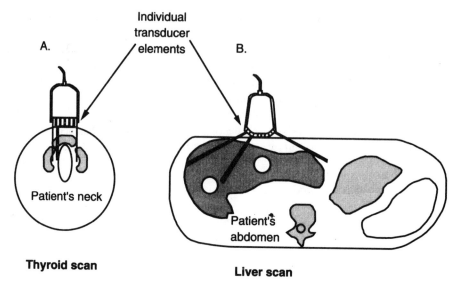

FIG. 11.4. Typical clinical transducers. **(A)** Linear phased array transducer. **(B)** A curvilinear phased array transducer.

–Image data are stored in a matrix that is typically 512×512, with a depth of 8 bits.
–One frame contains about 0.25 MB of information.
  –For color displays, the depth of a pixel can be as high as 3 bytes (24 bits).
–The transducer beam direction and echo delay time determine the pixel address that will store the echo data.

V. Clinical Aspects

A. Clinical transducers

–Low-frequency transducers have better tissue penetration.
–Transducers used for abdominal imaging are generally in the 2.5 to 5 MHz range.
  –Specialized high-resolution and shallow-penetration probes (8 to 20 MHz) have been developed for studying the eye.
  –In infants, 3.5 to 7 MHz transducers are used for echoencephalography.
  –Modern transducers can often operate at different frequencies.
–B-mode, M-mode, and Doppler systems are used to study the cardiovascular system.
–Special systems include **endovaginal** transducers for imaging the pelvic region and fetus, **endorectal** transducers for imaging the prostate, **transesophageal** transducers for imaging the heart, and **intravascular** probes for imaging inside blood vessels.
–Array transducers, which can be operated at high frame rates, are also better suited for Doppler imaging in which one image line must be sampled many times.
–**Table 11.4** lists types of ultrasound transducers and their clinical applications.

B. Harmonic imaging

–Harmonic frequencies are integral multiples of the fundamental ultrasound pulse frequencies.
–A high-frequency harmonic can be twice the central frequency of the initial ultrasound pulse.

–High frequencies arise from interactions with contrast agents (microbubbles) and tissues.

–Harmonic imaging enhances contrast agent imaging by tuning the receiver to the high (harmonic) frequency alone, thereby eliminating the lower frequencies (clutter).

–Harmonic imaging uses longer pulse lengths, which permits easier separation of the harmonic from the fundamental frequency.

–The first harmonic (twice the fundamental frequency) is often used for imaging.

–**Pulse inversion harmonic imaging** has recently been introduced, which improves the sensitivity of ultrasound to contrast agents.

  –Two pulses are used, standard plus inverted (phase reversed) along the same beam direction, which cancel out for soft tissues but not for microbubbles.

C. Resolution performance

–**Axial resolution** is the ability to separate two objects lying along the axis of the beam and is determined by the pulse length.

–Axial resolution is limited to half the pulse length and is therefore dependent on pulse frequency and duration.

–With a typical wavelength of 0.3 mm and three waves per pulse, the axial resolution is approximately 0.5 mm.

–**Axial resolution deteriorates** with increasing pulse length, decreasing frequency, and increasing wavelength.

–The use of damped (low-Q) transducers produces short pulses that improve axial resolution.

–**Lateral resolution** is the ability to resolve two adjacent objects and is determined by the width of the beam and line density.

–Lateral resolution is best in the Fresnel zone.

–A focused transducer produces a narrower beam at the focal zone and therefore has better lateral resolution than does an unfocused transducer of the same size (**Fig. 11.3**).

–Increased line density also results in improved lateral resolution but decreased frame rate.

–Lateral resolution is generally a few millimeters and is measured using phantoms.

TABLE 11.4. *Clinical transducers*

Transducer type	Frequency (MHz)	Body regions	Resolution		Comments
			Axial	Lateral	
Sector scanner or curvilinear array	3–6 (2.5 MHz) for obese patients)	Abdomen	Moderate	Moderate	Good depth penetration (grainy images at 2 MHz)
Linear array	5–13	Thyroid, testicles, carotids, breast, legs	Excellent	Very good	Poor depth penetration (used for superficial organs)
Curvilinear array	5–10	Pediatric abdomen; vascular imaging in very large patients	Very good	Good	Used for large superficial organs
Vaginal	3.75–7.5	Ovaries, uterus	Excellent	Very good	Limited range; may be accompanied by transadominal study
Endorectal	3.75–7.5	Prostate, rectal wall	Very good to excellent	Very good	Limited range

D. Ultrasound artifacts

–**Speckle** is a textured appearance that results from small, closely spaced structures that are too small to resolve as seen on images of solid organs.

–**Image noise** is the result of random signals produced in the electronic preamplifier of the transducer.

　–Noise reject controls can be adjusted to filter out weak noise, but this also eliminates weak echo signals.

–**Reverberation** echoes are the result of multiple reflections occurring from two adjacent interfaces.

　–Reverberation produces delayed echoes that are incorrectly localized as a more distant interface.

–The number of reverberations is limited by the power of the beam and sensitivity of the detector.

–**Acoustic shadowing** is the reduced echo intensity behind a highly attenuating or reflecting object, such as a stone creating a "shadow."

–**Acoustic enhancement** is the increased echo intensity behind a minimally attenuating object such as a fluid filled cyst.

–**Refraction** causes artifacts in the form of spatial distortions.

–**Speed displacement** artifacts are caused by the variability of the speed of sound in different tissues.

–**Side lobes** are emissions of ultrasound energy off axis and give rise to artifacts when echoes arise "off axis" but are placed as having occurred on the central axis.

–**Grating lobes** result from the division of a smooth transducer into a large number of small elements in multielement transducer arrays.

E. Ultrasound bioeffects

–At high power levels, ultrasound can cause **cavitation,** which is the creation and collapse of microscopic bubbles.

–Viscous stress can occur, resulting in small-scale fluid motions called microstreaming.

–**Tissue heating** occurs as a result of energy absorption and is the basis of using ultrasound for hyperthermia treatments.

–At low-megahertz frequencies, there have been no independently confirmed, significant biological effects in mammalian tissues at intensities below approximately 100 mW/cm^2 for unfocused beams or below 1 W/cm^2 for focused beams.

　–Typical intensities in clinical ultrasound are 1 to 10 mW/cm^2.

–The American Institute of Ultrasound in Medicine (AIUM) has established a Bioeffects Committee to review ultrasound safety.

–More than half the pregnant women in the United States undergo ultrasonic examinations with no real evidence of detrimental effects.

–Ultrasound is nonionizing and at diagnostic intensity levels is widely held to be biologically safe.

VI. Doppler Ultrasound

A. Doppler physics

–The **Doppler effect** refers to the **change in frequency that results from a moving sample** or ultrasound source.

–Objects moving toward the detector appear to have a higher frequency and shorter wavelength.

–Objects moving away from the detector appear to have a lower frequency and longer wavelength.

–Doppler ultrasound is used primarily to identify and evaluate blood flow in vessels based on the backscatter of blood cells.

–Because blood is a weak scatterer, Doppler systems run at lower frequencies to minimize attenuation.

–If the object is moving perpendicular to the ultrasound beam, there is no change in frequency or wavelength.

–By measuring the frequency shift, the speed and direction of movement can be determined.

–The shift in frequency is **$2f(v/c)\cos\theta$,** where f is the ultrasound frequency, c is the velocity of sound, v is the speed of the moving object, and θ is the angle between the ultrasound beam and the moving object.

–**Table 11.5** lists typical values of Doppler ultrasound frequency shift for moving blood.

–The Doppler shift is in the audio range.

–**Aliasing artifacts** can occur in pulsed Doppler, resulting in errors in estimating velocity.

–The range and distribution of flow velocities can be displayed as a spectrum or sonogram which is a plot of Doppler frequency (velocity) versus time **(Fig. 11.5).**

–**Spectral broadening** is the result of a mixture of velocities in the sample and produces a shaded area below the peak velocity value.

B. Continuous-wave Doppler

–In **continuous-wave Doppler,** one transducer continually transmits and another transducer continuously receives.

–The frequencies of the two signals are subtracted to give the Doppler shift.

–The Doppler signal contains very low frequency signals (clutter) from moving specular reflectors, such as blood vessel walls.

–The Doppler signal from the clutter is much greater than that from blood.

–A "wall filter" selectively removes these very low frequencies.

–The Doppler signal is amplified to an audible sound level and can also be recorded to track spectral changes as a function of time to assess transient pulsatile flow.

–Continuous-wave Doppler is inexpensive and does not suffer from aliasing but lacks depth resolution and provides little spatial information.

–Continuous-wave Doppler is good for measuring fast flow and assessing deep-lying vessels.

–Depth gain compensation is not used in continuous-wave Doppler.

C. Pulsed Doppler

–**Pulsed Doppler** allows both velocity and depth information (ranging) to be obtained.

TABLE 11.5. *Doppler frequency shift for a 3 MHz beam*

Blood velocity (cm/sec)	Doppler shift (Hz) when angle between transducer and flow direction is:		
	0 Degrees	30 Degrees	60 Degrees
5	190	170	100
10	390	340	190
20	780	670	390

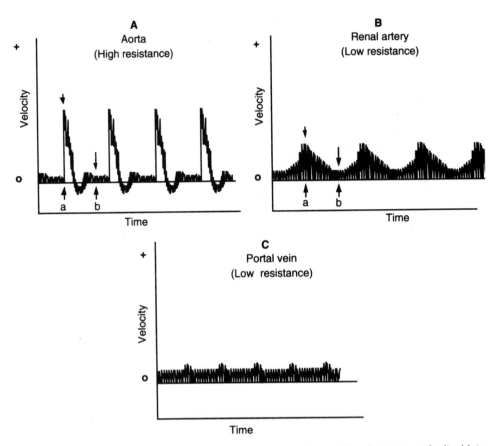

FIG. 11.5. A Doppler waveform is a tracing that shows the relation between velocity (determined from the Doppler shift frequency) and time and is unique to the flow pattern in the vessel. **(A)** A high-resistance arterial vessel demonstrates a rapid fall in velocity following systole. **(B)** A low-resistance artery shows flow during diastole as well. **(C)** Veins typically have a low velocity and low resistance. The maximum amplitude *(a)* represents peak velocity. The slowest forward flow measured in diastole is *b.* The resistive index is $(a - b)/a$, and the higher the resistance to blood flow, the higher the resistive index. Negative velocity represents flow away from the transducer.

–Longer pulse lengths are used in pulsed Doppler to improve sensitivity and the accuracy of the frequency shift, at the expense of axial resolution.

–To avoid **aliasing artifacts,** the PRF must be at least twice the highest Doppler frequency shift.

–A 1 kHz Doppler shift requires a PRF of at least 2 kHz.

–A clinical example of aliasing occurs when the highest velocities in the center of a vessel appear to have reverse flow.

–The maximum velocity that can be accurately determined by pulsed Doppler increases with PRF, lower operating frequency, and increasing angle.

–Large angles minimize aliasing artifacts but result in larger errors in the estimates of blood velocity.

–**Duplex scanning** combines B-mode imaging and pulsed Doppler acquisition.

–The Doppler information is provided only for a specific area (sampling volume).

–The Doppler signal can be represented by a spectrum of frequencies from a range of velocities contained at a given location.

–Laminar flow normally exists at the center of large smooth vessels.

–Turbulent flow occurs when the vessel is disrupted by plaque and stenoses.

–**Fig. 11.5** shows Doppler waveforms for a several types of blood vessels.

D. Color scanning

–**Color scanning** involves displaying color Doppler data on real time (B-mode) grayscale images.

–Acquisition of image information is interleaved with that of flow information.

–Color scanning allows velocity and position information to be obtained simultaneously.

–Colors (blue and red) are assigned, depending on motion toward or away from the transducer.

–Information is provided over a large area and superimposed on a grayscale image.

–Color Doppler can detect flow in vessels too small to be seen by imaging alone.

–**Real-time color flow imaging** maps the direction and velocity of movement in each pixel using an arbitrary color scale.

–Typically flow toward the transducer is assigned red and flow away from the transducer blue.

–Turbulent flow can be displayed as green or yellow.

–The color intensity varies with flow velocity, with a grayscale used to depict the absence of movement.

–One limitation of color scanning is that clutter of slow-moving solid structures and noise can overwhelm the smaller echoes from moving blood.

–**Spatial resolution** of the color image is much lower than that of the grayscale image.

E. Power Doppler

–Power Doppler uses the return Doppler signal strength alone.

–Power Doppler ignores the direction of frequency shift (phase), as in conventional color flow imaging.

–Power Doppler uses the same power levels as those of conventional color scanning; *energy* sometimes replaces the term *power*.

–Power Doppler is more sensitive than standard color flow imaging.

–The image signal does not vary with the direction of flow.

–Aliasing artifacts do not occur in power Doppler.

–Power Doppler permits detection and interpretation of slow blood flow.

–Power Doppler sacrifices directional and quantitative flow information.

–Power Doppler generally uses slower frame rates and has greater sensitivity to motion of the patient, tissues, and transducer ("flash artifacts").

Review Test

1. The velocity of an ultrasound beam is always:

(A) Constant for all solids
(B) Proportional to frequency cubed
(C) Equal to the velocity of the molecules of the medium
(D) Equal to frequency times wavelength
(E) 3×10^8 m/second

2. Sound waves are:

(A) Constant velocity
(B) Low-frequency electromagnetic radiation
(C) Ionizing radiation
(D) Audible at 1 MHz
(E) Longitudinal waves

3. A 2 MHz transducer has an approximate wavelength of:

(A) 0.01 mm
(B) 0.1 mm
(C) 1.0 mm
(D) 10 mm
(E) More than 10 mm

4. The wavelength of a 3 MHz sound beam is shortest in:

(A) Air
(B) Castor oil
(C) Fat
(D) Muscle
(E) Bone

5. Acoustic impedance (Z) is primarily dependent on tissue:

(A) Density
(B) Attenuation
(C) Atomic number
(D) Temperature
(E) Oxygenation

6. Which of the following has the highest acoustic impedance?

(A) Bone
(B) Fat
(C) Air
(D) Water
(E) Eye lens

7. The wavelength of a 1 MHz sound beam is *not:*

(A) The same in all solid media
(B) 0.3 mm in air

(C) 1.5 mm in soft tissue
(D) 4.1 mm in bone
(E) Velocity divided by frequency

8. If an ultrasound beam is attenuated by 99%, the attenuation is:

(A) 1 dB
(B) 3 dB
(C) 10 dB
(D) 20 dB
(E) Greater than 20 dB

9. The key factor determining the fraction of ultrasound reflected at a large interface is the:

(A) Depth of the interface
(B) Transducer diameter
(C) Transducer output intensity
(D) Differences in acoustic impedance
(E) Scan mode (A, B, or M)

10. What fraction of ultrasound is reflected from a liver (Z = 1.55) and soft tissue (Z = 1.65) interface?

(A) 1/2
(B) 1/10
(C) 1/100
(D) 1/500
(E) 1/1,000

11. Ultrasound shadowing artifacts are unlikely behind:

(A) Strong attenuators
(B) Bone
(C) Air
(D) Fluid-filled cysts
(E) Metallic clips

12. Reflections occur from all of the following *except:*

(A) Smooth surfaces
(B) Kidney interior
(C) Fat-kidney interfaces
(D) Bladder wall
(E) Bladder contents

13. Snell's law describes the relation between the:

(A) Angle of incidence and transmission
(B) Fraunhofer angle and wavelength
(C) Angle of incidence and angle of reflection

(D) Focus and transducer curvature
(E) Fresnel zone and wavelength

14. An ultrasound beam traveling through tissue *cannot* be:

(A) Absorbed
(B) Amplified
(C) Scattered
(D) Reflected
(E) Refracted

15. Higher-frequency transducers have increased:

(A) Thickness
(B) Intensity
(C) Attenuation
(D) Velocity
(E) Wavelength

16. The Q factor of a transducer refers to:

(A) Coupling efficiency
(B) Minimum intensity
(C) Maximum intensity
(D) Purity of the frequency
(E) Transducer dead time

17. The damping material behind the crystal transducer reduces:

(A) Pulse frequency
(B) Ring-down time
(C) Echo amplitude
(D) Lateral resolution
(E) PRF

18. The Fresnel zone length of an ultrasound beam increases with increasing:

(A) Transducer diameter
(B) Transducer thickness
(C) Wavelength
(D) Intensity
(E) TGC

19. TGC corrects for which of the following?

(A) Signal losses at skin interface
(B) Velocity of moving objects
(C) Intensity decrease with tissue penetration
(D) Transducer damping material
(E) Image fading on cathode ray tube

20. An echo received 65 microseconds after the signal is sent is from what depth?

(A) 2 cm
(B) 5 cm
(C) 7 cm
(D) 10 cm
(E) 15 cm

21. In B-mode ultrasound, the PRF does *not* affect:

(A) Pulses per second
(B) Frame rate
(C) Number of lines per frame
(D) Maximum penetration depth
(E) Ultrasound frequency

22. Choice of frequency in ultrasound is most likely a trade off between patient penetration and:

(A) Contrast
(B) PRF
(C) Noise
(D) Lateral resolution
(E) Axial resolution

23. Ultrasound signals are converted from digital data to a video monitor display using a:

(A) Log amplifier
(B) Photomultiplier tube
(C) Photocathode
(D) Scan converter
(E) Array processor

24. The best axial resolution is obtained using:

(A) 5.0 MHz phased array
(B) 5.0 MHz linear array
(C) 5.0 MHz continuous-wave Doppler
(D) 10 MHz sector scanner
(E) 10 MHz continuous-wave Doppler

25. Lateral resolution in ultrasound imaging would most likely be improved by:

(A) Increasing transducer focusing
(B) Imaging in the Fraunhofer zone
(C) Using fewer scan lines
(D) Increasing the frequency
(E) Reducing the pulse length

26. Below a structure, a very faint image of the structure is probably owing to:

(A) Reverberation artifact
(B) Side lobes
(C) Specular reflection
(D) Nonspecular reflection
(E) Incorrect TCG

27. All of the following may cause significant ultrasound artifacts *except:*

(A) Reverberation
(B) Side lobes
(C) Nonspecular reflections
(D) Refraction
(E) Speed displacement

28. Clinical ultrasound beams normally have an intensity of:

(A) 0.5 mW/cm^2
(B) 5 mW /cm^2
(C) 50 mW/cm^2
(D) 0.5 W/cm^2
(E) 5 W/cm^2

29. The Doppler shift from a moving object depends on all of the following *except:*

(A) Speed of ultrasound beam

(B) Frequency
(C) Angle between beam and object
(D) Object depth
(E) Object speed

30. Continuous-wave Doppler uses:

(A) One transducer
(B) High frequency transducers
(C) A low Q factor
(D) A scan converter
(E) Little spatial information

Answers and Explanations

1–D. The velocity *(v)* of any wave is always the product of the frequency *(f)* and wavelength (λ) (i.e., $v = f \times \lambda$).

2–E. In ultrasound, the displacement is along the direction of travel (electromagnetic waves are transverse, because the displacement is perpendicular to the direction of the wave motion).

3–C. Because $v = f \times \lambda$, and the velocity of sound is 1540 m/second, the wavelength is given by $[(1,540)/(2 \times 10^6)]$ m, or about 1 mm.

4–A. The wavelength (λ) is given by v/f, and because the speed of sound in air (330 m/second) is much less than in soft tissue (1,540 m/second), the wavelength is correspondingly shorter.

5–A. Acoustic impedance is dependent on tissue density and is obtained using the equation $Z = \rho \times v$, where ρ is the tissue density, and v is the velocity of sound in the tissue.

6–A. Acoustic impedance is the product of the density and velocity of sound, both of which are the highest for bone.

7–A. Wavelength generally changes with medium because frequency will be the same, but velocity depends on the medium.

8–D. Decibels are $10 \times \log_{10} (I_o/I)$, where I_o is 100 and I is 1; this corresponds to 20 decibels.

9–D. The difference in acoustic impedance between the two tissues (Z_1, Z_2) determines the fraction of incident energy reflected.

10–E. The reflected fraction of an ultrasound beam is given by $[(Z_1 - Z_2)/(Z_1 + Z_2)]^2$, which gives 1/1,000.

11–D. Shadowing artifacts occur because of a large loss of transmitted signal intensity caused by either attenuation or reflection; fluid-filled cysts transmit ultrasound and result in enhancement of echoes beyond the cyst.

12–E. There are no reflections from fluids in the bladder.

13–A. Snell's law describes the angle of refraction that occurs when an ultrasound beam passes from one medium to another.

14–B. There is no mechanism for amplifying ultrasound beams in patients. Echoes from tissue interfaces, however, can be amplified electronically.

15–C. The attenuation in tissue is about 1 dB/cm at 1 MHz and increases approximately linearly with frequency (there is no direct relationship between intensity and frequency).

16–D. Q is defined as the operating frequency (MHz) divided by the bandwidth, so that high Q values correspond to a pure frequency and vice versa.

17–B. The ring-down time is reduced and very short pulses of only two or three wavelengths are generated.

18–A. The Fresnel zone is given by r^2/λ, where r is the transducer radius and λ is the wavelength.

19–C. TGC corrects for normal attenuation in tissue, and is generally assumed to be 1 dB/cm per 1 MHz.

20–B. The equation to use is $d = c \times t$, where d is the total travel distance, c is the speed (1,540 m/second), and t is the time (65 microseconds); we obtain a round trip distance of 10 cm, which corresponds to depth of 5 cm.

21–E. Ultrasound frequency has no relationship to the PRF but is determined by the transducer crystal thickness.

22–E. As frequency increases, the wavelength is reduced, which improves resolution but reduces patient penetration.

23–D. Scan converters convert ultrasound data into an image that is displayed on a video monitor.

24–D. Highest frequency normally gives the best axial resolution. However, continuous-wave Doppler provides little spatial information and has the "worst" axial resolution.

25–A The lateral resolution improves with focussing

26–A. Reverberation artifact is produced by the beam bouncing off the posterior interface, then off the anterior interface, then back off the posterior interface, and finally being recorded as a faint image further away from the actual structure.

27–C. Nonspecular reflection will result in the beam being scattered in all directions and is unlikely to be the direct cause of image artifacts.

28–B. Diagnostic ultrasound uses 1 to 10 mW/cm^2.

29–D. The depth of the moving object is immaterial.

30–E. Continuous-wave Doppler provides little spatial information because the beam is continuously on, which permits detection of the frequency differences between emitted and reflected signals.

12

Magnetic Resonance

I. Basic Physics

A. Magnetic nuclei

–As a result of their nuclear spin and charge distribution, protons and neutrons have a magnetic field called a **magnetic dipole.**

–Although neutrons have no net charge, they do have a charge distribution.

–**Magnetic moment** is a vector that represents the strength and orientation of a magnetic dipole.

–Nuclei with an even number of protons and neutrons have no net magnetic moment.

  –The protons and neutrons pair up with their magnetic moments aligned in opposite directions and cancel each other.

–Nuclei with an odd number of protons or neutrons have a net magnetic moment and behave like a bar magnet.

–These nuclei are candidates for magnetic resonance (**Table 12.1**).

–The hydrogen nucleus has a large magnetic moment, and its abundance in the body makes it the basis of most clinical **magnetic resonance (MR)** imaging.

B. Tissue magnetization

–There are more than 10^{20} hydrogen protons in each cubic centimeter of tissue.

–Nuclear spins of these protons are normally randomly oriented and thus produce no net magnetic moment (**magnetization vector).**

–In a magnetic field, hydrogen nuclei (protons) may be orientated either **spin up** (i.e., aligned along the **field**) or **spin down** (i.e., aligned opposite to the field).

–Spin-down alignment has slightly more energy.

–A small excess of protons go into the spin-up alignment.

–The magnetic fields of the remaining spin-up and spin-down nuclei cancel.

–Any tissue placed in a large magnetic field therefore has a small net **magnetization vector** of unpaired hydrogen protons aligned in the direction of the external field.

–Only the excess nuclei in the lower-energy (spin-up) state generate the MR signal.

  –This excess is approximately three per million proton nuclei at a magnetic-field strength of 1 tesla (T).

–MR signals are weak and considerable technical ingenuity is required to maximize signal-to-noise ratios (SNRs).

C. Larmor frequency

–When magnetic moments are placed into a magnetic field, a torque causes the magnetic moments to perform a precession motion similar to a spinning top.

–The **Larmor frequency** (f_L) is the precession frequency (MHz) of nuclei in a magnetic field (B). $f_L = \gamma B$, where the gyromagnetic ratio (γ) is a constant for a given nucleus.

TABLE 12.1. *Nuclei used for magnetic resonance in radiology*

Nucleus	Natural abundance (%)	Relative sensitivity*
^{1}H	99.985	1.00
^{19}F	100	0.833
^{23}Na	100	0.093
^{31}P	100	0.066

*Includes differences in natural abundance and innate sensitivity per nucleus.

–Protons have a Larmor frequency of 21 MHz at 0.5 T, 42 MHz at 1 T, and 63 MHz at 1.5 T.

–For comparison, ^{19}F has a Larmor frequency of 40 MHz at 1 T, and ^{23}Na has a Larmor frequency of 11 MHz at 1 T.

D. Resonance

–Resonance occurs when the net magnetization vector is perturbed from its equilibrium orientation.

–Electromagnetic radiation applied at the Larmor frequency (f_L) and perpendicular to the external magnetic field (z axis) causes the magnetization vector to rotate out of alignment with the field toward the x-y plane.

  –This electromagnetic radiation is in the radiofrequency (RF) part of the electromagnetic spectrum.

–The component of the net magnetization vector parallel to the magnetic field is called the **longitudinal magnetization.**

–The component perpendicular to the magnetic field is called the **transverse magnetization.**

–The rotation angle (flip angle) depends on the strength of the applied RF field and the total time that it is switched on (**pulse duration).**

–A **180 degree RF pulse** reorients the magnetization vector in a direction opposite to the equilibrium orientation, but still parallel to the external magnetic field.

–A **90 degree RF pulse** reorients the magnetization vector into the plane perpendicular to the external magnetic field.

–A 90 degree RF pulse duration is half as long as a 180 degree RF pulse.

E. Free induction decay

–After a 90 degree RF pulse, longitudinal magnetization is converted to transverse magnetization, which then precesses at the Larmor frequency about the external magnetic field.

–This rotation gives rise to the **free induction decay (FID)** signal.

–FID signals can be detected as an oscillating voltage, at the Larmor frequency (f_L), in a receiver coil placed around the sample.

  –The FID signal is weak because of the small number of nuclei that contribute to the signal (three per 10^6) and the small size of the nuclear magnetic moments.

  –The receiver coil may be the same as the RF transmitter coil.

–FID signals are detected, digitized, stored in a computer, and—through use of Fourier analysis—transformed into MR images.

F. T1 relaxation

–Protons placed into a strong magnetic field produce a net magnetization *(M)* parallel to the magnetic-field axis.

   –This magnetization grows exponentially from the initial value of zero to the equilibrium value of *M* with a time constant T1.

   –At time equal to T1, 63% of the signal has returned and at 3 × T1, 95% has returned.

   –Equilibrium to full magnetization *M* occurs after a time interval of approximately 4 × T1.

–If the field is switched off, magnetization *M* decays exponentially with the same time constant T1 (i.e., as $e^{-t/T1}$), where t is the elapsed time.

–T1 relaxation is called **longitudinal** or **spin-lattice relaxation.**

–**Fig. 12.1A** shows the T1 relaxation curve for two different tissues.

–For most tissues, T1 times are a few hundred milliseconds **(Table 12.2)**

   –**T1 is long** in small molecules such as water and in large molecules such as proteins.

   –**T1 is short** in fats and in intermediate-sized molecules.

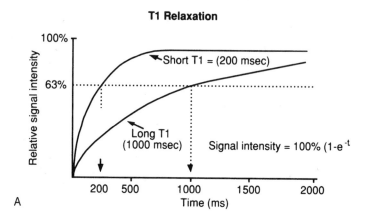

A

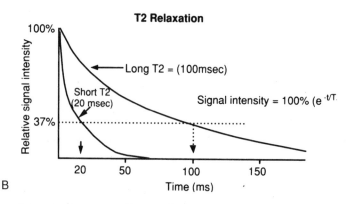

B

FIG. 12.1. T1 and T2 relaxation times. **(A)** The T1 relaxation is represented as a return to equilibrium of the longitudinal component of magnetization. At time T1, the signal has grown to 63% of its maximum value. **(B)** The T2 relaxation is represented as a decrease in the transverse component of magnetization due to dephasing. At time T2, the signal has decayed to 37% of its maximum.

TABLE 12.2. *T1 and T2 relaxation times*

Tissue	T1 (msec) at field of:		T2 (msec)
	0.5 T	1.5 T	
Fat (adipose)	200	260	80
Liver	320	490	45
Kidney	500	650	60
White matter	530	780	90
Gray matter	650	920	100
Cerebrospinal fluid	2,000	2,400	180

–Contrast agents such as gadolinium—diethylenetriaminepentaacetic acid (Gd-DTPA) can cause T1 shortening.

–In general, T1 increases with increasing magnetic-field strength.

G. T2 relaxation

–After a 90 degree pulse, the transverse magnetization vector rotates at the Larmor frequency in a plane perpendicular to the external magnetic field.

–The FID signal produced is proportional to this magnetization vector, which decays exponentially.

–In perfectly uniform magnetic fields, the decay rate constant is T2, and the induced FID signal decays as $e^{-t/T2}$.

   –At a time equal to T2, the signal has decayed to 37% of its maximum.

   –At $3 \times T2$, the signal has decayed to 5%, and at approximately $4 \times T2$, the signal has almost completely decayed.

–**Fig. 12.1B** shows the T2 decay curves for two different tissues.

–T2 relaxation is called **transverse** or **spin-spin relaxation.**

–For most tissues, T2 times are typically tens of milliseconds (**Table 12.2).**

   –T2 decreases with increasing molecular size and decreased molecular mobility.

   –Liquids generally have **long T2 times,** whereas large molecules and solids generally have **short T2 times.**

–Values of T2 for tissues are approximately independent of magnetic-field strength.

H. T2*

–Normal magnets have magnetic-field inhomogeneities of a few parts per million (ppm) or a few μT in fields of 1 T.

–The non-symetric shape of humans, as well as bone/tissue and air/tissue interfaces, can also distort magnetic fields leading to magnetic inhomogeneitieis.

–Decay of transverse magnetization caused by both **spin dephasing,** owing to inhomogeneities in the main magnetic field, and T2 is called T2*.

   –Spins that are in slightly higher fields rotate slightly faster and vice versa, resulting in dephasing of the spins.

   –This dephasing results in a decrease in magnetization vector intensity.

–The observed FID signal falls exponentially with a decay rate constant T2* (i.e., $e^{-t/T2*}$).

   –The relationship between T2, T2*, and spin dephasing due to inhomogeneities ($T2_{inhomogeneity}$), is given by $1/T2* = 1/T2 + 1/T2_{inhomogeneity}$.

–T2* is a few milliseconds and is always shorter than T2.

–Dephasing owing to the inhomogeneity contribution to T2* can be overcome by generating spin-echoes (SEs), whereas signal loss owing to true T2 relaxation is irreversible.

–Materials such as paramagnetic and ferromagnetic contrast agents disrupt the local magnetic-field homogeneity and shorten T2*.

–For all tissues, **T2* ≤ T2 ≤ T1.**

II. Instrumentation

A. Magnets

–Powerful magnets capable of generating strong, stable, spatially uniform magnetic fields are essential for MR.

–Magnetic fields are measured in tesla, where 1 T = 10,000 gauss (G).

–The Earth's magnetic field is weak (50 μT, or 0.5 G).

–To perform MR, the magnetic field must have a high homogeneity of only a few part per million.

  –**Shim coils** superimpose small corrective field differences on the main field to improve the magnetic-field uniformity.

–The large whole-body magnets used in MR scanners can be **resistive, permanent, or superconducting.**

  –Permanent magnets have low operating costs and small fringe fields but are heavy and can only generate fields up to approximately 0.35 T.

  –Resistive magnets can generate magnetic fields up to approximately 0.5 T.

  –Resistive magnets can be turned on and off, but consume a large amount of electrical power and need cooling because of the heat generated.

–As **MR field-strength increases,** so does the T1 relaxation time, the SNR, certain image artifacts, and RF energy deposition in the patient.

B. Superconducting magnets

–The best MR images are achieved at field strengths higher than those of resistive and permanent magnets.

  –Field strengths of several tesla can be generated by superconducting magnets.

–**Superconductivity** is the ability of certain materials to conduct electrical current without any resistance.

–Superconductors use a wire-wrapped cylinder (i.e., a solenoid) to generate the magnetic field.

–Superconducting magnets are generally kept cool using liquid helium (4.2 K).

  –A constant electric current creates the magnetic field, which is on at all times.

–If the wire temperature rises accidentally, the system loses its superconducting properties, and the energy stored in the magnetic field is converted to heat, resulting in a magnet **quench.**

–**Fig. 12.2** is a cutaway view of a superconducting MR imaging system.

C. Gradient coils

–Magnetic gradients are used to code the spatial location of the MR signal and are essential for generating MR images.

–MR systems have magnetic-field gradients in the *x, y* and *z* orientations.

  –When activated, these gradients superimpose a small field gradient on the main magnetic field.

  –With gradients superimposed on the main magnetic field, each magnetic-field location corresponds to a slightly different Larmor frequency, which alters the precession frequency of nuclei in this specific region.

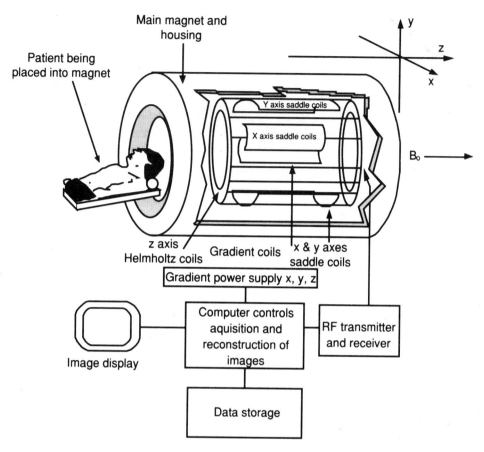

FIG. 12.2. Superconducting magnetic resonance system showing the main magnetic field (Bo) produced by the superconducting magnet, which is cooled by liquid helium. Three paired coils apply the gradients. A radiofrequency coil transmits and receives the radiofrequency signal.

–Combinations of three orthogonal sets of gradients allow the gradient field to be oriented in any direction.

–Gradient strengths range up to 60 mT/m (6 G/cm).

–Axial gradients (z) are produced using **Helmholtz coils.**

–**Fig. 12.3** shows a pair of Helmholtz coils being used to produce a gradient along the z axis for section selection.

–Gradients which change the main field as a function of x or y distance are normally produced by **saddle coils.**

–Gradients may need to be switched on and off rapidly (within less than 500 microseconds).

–Gradients generate small, rapidly decaying eddy currents in other coils or metal structures nearby; these currents impair scanner performance and may create image artifacts.

D. Radiofrequency coils

–RF is electromagnetic radiation with frequencies in the range of approximately 1 MHz to 10 GHz.

–**Transmitter coils** are used to send in RF pulses.

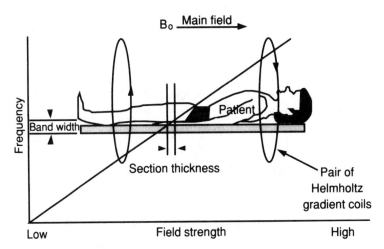

FIG. 12.3. Section selection along the *z* axis using a pair of Helmholtz gradient coils that superimpose a magnetic field on the main field. The resultant variation in Larmor frequency along the gradient allows a section of tissue perpendicular to the gradient to be selected.

　　–The same or separate coils are used as **receivers** to detect FID signals from the patient.
　–Small RF detection coils maximize the SNR of the weak FID signals.
　　–Small coils generally increase the SNR but restrict the region or volume being imaged.
　　–The SNR may also be improved by using **quadrature** coils designed for particular anatomic regions (e.g., knee).
　–Surface coils have increased sensitivity, but the detected signal intensity falls off rapidly with distance from the coil.
　–**Phased array coils** also be used to improve SNR performance.

E. Shielding
　　–The **magnetic flux lines** from the main magnetic field can extend out to a large distance from the magnet.
　　–The peripheral magnetic field is called the **fringe field** and can affect magnetically sensitive devices **(Table 12.3).**
　　–Nearby, large metallic objects (e.g., elevators and ferromagnetic structures) can disrupt the uniformity of the main magnetic field and degrade MR image quality.
　　–**Magnetic shielding** usually consists of steel plates or layers of sheet metal placed around the MR magnet.
　　–MR imaging units also require **RF shielding** to prevent RF signals from entering or escaping to the outside world.
　　　–The RF shielding is a **faraday cage,** which consists of copper sheet metal or screen lining the MR imager or room.

TABLE 12.3. *Limiting fields close to magnets*

Field limit	Object
0.5 mT (5 G)	Pacemakers, cathode ray tubes
1 mT (10 G)	Credit cards, watches
2 mT (20 G)	Floppy disks
5 mT (50 G)	Power supplies

TABLE 12.4. *United States Food and Drug Administration guidelines for radiofrequency power*

Parameter	Limit
Average radiofrequency absorption rate (W/kg)	
Whole body	<0.4
Head	<3.2
Any gram of tissue	<8.0
Temperature (°C)	
Core body temperature rise	<1
Head	<38
Body	<39
Extremities (local heating)	<40

–RF shielding is also essential in limiting outside interference from sources such as radio broadcasts.

F. MR safety

–Detrimental biological effects from exposure to static magnetic fields are not evident below 10 T.

–One of the greatest potential hazards around a magnet is the **missile effect.**

  –Ferromagnetic objects such as pens, scissors, screwdrivers, oxygen cylinders, and other metallic devices can be pulled into the magnet.

  –Pacemakers may be deactivated by magnetic fields.

–Because of the torque produced by the magnetic field, hazards also exist for patients who have ferromagnetic devices implanted in their bodies, including aneurysm clips, cochlear implants, implanted electrodes, and internal drug infusion pumps.

–The **time-varying magnetic fields** created by the gradients are a safety concern.

  –Time-varying magnetic fields induce currents in the patient and can induce mild cutaneous sensations, involuntary muscle contractions, and cardiac arrhythmias.

  –The FDA recommends a limit of 3 T/second to prevent peripheral nerve stimulation.

  –Time-varying magnetic fields can also produce magnetophosphenes (light flashes).

–There are no hazards beyond the 0.5 mT (5 G) fringe field of an MR magnet.

  –General access is restricted in areas having magnetic fields above 0.5 mT (5 G).

  –Warning signs must be posted in areas with magnetic fields above 1.5 mT (15 G).

–The measure of **dose** of RF fields is the **specific absorption rate (SAR)** in watts per kilogram (W/kg) and is a measure of power absorbed per unit of mass, or tissue.

  –Absorption of RF power will increase tissue temperature.

  –Limits are imposed on the average and maximum power deposition rates in any gram of tissue, and on the rise in tissue temperature.

–U.S. Food and Drug Administration (FDA) guidelines for magnet and RF power levels are listed in **Table 12.4.**

–The noise level in MR systems ranges from 65 to 120 dB, and there have been anecdotal reports of temporary hearing loss.

III. Imaging

A. Magnetic resonance signal localization

–Signal localization for image construction is based on adding a magnetic-field gradient onto the main (constant) magnetic field.

–Along the gradient, a unique magnetic-field strength corresponds to each location.

–Each field strength location corresponds to a specific Larmor frequency in the detected signal.

–A frequency analysis of the MR signal permits the origin of each signal to be determined.

–To identify the location of the MR signal, frequency analysis of FID signals is performed using Fourier techniques.

–Image reconstruction is performed digitally by computers using two- (2D) or three-dimensional (3D) **Fourier transform algorithms.**

B. Two-dimensional image formation

–Pulse sequences are repeated n times using a repetition time interval of TR to obtain phase-encoding.

–The number of **phase-encoding steps** *(n)* determines the number of pixels in the y direction, with n typically ranging from 128 to 256.

–The number of pixels in the read-direction is related to the number of samples in FID acquired and is typically 256.

–For a constant field of view (FOV), increasing the number of pixels in the read-direction increases resolution and reduces signal strength.

–The time to complete an imaging sequence is $N_{ex} \times n \times$ TR, where n is the number of phase-encoding steps; TR, the repetition time; and N_{ex}, the number of repeat acquisitions.

–For a typical sequence of TR = 500 milliseconds, N_{ex} = 2, and n = 128, imaging time is 128 seconds (approximately 2 minutes).

–Multiple images are usually obtained during an acquisition by interrogating several slices during each TR interval in an interleaved fashion.

–A variety of **pulse sequences** are used to generate signal intensities from a given region.

–Pulse sequences are the **strength, order, duration,** and **repetition and detection of RF pulses** and **magnetic gradients** used to generate an image.

–The most commonly used pulse sequences in clinical imaging are **SE, inversion recovery (IR),** and **gradient recalled echo (GRE).**

C. Spin-echo

–**SE** pulse sequences commence with 90 degree pulses to rotate the magnetization vector into the transverse plane where the transverse magnetization rapidly dephases (T2* effects).

–**Spin rephasing** is achieved by using a 180 degree RF pulse at a time TE/2 that generates an echo at time **TE.**

–The intensity of the spin-echo at time TE is reduced by a factor of $e^{-TE/T2}$ because of T2 effects.

–The 180 degree pulse can be repeated to generate **multiple echoes** with progressively longer TE values.

–The sequence is repeated with a **repetition time (TR),** which is the time interval between successive 90 degree pulses.

–For TR values less than $4 \times$ T1, the tissue longitudinal magnetization vector is unable to fully recover after a 90 degree pulse.

–An equilibrium tissue magnetization vector size is generally reached after a few successive 90 degree pulses; the size of this magnetization is reduced in intensity for longer T1 values.

–**Fig. 12.4A** shows the specific components of an SE pulse sequence.

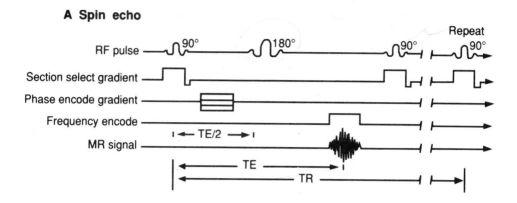

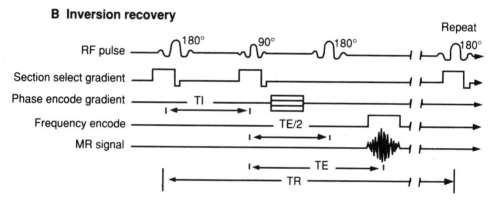

FIG. 12.4. Spin-echo **(A)** and inversion recovery pulse **(B)** sequences.

–SE sequences can be modified to emphasize T1 differences (T1 weighting), T2 differences (T2 weighting), or proton density differences.

D. T1 and T2 weighting

–T1-weighted images are obtained with a short TR (less than 600 milliseconds) to emphasize T1 differences and a short TE (less than 20 milliseconds) to minimize T2 differences.

–Short-T1 tissues have a high signal intensity because of their complete relaxation.

–T2-weighted images are obtained with a long TR (more than 2,000 milliseconds) to minimize T1 differences, because all tissues exhibit full relaxation, and a long TE (more than 60 milliseconds) to emphasize T2 differences.

–For long TEs, tissues with long T2s appear bright, and tissues with short T2s appear dark.

–Proton density-weighted images are obtained with a long TR (more than 2,000 milliseconds) to minimize T1 differences and a short TE (less than 20 milliseconds) to minimize T2 differences.

–**Table 12.5** summarizes the influence of TE and TR times on the type of contrast obtained in MR images.

–**Fast SE (FSE)** techniques resemble multiecho SE sequences but change the phase-encoding gradients for each echo.

TABLE 12.5. *Effects of TE and TR Parameters on spin-echo images*

TR	Short TE	Long TE
Short	T1-weighted	Mixed
Long	Proton density	T2-weighted

TE, echo time; TR, repetition time.

–In FSE, the number of repeat pulses separated by time TR is greatly reduced with a corresponding reduction in imaging time.

–FSE shortens acquisition time by applying multiple phase-encoding steps and 180 degree echoes after every 90 degree pulse.

  –T1-weighted images acquired in this way have more T2 weighting than do conventional SE images.

–Compared with conventional SE imaging, FSE techniques decrease the number of interleaved slices that can be obtained because there is a greater fraction of the TR interval used to obtain MR signals.

E. Inversion recovery

–**IR** uses 180 degree pulses to invert the magnetization vector.

–The longitudinal magnetization vector recovers with a time constant T1, and complete recovery occurs after a time of $4 \times$ T1.

–The 180 degree pulse is followed by a 90 degree (readout) pulse after time **TI (inversion time)** to flip the relaxed spins into the transverse plane.

–A second 180 degree pulse at time TE/2 produces an echo at time TE, which is the detected signal intensity.

–The size of the signal obtained with the readout pulse is strongly dependent on the value of T1 and TI.

–IR emphasizes T1 differences, and tissues with short T1 values produce high-intensity signals.

–**Fig. 12.4B** shows the specific components of an IR pulse sequence.

–IR is the basis of **short-time IR (STIR)** sequences for fat suppression, in which TI is selected to null the signal from fat.

–In **fluid-attenuated IR (FLAIR)** sequences, TI is set to attenuate cerebrospinal fluid signal.

F. Gradient recalled echoes

–**GRE** techniques make use of short TRs, short TEs, and low flip angles.

  –This combination permits fast acquisition times and permits 3D imaging within reasonable times.

  –Sequences may use TRs of only 5 milliseconds, and 256 phase encoding steps can be acquired in 1.3 seconds.

–GRE imaging relies on reversing the polarity of the magnetic-field gradients instead of 180 degree refocusing of RF pulses to generate echoes.

  –This is accomplished by reversing the polarity of the magnetic gradient to rephase the spins and generate an echo FID signal.

–Short TE values emphasize T1 differences between tissues.

–Examples of fast imaging include fast low-angle shot **(FLASH),** fast imaging with steady-state precession **(FISP),** and gradient recalled acquisition in the steady state **(GRASS).**

–Parameters can be adjusted to emphasize blood flow, and angiographic images can therefore be constructed.

G. Three-dimensional imaging

–3D Fourier transform (3DFT) imaging techniques are possible to image relatively small volumes such as knees.

–In 3D imaging, two sets of orthogonal phase-encoding gradients are used in addition to the frequency-encoding gradient.

–A nonselective RF pulse simultaneously excites the entire sample volume.

–3DFT is applied along all three axes for image reconstruction.

–After the volume data are reconstructed, 2D images in any selected plane can be constructed.

–3D imaging times are $N_{ex} \times n_1 \times n_2 \times$ TR, where n_1 is the number of phase-encoding steps in one plane, and n_2 is the number in the orthogonal plane.

–**Disadvantages** of 3DFT techniques include longer acquisition times and susceptibility to motion artifacts.

–**Advantages** of 3DFT include the high resolution in all three orientations and the availability of contiguous sections.

–3D also permits the generation of arbitrary oblique slices using postprocessing.

IV. Image Quality

A. Magnetic resonance images

–MR images typically have matrix sizes between 128×128 and 256×256.

–Each pixel needs 12 to 16 bits to code the pixel intensity level, which is achieved using 2 bytes.

–A single MR image (256×256) has a file size of 0.125 MB.

–The MR imaging parameters selected determine the tradeoffs that influence contrast, noise, resolution, and acquisition time.

–Regular quality control measurements should be taken to ensure that the MR system is functioning optimally.

–Quality control tests may measure section thickness, resolution, SNR, field uniformity, gradient linearity, spatial distortion, and image contrast.

B. Image contrast

–The pulse sequence chosen determines the type of contrast observed in the resultant MR image.

–Image contrast is markedly influenced by tissue differences in T1, T2, and proton density.

–Tissues with short T1 values appear bright on T1-weighted images.

–Tissues with long T2 values appear bright on T2-weighted images.

–Proton density–weighted images demonstrate little intrinsic contrast because of the small variations (approximately 10%) in proton density for most tissues.

–Flow can also affect image contrast and is the basis for MR angiography.

–Image contrast can be modified by the administration of contrast agents, such as Gd-DTPA.

C. Signal-to-noise ratio

–The inherent contrast of MR is high because of the large differences in the relaxation properties of different tissues.

–The **SNR** affects the acquired image quality.

–The SNR is increased by increasing slice thickness, decreasing matrix size, and reducing RF bandwidth during signal detection.

–High magnetic-field strength also increases the SNR.

–SNR increases as the square root of the number of image acquisitions: $\sqrt{N_{ex}}$.

–The tradeoff for increased SNR and the resultant improved image quality is an increase in imaging time.

D. Resolution

–The spatial resolution achieved on MR systems is determined by the FOV and data collection matrix size, which is typically between 128^2 and 256^2.

–Pixel size equals the FOV divided by the matrix size and is approximately 1 mm for head images and 1.4 mm for body images.

–MR resolution is about 25% to 50% of that achieved by computed tomography and is generally no better than approximately 0.3 lp/mm.

–Higher resolution can be achieved by using stronger gradients and more phase-encoding steps.

–The tradeoffs for improved resolution include loss of signal intensity and increases in image acquisition time.

E. Chemical shift artifacts

–Artifacts are areas of high or low signal intensity or distortion in the image that can simulate or mask anatomic structures or pathologic conditions.

–**Chemical shift artifacts** are caused by the slight difference in resonance frequency of protons in water and in fat.

–Molecular structure and local magnetic environment differences cause protons in fat and water to have slightly different resonance frequencies.

–This difference is noticeable at fat/water interfaces with high magnetic-field strength and results in misregistration of the signal from the two proton groups.

–Chemical shift artifacts can result in light and dark bands at the edges of the kidney or the margins of vertebral bodies.

–**Fat-suppression** techniques can be used to eliminate unwanted signals from fat in breast and brain imaging.

–Fat-suppression techniques work best on high field systems with good uniformity.

F. Miscellaneous artifacts

–**Patient motion** is common because of the long image acquisition times.

–Patient motion results in **ghost images** that appear in the phase-encode direction because of mismapping of measured signals.

–Cardiac, respiratory gating, or phase reordering can be used to minimize motion artifacts in body imaging.

–Flowing blood and cerebrospinal fluid can also result in MR image artifacts.

–Truncation artifacts in the spinal cord may simulate a syrinx.

–Inhomogeneities in the main magnetic field have a significant impact on GRE and other fast imaging techniques.

–**Wraparound artifact** occurs when the FOV is smaller than the structure, and imaged objects outside the FOV are mapped to the opposite side of the image.

–Wraparound is caused by undersampling (aliasing) and can be corrected by increasing the sampling rate (e.g., increase number of phase-encode steps).

–There are many other sources of MR artifacts, including **truncation, zipper,** and **central point.**

V. Contrast Agents

A. Introduction

–Contrast agents can result in image enhancement in anatomic regions that are perfused by these agents.

–**Paramagnetism, superparamagnetism,** and **ferromagnetism** all act as sources of local magnetic-field inhomogeneity.

–These types of materials produce affect T2* and/or T1, and can be used as contrast agents.

–Contrast agents that reduce T1 more than T2 produce hyperintensity on T1-weighted images and are called **positive contrast agents.**

–Contrast agents that reduce T2 more than T1 produce hypointensity on T2-weighted images and are called **negative contrast agents.**

B. Diamagnetism

–**Magnetic susceptibility** is the extent to which matter becomes magnetized when placed in an external magnetic field *(B)*.

–The local (internal) magnetic field is $B \times (1 + X)$, where X is the susceptibility.

–**Diamagnetic** materials result in small decreases in magnetization relative to the external field and therefore have small **negative values of susceptibility.**

–Most tissues are diamagnetic with a negative X in the range 10^{-4} to 10^{-6}.

–At tissue interfaces, especially between air and bone, changes in magnetic susceptibility result in changes in the local field, which can result in imaging artifacts.

C. Paramagnetism

–Paramagnetism is caused by the presence of **unpaired atomic electrons** or molecular electrons.

–When paramagnetic atoms are placed in an external magnetic field, the local (internal) magnetic field is increased.

–Paramagnetic materials thus have **positive values of susceptibility,** which are typically approximately 10^{-3}.

–Paramagnetism has a much larger effect than diamagnetism and results in an enhancement of the local (internal) field.

–Paramagnetism occurs with chelates of metals such as Cr, Fe, Mn, Co, Ni, Cu, Gd, and Dy, as well as with deoxyhemoglobin.

D. Ferromagnetism

–Ferromagnetism is a property of a **large group of atoms,** whereas diamagnetism and paramagnetism are properties of individual atoms or molecules.

–The group of atoms in ferromagnetic substances is called a **domain.**

–Ferromagnetic substances such as Fe, Ni, and Co have unpaired electrons that are strongly coupled, resulting in large local fields and **high positive susceptibilities.**

–Ferromagnetic materials generally consist of large numbers of domains with relative orientations that depend on the external magnetic fields.

–Ferromagnets may have residual magnetization even after the external field is removed.

E. Superparamagnetism

–Small particles of Fe_3O_4, less than approximately 350 Å and thus consisting of a **single domain,** are termed superparamagnetic.

–When placed in an external magnetic field, superparamagnetic particles develop a strong internal magnetization.

–Superparamagnetism differs from ferromagnetism in that superparamagnets have a single domain, no magnetic memory, and a moderate degree of induced magnetism.

–Superparamagnetic crystals of iron oxide are used for imaging the liver and reticuloendothelial system.

F. Clinical contrast agents

–**Gd-DTPA** is an example of a **paramagnetic contrast agent.**

–Gadolinium has **seven unpaired electrons** with magnetic moments approximately 1,000 times stronger than the proton magnetic moment.

–Gadolinium acts as a relaxation agent of nearby protons and reduces T1 significantly and T2 slightly. The overall effect is highly dependent on the concentration of gadolinium.

–Contrast agents under investigation include complexes of transition elements and rare earth elements such as Fe and Mn.

–Contrast agents are useful for evaluating blood-brain barrier breakdown and renal lesions.

VI. Advanced Techniques

A. Flow effects

–Flowing blood changes position between excitation by the RF pulses and signal reception, resulting in signal void on SE images.

–The opposite phenomenon is known as **flow enhancement,** which occurs when unsaturated protons enter the first section and generate a greater signal intensity than stationary, partially saturated tissues.

–Depending on the sequences used, signal is affected by the direction, speed, and pattern of blood flow.

–The presence of unsaturated protons from fluid moving perpendicular to the image slice will make these materials appear bright.

–The degree of enhancement depends on the TR, slice thickness, and flow velocity.

B. Magnetic resonance angiography

–Noninvasive MR angiography is quickly being established in the clinical setting.

–MR angiographic techniques include time-of-flight and phase-contrast.

–**Time-of-flight** techniques rely on bright signal from unsaturated protons in flowing blood entering the imaging section.

–**Phase-contrast** techniques use bipolar gradients to produce phase changes in moving blood.

–The surrounding tissues, which are stationary, exhibit no net phase change.

–The phase change is related to the time between bipolar gradients and flow velocity, which provides a correlation between signal intensity and blood flow velocity.

–MR angiographic images are produced by projecting the stack of sections onto a single 2D image because display of tortuous blood vessels is inadequate on thin-section images.

–A common display technique is **maximum intensity projection (MIP).**

–MR angiography is useful in patients who cannot tolerate iodinated contrast agents.

C. Echo planar imaging and diffusion-weighted imaging

–**Echo planar imaging (EPI)** uses rapidly switching gradients to refocus echoes.

–Frequency-encode gradients that rapidly change polarities are paired with an applied phase-encode gradient.

–EPI can generate MR images in 50 milliseconds but with limited resolution (64^2 or 128^2 matrix).

–Special high gradients between 20 and 60 mT/m (2 and 6 G/cm) are required to perform EPI.

–Diffusion depends on the random motion of water molecules in tissues.

–Structural integrity of tissues can be assessed by **diffusion-weighted imaging (DWI).**

–Water diffusion characteristics can be displayed using **apparent diffusion coefficient** maps.

   –Apparent diffusion coefficient maps of the spine can evaluate pathophysiology, and DWI is used to detect ischemic injury.

   –Apparent diffusion coefficient maps are also useful in the early detection of stroke.

–Standard SE and EPI pulse sequences with diffusion gradients are used in DWI.

   –One limitation of DWI is sensitivity to motion, which can be minimized by the use of electrocardiographic gating and other motion compensation methods.

D. Magnetization transfer

–**Magnetization transfer contrast (MTC)** techniques modulate image contrast by saturating a pool of protons in macromolecules and their associated bound water.

–Narrow-band RF pulses, shifted slightly away from the water resonance frequency, are used to selectively excite the protons in macromolecules.

–Some of this magnetization is transferred from the macromolecules to water. These water molecules, which have a reduced signal intensity, are then imaged using reduced conventional MR pulse sequences.

–MTC is useful in reducing background signal in MR angiography and can also have applications in breast imaging.

E. Magnetic resonance spectroscopy

–**MR spectroscopy** makes use of the slight difference in resonance frequency of protons or other nuclei bound in different molecular structures.

–^{1}H and ^{31}P are the nuclei most often used for *in vivo* spectroscopy.

–Phosphorus spectroscopy can be used to evaluate cellular metabolism by identifying the relative concentration of inorganic phosphate, phosphocreatine, and adenosine triphosphate.

–MR spectroscopy requires a stronger and more uniform field than conventional hydrogen imaging.

–A typical minimum voxel size used in MR spectroscopic studies is approximately 1 cm^3 for ^{1}H and 8 cm^3 for ^{31}P.

F. Functional imaging

–**Functional imaging** relies on local blood flow and blood oxygenation changes in the brain associated with activation of visual, motor, auditory, or other brain system.

–Cerebral stimulation of specific regions of the brain increases local venous blood oxygenation. This enhances the detected MR signal intensity from regions with increased blood flow.

   –Functional images are obtained from the difference of images obtained before and during the cerebral activity.

–Functional imaging maps the areas of cerebral stimulation with better temporal and spatial resolution than positron emission tomography.

–Functional imaging is best performed at high field strengths (1.5 T or higher) using EPI or other fast techniques.

–Functional imaging is becoming a powerful tool in brain research.

Review Test

1. Which would *not* be useful for medical MR imaging?

(A) ^{1}H
(B) ^{13}C
(C) ^{16}O
(D) ^{23}Na
(E) ^{31}P

2. The Larmor frequency is the frequency of:

(A) Pulse repetition
(B) Nuclear precession
(C) Phase encoding
(D) Spatial encoding
(E) Gradient switching

3. The resonance frequency for ^{1}H in a 1.5 T magnetic field is:

(A) 63 H$_3$
(B) 63 kH$_3$
(C) 63 MH$_3$
(D) 63 GH$_3$
(E) 63 TH$_3$

4. The maximum MR signal is obtained by using a:

(A) 90 degree RF tip, short TE, and short TR
(B) 45 degree RF tip, short TE, and short TR
(C) 90 degree RF tip, short TE, and long TR
(D) 90 degree RF tip, long TE, and short TR
(E) 45 degree RF tip, long TE, and short TR

5. For most tissues, which of the following is *false*?

(A) T1 is of the order of a few seconds.
(B) T2 is of the order of tens of milliseconds.
(C) T2 is relatively independent of field strength.
(D) T1 increases as field strength increases.
(E) T1 and T2 often increase with malignancy.

6. The small amount of bound water produces no detected MR signal because:

(A) T1 is too short
(B) T2 is too short
(C) T2* is very long
(D) T2 is longer than T1
(E) T2* is longer than T2

7. For most biological tissues, T2 is:

(A) Less than T1
(B) More than T1
(C) Less than T2*
(D) More than 100 milliseconds
(E) Less than 5 milliseconds

8. MR "shimming" is used to:

(A) Minimize noise in RF coils
(B) Correct for magnetic-field inhomogeneities
(C) Reduce the noise level in MR systems
(D) Minimize the possibility of quenches
(E) Increase signal phase

9. The superconducting magnets used in MR normally have:

(A) No magnetic-field inhomogeneities
(B) Water cooling to dissipate heat production
(C) Coils with alternating electric currents
(D) Magnetic fields perpendicular to the bore axis
(E) Liquid helium coolant

10. Gradient fields in MR are used most commonly to:

(A) Increase T2
(B) Shorten T1 values
(C) Localize MR signal source
(D) Increase signal in large patients
(E) Reduce electronic noise

11. Which of the following is generally acceptable for MR at 1.5 T?

(A) Cochlear implants
(B) Pacemakers
(C) Ferromagnetic aneurysm clips
(D) Claustrophobic patients
(E) Pregnant patients

12. Which line is an exclusion zone for persons with pacemakers?

(A) 0.5 G
(B) 5 G
(C) 50 G
(D) 500 G
(E) Over 500 G

13. Safety concerns for 1.5 T MR include all of the following *except:*

(A) Fringe magnetic fields
(B) Electrical stimulation neurons
(C) RF heating effects
(D) Ferromagnetic surgical slips in patients

(E) Flying metallic objects

14. The FDA limit on power deposition in patients undergoing MR does *not* include:

(A) 3.2 W/kg averaged over the head
(B) 8 W/kg peak value
(C) 0.4 W/kg averaged over body
(D) A less than 3°C temperature rise in the heart
(E) A less than 1°C core body temperature rise

15. The most common reconstruction method for MR units is:

(A) 2DFT
(B) 3DFT
(C) Algebraic reconstruction
(D) Back projection
(E) Filtered back projection

16. Which does not generally affect the total patient examination time in MR?

(A) Read encode matrix size
(B) Number of phase-encoding steps
(C) Number of pulse sequences used
(D) Acquisitions (N_{ex})
(E) TR

17. In spin-echo imaging, the echo signal normally is measured:

(A) Immediately ($t = 0$)
(B) After time TE
(C) After time $4 \times T1$
(D) After time T2
(E) After time TR

18. In IR sequences, the TI value is the time:

(A) Of the complete scan
(B) To the interval echo
(C) Between successive 90 degree pulses
(D) Between successive 180 degree pulses
(E) Between an initial 180 degree and subsequent 90 degree pulse

19. Increased signal intensity in MR *cannot* arise as a result of:

(A) Short T1
(B) Long T2
(C) Flow effects
(D) Spin density
(E) Dephasing effects

20. MR SNR cannot be improved by increasing the:

(A) Matrix size
(B) Number of acquisitions
(C) Static magnetic-field strength

(D) Section thickness
(E) RF coil sensitivity

21. Chemical shift artifacts are caused by:

(A) Different resonant frequencies of ^{1}H in water and fat
(B) Foreign chemicals agents in the patient
(C) Magnetic-field gradients
(D) Contrast agents
(E) Spin-lattice interactions

22. In MR, motion results in ghost images that appear in which direction?

(A) Read encode
(B) Phase encode
(C) Slice selection axis
(D) PA
(E) Lateral

23. All of the following are MR artifacts *except:*

(A) Chemical shift
(B) Bounce point
(C) Zipper
(D) Susceptibility
(E) Reverberation

24. Superparamagnetic materials are *not:*

(A) Small particles (smaller than 350 Å)
(B) Single domains
(C) Strongly magnetic
(D) Related to ferromagnetic materials
(E) Superconductors

25. Contrast in MR can be due to all the following differences *except:*

(A) Presence of flow
(B) Proton density
(C) T1
(D) Atomic number
(E) T2

26. Proton relaxation by Gd-DTPA is owing mainly to the effect of the:

(A) Gadolinium nucleus
(B) DTPA
(C) Unpaired gadolinium electrons
(D) Gadolinium K-edge energy
(E) K-shell electrons

27. Common MR angiography techniques are based on:

(A) Phase contrast
(B) Phase encoding
(C) T1 contrast

(D) Time to inversion
(E) FSE imaging

28. EPI generally requires all of the following *except:*

(A) Gradient-recalled echoes
(B) Gradients between 20 and 60 mT/m
(C) Rapid gradient switching
(D) High magnetic fields
(E) Rapid repetition of 180 degree RF pulses

29. MR spectroscopy is used to detect all the following except:

(A) ^{31}P

(B) ^{32}P
(C) Inorganic phosphate
(D) Phosphocreatinine
(E) adenosine triphosphate

30. Functional imaging using magnetic resonance does *not* show:

(A) Brain activation sites
(B) Increased venous oxygenation
(C) Increased spin density sites
(D) Superior temporal resolution to positron emission tomography (PET)
(E) superior spatial resolution to PET

Answers and Explanations

1–C. ^{16}O is an example of an even-even nucleus (eight neutrons and eight protons), which has no magnetic moment and thus cannot be used for MR.

2–B. Magnetic nuclei precess at the Larmor frequency when placed into a magnetic field.

3–C. 63 MHz.

4–C. Maximum signal strength is obtained by using a 90 degree pulse to maximize the magnetization in the transverse plane, starting with the maximum longitudinal magnetization (i.e., long TR) and minimizing dephasing (i.e., short TE).

5–A. T1 is of the order of hundreds of milliseconds, not a few seconds.

6–B. The T2 is too short (microseconds) to give rise to a detected signal from all solids including bone.

7–A. T2 is generally of the order of tens of milliseconds, whereas T1 is on the order of hundreds of milliseconds.

8–B. Shimming is used to reduce field inhomogeneities to a few parts per million.

9–E. Superconductors normally require liquid helium coolant.

10–C. Gradients define the MR image plane and are used for frequency and phase encoding to determine the spatial origin of the detected signals.

11–E. Pregnant patients can undergo MR scans (no ionizing radiation).

12–B. Areas with magnetic fields greater than 5 G (0.5 mT) should be restricted to individuals with pacemaker implants.

13–B. For magnetic-field strengths below 2 T, the effect of magnetic field–induced electrical potentials in neurons has not been observed.

14–D. There are no specific temperature rise limits set for the heart by the FDA in MR.

15–A. 2DFT is standard on virtually all commercial MR units.

16–A. The number of pixels in the read-direction is related only to the number of samples in FID acquired and will not affect image acquisition time.

17–B. A phase-refocusing 180 degree pulse is applied at time TE/2, which results in an echo at time TE.

18–E. An IR sequence starts with a 180 degree inversion pulse followed by a 90 degree readout pulse after time TI.

19–E. Dephasing effects always reduce signal intensities (they may increase contrast, but not signal intensity per se).

20–A. Increasing the matrix size will not increase SNR but will reduce the SNR per pixel.

21–A. Chemical shift artifacts arise because of the slightly differing resonance frequencies of proton in different molecules.

22–B. Motion usually appears as a series of ghost images of reduced intensity displaced in the phase-encoding direction.

23–E. Reverberation artifacts occur in ultrasound.

24–E. Superparamagnetism has no relation to superconductivity.

25–D. Atomic number *(Z)* does not give rise to image contrast in MR but does give rise to image contrast in x-ray imaging.

26–C. The seven unpaired electrons in Gd result in the relaxation of adjacent nuclei.

27–A. Phase-contrast and time-of-flight are the two common methods used in MR angiography.

28–E. No MR sequences require a rapid set of RF pulses.

29–B. ^{32}P is a radioactive beta emitter used as a tracer in biomedical research, as is not used for MR spectroscopy.

30–C. Functional MR has no direction relation to spin density.

EXAMINATION GUIDE

Education is what survives when what has been learnt has been forgotten.
–*B.F. Skinner*

Following are two practice examinations, each consisting of 120 questions and answers. These questions cover all the material summarized in this book, with the first 10 questions pertaining to Chapter 1, the second 10 questions to Chapter 2, and so on. The examinations provided should be taken without consulting textbooks, with a single practice examination requiring no more than 2 hours. Taking practice examinations under realistic test conditions serves several useful purposes, including the following:

Practice for the real examination. Taking these practice examinations will enable you to learn whether you are taking too long to read and answer questions. It is also an excellent opportunity for you to develop a strategy for dealing with difficult questions, such as guessing *after* eliminating all "wrong" answers or by temporarily skipping difficult questions and returning to complete them at a later time.

Highlighting areas of weakness. Once the examinations have been completed, you should have a very good idea of your areas of weakness. Weaknesses should be corrected by consulting the appropriate chapter in this review book or, if greater depth is required, by reading an appropriate textbook.

Building confidence. Successful completion of the examinations demonstrates that the material has been satisfactorily covered, which may help to ease any preexamination nervousness.

It is recommended that you first read the appropriate material in selected textbooks to ensure sufficient knowledge of the subject. You should then review the material in each chapter of this book and answer the appended questions. Having completed these steps, you should be ready to take these mock examinations. The following is a list of guidelines for successfully completing examinations.

1. *Read and follow all examination instructions.*
2. Read each question *carefully.*
3. Do not assume information; focus on key words (e.g., almost, never, most, not).
4. Eliminate obviously incorrect answers and focus on remaining answers.
5. Do not spend more than 2 minutes on any question.
6. Check the time every 30 minutes.
7. Should time permit, reread the questions and verify your answers.
8. Answer *all* questions, even if you have to guess; you have nothing to lose but you may gain.

A1. Which of the following is *not* an example of a fundamental type of force in nature?

(A) Gravitational
(B) Electrostatic
(C) Weak
(D) Electric current
(E) Strong

A2. Which quantity measures power?

(A) Joule
(B) Erg
(C) Watt
(D) Electron-volt
(E) Newton

A3. Which of the following refers to the total number of nucleons in the nucleus of an atom?

(A) Mass number
(B) Atomic number
(C) Avogadro's number
(D) Atomic mass unit
(E) Nucleon binding energy

A4. Which element has an atomic number of 56 and a K-shell binding energy of 37 keV?

(A) Calcium
(B) Iodine
(C) Barium
(D) Tungsten
(E) Lead

A5. The electron binding energy is:

(A) independent of the electron distance from the nucleus
(B) independent of the nuclear charge
(C) several MeV
(D) overcome for the electron to be ejected from the atom
(E) a result of the strong interaction

A6. All of the following are examples of electromagnetic radiation except:

(A) Radio waves
(B) Visible light
(C) Ultraviolet
(D) X-rays
(E) Cosmic radiation

A7. Ionizing radiations include all of the following *except:*

(A) photons
(B) electrons
(C) neutrons
(D) alpha particles
(E) pulsed ultrasound waves

A8. Which is *not* true regarding radioactivity?

(A) The curie is a non-SI unit.
(B) One curie is 7.3×10^7 disintegrations per second.
(C) The curie is based on the activity of 1 g of ^{226}Ra.
(D) One becquerel is equal to 1 transformation per second.
(E) One mCi is 37 MBq.

A9. Which of the following particles has no rest mass?

(A) Electron
(B) Positron
(C) Proton
(D) Alpha particle
(E) Photon

A10. Electron capture does not:

(A) result in the emission of a neutrino
(B) can compete with positron emission
(C) result in characteristic x-ray emission
(D) result in Auger electron emission
(E) Result in internal conversion electron emission

A11. A typical x-ray generator has a power level of about:

(A) 0.1 kW
(B) 1 kW
(C) 10 kW
(D) 100 kW
(E) more than 100 kW

A12. Transformers in x-ray tubes do not use:

(A) electromagnetic induction
(B) mechanical motion
(C) alternating current
(D) oil for insulation
(E) primary and secondary circuits

A13. 90 keV electrons striking a tungsten target lose energy mainly by:

(A) characteristic x-ray production
(B) bremsstrahlung x-ray production
(C) excitation and ionization of K-shell electrons
(D) excitation and ionization of *outer*-shell electrons
(E) photoelectric effect

A14. Increasing the x-ray tube voltage (kVp) will *not* increase:

(A) x-ray beam intensity
(B) patient penetration
(C) x-ray beam half-value layer
(D) x-ray beam filtration
(E) heat produced in the anode

A15. 100 keV electrons incident on a tungsten target can produce:

(A) bremsstrahlung x-rays with a maximum energy of 100 keV
(B) bremsstrahlung x-rays with an average energy of 100 keV
(C) characteristic x-rays of 100 keV
(D) 1% energy deposition (heat) in the target
(E) 100 keV photoelectrons

A16. The maximum photon energy in x-ray beams is determined by the:

(A) atomic number of the target
(B) atomic number of the filament
(C) voltage across the filament
(D) voltage between anode and cathode
(E) tube current

A17. At 65 kV and a tungsten target, what amount of the x-rays is from K shell characteristic x-rays?

(A) 0%
(B) 1%
(C) 10%
(D) 50%
(E) 99%

A18. Tungsten ($Z = 74$) is used for the x-ray target rather than lower-Z materials because:

(A) higher energy x-rays are produced
(B) the intensity of the resulting x-ray beam is high
(C) there is no characteristic radiation from tungsten
(D) x-rays are preferentially emitted at 90 degrees
(E) the heel effect is minimized

A19. A constant potential generator operated at 100 kV and 1,000 mA for 0.1 second deposits:

(A) 1,000 heat units
(B) 1,350 heat units
(C) 10,000 heat units
(D) 13,500 heat units
(E) 100,000 heat units

A20. The heel effect is more pronounced:

(A) further from the focal spot
(B) with a large focal spot
(C) with a small cassette
(D) with a small target angle
(E) near the central axis

A21. After photoelectric interactions, the following emission *cannot* occur.

(A) Photoelectrons
(B) Scattered photons
(C) K-characteristic x-rays
(D) Auger electrons
(E) L-characteristic x-rays

A22. Backscattered photons in fluoroscopy are most likely caused by:

(A) compton scatter
(B) isomeric transitions
(C) coherent interactions
(D) k-shell interactions
(E) photodisintegration interactions

A23. In water, the photoelectric and Compton effects are equal at what energy?

(A) 0.5 keV
(B) 4 keV
(C) 25 keV
(D) 69.5 keV
(E) 88 keV

A24. In diagnostic radiology, the attenuation does *not* increase with increasing:

(A) mass density (ρ)
(B) atomic number (Z)
(C) photon energy
(D) thickness
(E) electron density

A25. Three tenth-value layers have approximately the same attenuation as how many half-value layers?

(A) 5
(B) 10
(C) 15
(D) 20
(E) 25

A26. The x-ray beam HVL does *not* depend on the:

(A) radiation intensity
(B) tube voltage
(C) voltage waveform
(D) filtration
(E) anode material

A27. Decreasing x-ray beam filtration generally results in increased:

(A) maximum photon energy
(B) average photon energy
(C) entrance skin exposure
(D) importance of the Compton effect
(E) patient penetration

A28. All the following are related to exposure *except:*

(A) linear energy transfer (LET)
(B) ability to ionize air
(C) ionization chambers
(D) roentgen
(E) output of an x-ray tube

A29. The f-factor, which converts exposure to absorbed dose, is generally:

(A) independent of photon energy
(B) independent of atomic number *(Z)*
(C) much greater than 1.0 at high photon energy levels
(D) about 4 for bone for diagnostic x-rays
(E) numerically the same in SI and non-SI units

A30. A Geiger-Muller detector would be best employed to:

(A) detect low-level ^{99m}Tc contamination
(B) measure the output of an x-ray tube
(C) monitor patient exposures
(D) estimate a skin dose
(E) measure x-ray leakage exposure

A31. Reducing the film processor temperature from 95° to 90°F will likely increase:

(A) contrast
(B) fog
(C) quantum mottle
(D) screen blur
(E) patient dose

A32. Using a screen/film combination rather than film on its own will *not* reduce:

(A) patient dose
(B) x-ray tube loading
(C) patient motion artifacts

(D) exposure times
(E) image contrast

A33. Absorption of a 30 keV photon by a screen with a 10% conversion efficiency will emit how many blue 3 eV light photons?

(A) 1
(B) 10
(C) 100
(D) 1,000
(E) 10,000

A34. X-ray grids are designed to attenuate mainly:

(A) Compton scatter
(B) Coherent scatter
(C) Backscatter
(D) Characteristic x-rays
(E) Annihilation photons

A35. Which examination would most likely be performed without a scatter removal grid?

(A) Extremity radiography
(B) Skull x-ray
(C) Abdomen radiography
(D) Portable abdomen
(E) Fluoroscopy

A36. The photocathode of an image intensifier converts:

(A) electrons to light
(B) x-rays to light
(C) x-rays to electrons
(D) electrons to x-rays
(E) light to electrons

A37. If the image intensifier output brightness is 20 cd/m^2, the input exposure rate is most likely about:

(A) 0.1 μGy/s (10 μR/s)
(B) 1 μGy/s (100 μR/s)
(C) 10 μGy/s (1 mR/s)
(D) 100 μGy/s (10 mR/s)
(E) 1 mGy/s (100 mR/s)

A38. The limiting spatial resolution in fluoroscopy can be improved by increasing the:

(A) grid ratio
(B) image intensifier input size
(C) radiation dose level
(D) tube voltage
(E) number of TV lines

A39. All are image intensifier artifacts *except:*

(A) LAG
(B) beam hardening
(C) pin cushion distortion
(D) vignetting
(E) veiling glare

A40. A noisy fluoroscopic image is most likely to be improved by increasing the:

(A) focal spot size
(B) x-ray beam filtration
(C) grid ratio
(D) exposure level
(E) monitor gain

A41. Subject contrast depends on:

(A) kVp
(B) tube current (mA)
(C) type of film
(D) development time and temperature
(E) film density

A42. Film contrast, as opposed to *subject* contrast, is affected primarily by the:

(A) kVp
(B) beam filtration
(C) presence of contrast agents (iodine, barium)
(D) tissue density differences
(E) film optical density level

A43. Films with high contrast *cannot* have:

(A) low fog
(B) low noise
(C) wide latitude
(D) high speed
(E) high resolution

A44. Limiting spatial resolution in contact radiography can be improved by reducing the:

(A) focal spot size
(B) tube voltage
(C) filtration
(D) grid ratio
(E) screen thickness

A45. The likely cause for the left lung being consistently blurry on a chest radiographs is:

(A) patient motion
(B) enlarged focal spot
(C) film/screen contact
(D) incorrect screen thickness
(E) bad rollers in processor

A46. The MTF of a fluoroscopy imaging system is primarily determined by the:

(A) focal spot
(B) input phosphor
(C) output phosphor
(D) optical lens
(E) TV system

A47. If an average of 10,000 photons are detected per mm^2, the chance of detecting between 9,700 and 10,300 counts in any exposed mm^2 is:

(A) 67%
(B) 90%
(C) 95%
(D) 99%
(E) Insufficient data to perform calculation

A48. Increasing the sensitivity will normally result in an increase in the:

(A) area under the receiver operator characteristic curve
(B) false-positive fraction
(C) specificity
(D) accuracy
(E) true negative fraction

A49. During fluoroscopy the typical patient entrance skin exposure rate is:

(A) less than 2 μGy/minute (0.2 mR/minute)
(B) 2 μGy/minute (0.2 mR/minute)
(C) 20 μGy/minute (2 mR/minute)
(D) 200 μGy/minute (20 mR/minute)
(E) more than 200 μGy/minute (20 mR/minute)

A50. The medical genetically significant dose is:

(A) likely to cause genetic defects
(B) an estimate of an individual's genetic risk
(C) a population index of potential genetic damage
(D) about 3 mSv/year
(E) increasing steeply

A51. Basic computation in a computer is performed by the:

(A) random access memory (RAM)
(B) read-only memory (ROM)
(C) central processing unit (CPU)
(D) small computer system interface (SCSI)
(E) dynamic RAM (DRAM)

A52. Which statement is true regarding computer memory?

(A) RAM is used for permanent memory.
(B) Buffer memory is used for temporary storage.

(C) Floppy disks hold more data than do hard disks.
(D) Magnetic tapes have access times shorter than 1 millisecond.
(E) Optical jukeboxes cannot store more than 1 GB.

A53. A computed tomography examination (512^2 matrix, 2 bytes per pixel), consisting of 20 images, involves:

(A) less than 1 MB
(B) 2 MB
(C) 5 MB
(D) 8 MB
(E) over 8 MB

A54. What is the pixel size if a 256^2 matrix is used to image a 25 cm wide field?

(A) 0.1 mm
(B) 0.5 mm
(C) 1 mm
(D) 2 mm
(E) Greater than 2 mm

A55. Which of the following is *not* used to detect x-rays?

(A) Photoconductor
(B) Scintillating crystal
(C) Charged couple device
(D) Photostimulable phosphor
(E) Screen phosphor

A56. In comparison with a medium-speed screen/film system, the speed of a computed radiography (CR) system is:

(A) less than 100
(B) 100
(C) 200
(D) 400
(E) indeterminate

A57. The typical luminance of soft copy display monitors in a diagnostic workstation is:

(A) below 10 cd/m^2
(B) 10 cd/m^2
(C) 100 cd/m^2
(D) 1,000 cd/m^2
(E) over 1,000 cd/m^2

A58. Lesion visibility in a digital radiograph would best be improved by increasing the:

(A) kVp
(B) exposure time
(C) filtration
(D) contrast-to-noise ratio
(E) display luminance

A59. A typical technique for digital subtraction angiography would *not* include:

(A) 75 kVp
(B) 200 mA
(C) 50 millisecond exposure
(D) 3 frames/second
(E) 256^2 matrix size

A60. Which of the following has the highest data transmission rate?

(A) Modem
(B) Ethernet
(C) Token ring
(D) Fiber distributed data interface
(E) Asynchronous transfer mode

A61. Calcifications are seen on mammograms *primarily* because of their:

(A) atomic number
(B) physical density
(C) electrons density
(D) size
(E) breast location

A62. Molybdenum, and not tungsten, is the mammography target because it has:

(A) higher melting point
(B) higher efficiency for x-ray production
(C) characteristic x-rays of about 18 keV
(D) less high-voltage arcing
(E) less leakage radiation

A63. Grids in mammography can increase all the following *except:*

(A) breast dose
(B) image contrast
(C) x-ray tube loading
(D) object contrast
(E) exposure time

A64. Grids in screen/film mammography do *not:*

(A) improve contrast
(B) increase the radiation dose
(C) have grid ratios of about 5:1
(D) improve spatial resolution
(E) increased mAs used

A65. Mammography resolution can be reduced by all *except:*

(A) thick screens
(B) large focal spot
(C) no breast compression
(D) slower film
(E) dual screen cassettes

A66. Magnification mammography requires:

(A) reduced kVp
(B) high ratio grids
(C) increased exposure time
(D) high-resolution film
(E) higher film densities

A67. Breast average glandular tissue dose does not depend on:

(A) breast thickness
(B) half-value layer
(C) kVp
(D) mAs
(E) source-to-image distance

A68. American College of Radiology (ACR) accreditation of breast imaging centers involves all the following except:

(A) documentation of a quality-control program
(B) assessment of image quality using a phantom
(C) independent evaluation of clinical images
(D) weekly measurement of kVp
(E) annual evaluations by a medical physicist

A69. Advantages of MR for breast imaging include all of the following except:

(A) no ionizing radiation
(B) three-dimensional imaging
(C) fat suppression
(D) spatial resolution comparable to screen/film
(E) excellent soft tissue contrast

A70. All the following are true of light diaphanography for breast imaging except:

(A) involves detection of light
(B) has been associated with poor clinical results
(C) has a problem with too much light scatter
(D) primarily detects increases in vascularity
(E) has radiation doses higher than mammography

A71. A material with an attenuation 5% greater than that of water has a Hounsfield unit value of:

(A) −50
(B) −5
(C) +5
(D) +50
(E) +500

A72. The common reconstruction algorithm for computed tomography (CT) is:

(A) two-dimensional Fourier transform (2DFT)
(B) three-dimensional Fourier transform (3DFT)
(C) algebraic (ART)

(D) iterative summation
(E) filtered back projection

A73. For a CT window width of 1,000 and a window center of 500, which CT numbers appear black?

(A) Greater than 500
(B) Less than 500
(C) Greater than 500
(D) Less than 0
(E) Less than 1,000

A74. The collimators of a CT scanner are not designed to:

(A) reduce scatter into the detectors
(B) determine one dimension of the voxel
(C) be located near the x-ray tube and the detectors
(D) be variable for different slice thicknesses
(E) improve in plane spatial resolution

A75. Increasing the CT image matrix from 256^2 to 512^2 can be expected to increase the:

(A) patient throughput
(B) x-ray tube loading
(C) patient dose
(D) limiting spatial resolution
(E) film printing time

A76. Detecting large, low-contrast objects by CT is affected by all of the following *except:*

(A) focal spot size
(B) mA
(C) slice thickness
(D) scan time
(E) reconstruction filter

A77. Increasing the kVp at a constant mAs in CT scanning generally reduces:

(A) anode loading
(B) subject contrast
(C) partial volume effects
(D) reconstruction time
(E) spatial resolution

A78. Use of intravascular contrast in CT will significantly increase the:

(A) Hounsfield units of blood vessels
(B) required kVp
(C) required mA
(D) patient radiation dose
(E) image noise

A79. Which of the following artifacts does *not* appear in CT images?

(A) Motion artifacts
(B) Phase-encoding artifacts
(C) Streak artifacts
(D) Ring artifacts
(E) Beam-hardening artifacts

A80. The typical dose to the eye lens from a CT scan of the head is:

(A) <0.4 mGy (<40 mrad)
(B) 0.4 mGy (40 mrad)
(C) 4 mGy (400 mrad)
(D) 40 mGy (4 rad)
(E) >40 mGy (>4 mrad)

A81. Which radionuclide has a primary photopeak energy of 365 keV?

(A) Oxygen 15
(B) Technetium 99m
(C) Iodine 131
(D) Thallium 201
(E) Fluorine 18

A82. An ideal therapeutic radionuclide would *not* have:

(A) high uptake in the organ of interest
(B) high-energy beta decay
(C) high-energy gamma rays
(D) a long biologic half-life in the organ of interest
(E) rapid blood clearance

A83. The exposure by a week-old ^{99m}Tc generator depends on all of the following *except* the:

(A) initial activity of ^{99}Mo
(B) number of times the generator was milked
(C) amount of Pb shielding around the generator
(D) amount of ^{99}Mo remaining
(E) distance from the generator

A84. The sensitivity of a gamma camera can be improved by increasing the:

(A) photomultiplier tube gain
(B) distance to the patient
(C) collimator thickness
(D) collimator hole diameter
(E) septal thickness

A85. In photomultiplier tubes, energy is converted from:

(A) x-rays to electrons
(B) light to electrons
(C) gamma rays to electrons
(D) electrons to light
(E) light to gamma rays

A86. Increasing the distance between the patient and a parallel hole collimator results in:

(A) reduced resolution
(B) reduced field of view
(C) increased patient dose
(D) image distortion
(E) increased sensitivity

A87. Parallel hole collimator resolution improves with increased collimator:

(A) hole size
(B) thickness
(C) diameter
(D) distance to patient
(E) sensitivity

A88. Pixel values in single positron emission computed tomography (SPECT) images represent:

(A) densities
(B) absorption factors
(C) attenuation factors
(D) radioisotope concentrations
(E) projection data

A89. Advantages of PET over SPECT imaging include all of the following *except:*

(A) shorter imaging time
(B) better resolution
(C) lower image noise
(D) rapid radiopharmaceutical decay
(E) much lower patient doses

A90. The biological half-life of a radionuclide depends on the:

(A) physical decay mode
(B) administered activity
(C) biological clearance
(D) physical half-life
(E) efficiency of detection system

A91. The radiation weighting factor (w_R) is used to convert:

(A) rems to sieverts
(B) absorbed dose to equivalent dose
(C) linear energy transfer to relative biological effectiveness
(D) exposure to absorbed dose
(E) Kerma to absorbed dose

A92. After an acute whole body dose of 1 Gy (100 rad), which is likely to be observed?

(A) Erythema
(B) Diarrhea
(C) Reduced lymphocyte count

(D) Permanent sterility
(E) Death within 60 days

A93. The chance of a radiation-induced cataract after four head CT examinations is about:

(A) 0%
(B) 0.2%
(C) 1%
(D) 5%
(E) over 5%

A94. Radiation doses in diagnostic radiology are likely to result in a significant:

(A) increase of temperature
(B) number of chromosome breaks
(C) production of ionization
(D) number of cell membranes broken
(E) number of cells killed

A95. A fetal radiation dose of 10 mGy (1 rad):

(A) is very unlikely during any diagnostic examination
(B) is less than annual natural background
(C) could occur during 1 minute of fluoroscopy
(D) would need a therapeutic abortion
(E) could kill the fetus

A96. Regulatory dose limits for a technologist include doses from:

(A) Chernobyl disaster
(B) high-altitude airplane flight
(C) domestic radon
(D) screening mammograms
(E) occupational exposure

A97. The ALARA concept requires that design of an x-ray facility should ensure all except:

(A) doses be as low as reasonably achievable
(B) unnecessary exposures be avoided
(C) account taken of social and economic factors
(D) patient doses be minimized
(E) patient doses do not exceed 50 mSv (5 rem)

A98. If both occupancy factor and workload are doubled, personnel doses are likely to:

(A) be halved
(B) stay the same
(C) double
(D) triple
(E) quadruple

A99. At 1 meter, the x-ray tube leakage should be less than:

(A) 10 μGy/hour (1 mR/hour)
(B) 30 μGy/hour (3 mR/hour)

(C) 0.1 mGy/hour (10 mR/hour)
(D) 0.3 mGy/hour (30 mR/hour)
(E) 1 mGy/hour (100 mR/hour)

A100. Which particle is emitted in the decay of ^{222}Rn (radon)?

(A) Proton
(B) Alpha particle
(C) Neutrino
(D) Beta particle
(E) 140 keV photon

A101. Which material has the highest ultrasound propagation velocity?

(A) Air
(B) Fat
(C) Soft tissue
(D) Bone
(E) Metal

A102. Acoustical impedance (Z) is:

(A) density × velocity of sound
(B) linearly dependent on frequency
(C) velocity divided by medium density
(D) transducer electrical resistance
(E) computed using Snell's Law

A103. Signal attenuation in ultrasound is *not:*

(A) normally measured in decibels
(B) very high in the lung
(C) proportional to frequency
(D) about 1 dB/cm at 1 MHz in soft tissue
(E) dependent on the intensity

A 104. The largest ultrasound reflections occur between:

(A) kidney and water
(B) brain and water
(C) water and muscle
(D) blood and brain
(E) fat and kidney

A105. The resonant frequency of an ultrasound transducer is determined primarily by the:

(A) crystal thickness
(B) refraction law (Snell's law)
(C) Q factor
(D) applied voltage
(E) acoustic impedence

A106. The Q factor of a transducer is all the following *except:*

(A) the maximum transducer intensity
(B) a measure of the frequency purity

(C) high for continuous-wave Doppler
(D) low for short pulse lengths
(E) operating frequency divided by bandwidth

A107. How long will it take to receive the ultrasound echo from an object 10 cm away?

(A) 1.3 μs
(B) 13 μs
(C) 130 μs
(D) 1.3 ms
(E) 13 ms

A108. Clinical ultrasound beams can have all the following *except:*

(A) frequencies of several MHz
(B) velocities of 1540 m/second in tissue
(C) wavelengths of about 0.5 mm
(D) pulse repetition frequencies (PRF) of 100 kHz
(E) pulses that contain only a few wavelengths

A109. Ultrasound with a short pulse length is most likely to result in improved:

(A) axial resolution
(B) fresnel zone length
(C) echo intensity
(D) tissue penetration
(E) pulse repetition frequency

A110. Cavitation is most likely to occur at:

(A) frequencies above 10 MHz
(B) depths beyond the Fresnel zone
(C) low pulse repetition frequencies
(D) interfaces with large acoustic impedance differences
(E) high ultrasound intensities

A111. Which of the following nuclei have *not* been used in biomedical MR?

(A) ^{2}H
(B) ^{19}F
(C) ^{23}Na
(D) ^{31}P
(E) ^{40}K

A112. After 90 degree radiofrequency (RF) pulses, spins lose their phase coherence in a time most comparable to:

(A) T1
(B) T2
(C) TE
(D) TI
(E) TR

A113. Which of the following is *unlikely* to affect the MR signal intensity?

(A) Proton spin density
(B) Atomic number (Z)
(C) T1 relaxation time
(D) T2 relaxation time
(E) Blood flow

A114. The magnetic field of resistive MR magnets is normally limited by the:

(A) field inhomogeneities
(B) need for shielding
(C) magnet weight
(D) fringe fields
(E) magnet heating

A115. Increasing the main magnetic field will generally increase all of the following *except:*

(A) T1
(B) T2
(C) signal-to-noise ratio
(D) MR imaging system cost
(E) proton resonance frequency

A116. The radiofrequency (RF) coils used in 1 T proton MR imaging do *not:*

(A) use 42 MHz
(B) emit RF pulses
(C) detect RF signals
(D) include quadrature coils
(E) have strengths up to 60 mT/m

A117. The bioeffects of static magnetic fields used in MR include:

(A) magnetophosphes
(B) DNA breaks
(C) displacement of aneurysm clips
(D) tissue heating
(E) induction of amnesia

A118. The appearance of cerebrospinal fluid on a conventional spin-echo image with T2 weighting is:

(A) similar to gray matter
(B) darker than white matter
(C) bright
(D) dark
(E) variable

A119. MR signal-to-noise ratio depends on all of the following *except:*

(A) strength of the magnetic field
(B) number of excitations (N_{ex})
(C) image reconstruction algorithm

(D) voxel size
(E) nucleus being imaged

A120. All of the following effects give rise to artifacts in MR *except:*

(A) susceptibility changes
(B) motion
(C) chemical shifts
(D) refraction
(E) undersampling

Answers And Explanations

A1–D. An electric current is the flow of charge in a circuit and not a force; electric currents are measured in amperes (A), whereas force is measured in newtons (N).

A2–C. Power is measured in watts (W), where 1 W is 1 J/second.

A3–A. The mass number (A) is the number of nucleons in a nucleus.

A4–C. Barium has an atomic number of 56 (calcium, 20; iodine, 53; tungsten, 74; lead, 82).

A5–D. The electron binding energy is the energy that must be supplied to pull the electron away from the atom. It decreases with increasing distance from the nucleus, increases with Z, is never more than about 100 keV, and is caused by electrostatic forces between the positive nucleus and negative electron.

A6–E. Cosmic rays are energetic particles.

A7–E. Ultrasound is not ionizing radiation. Photons and neutrons are indirectly ionizing radiations, whereas charged particles like electrons and alpha particles are directly ionizing.

A8–B. One curie 5 3.7 3 1010 disintegrations per second.

A9–E. Photons have no rest mass.

A10–E. A proton usually combines with a K-shell electron to create a neutron (and emit a neutrino). In filling the resultant K-shell vacancies, characteristic x-rays and Auger electrons are emitted, but not internal conversion electrons.

A11–D. Most x-ray generators produce 80 to 100 KW.

A12–B. There is no mechanical motion in transformers.

A13–D. X-ray production is relatively inefficient with 99% of the energy being lost as heat via outer shell electron "interactions."

A14–D. Beam filtration depends on the x-ray tube window and added filters, and is therefore independent of x-ray tube voltage.

A15–A. Most of the x-rays are produced by bremsstrahlung, the spectrum of which has a maximum photon energy of 100 keV.

A16–D. The maximum kinetic energy of electrons incident on the target is numerically equal to the maximum voltage, and it is possible for electrons to lose all this energy in a bremsstrahlung process.

A17–A. At 65 kV, the electrons striking the tungsten target will only have an energy of 65 keV, which is insufficient to eject K-shell electrons (binding energy of 69.5 keV).

A18–B. The intensity of x-ray production is approximately proportional to the atomic number.

A19–D. For constant potential units, the energy deposited in joules is kVp $\times$ mA $\times$ seconds; to get the heat unit, the energy in joules must be multiplied by 1.35.

A20–D. Focal spot size is irrelevant; other factors decrease the heel effect.

A21–B. Scattered photons are generally produced in Compton processes. The incident photon is completely absorbed during the photoelectric effect.

A22–A. Compton scatter is the major interaction in fluoroscopy, and the only one that results in backscattered x-rays.

A23–C. In water, photoelectric processes dominate below 25 keV, whereas Compton scatter is more important above 25 keV.

A24–C. Attenuation decreases with increasing photon energy.

A25–B. Three tenth-value layers will reduce the exposure by a factor of 1,000 (10^3) and 10 half-value layers will reduce the exposure by a factor of 1,024 (2^{10}).

A26–A. The half-value layer expressed in mm of aluminum depends only on the x-ray spectrum; it is thus independent of the intensity of the beam as measured by the exposure.

A27–C. The entrance skin exposure is always increased as the kVp or filtration is reduced (the x-ray beam becomes less penetrating and more intensity is required to achieve the same exposure level at the screen/film).

A28–A. The LET determines the radiation weighting factor for computing equivalent dose.

A29–D. The f-factor (rad/R) is about 4 for bones and about 1 for soft tissues at diagnostic x-ray energies.

A30–A. Geiger-Müller detectors are very sensitive and ideal for detecting low-level contamination in a nuclear medicine department.

A31–E. Patient dose is increased because as the temperature is reduced, the film speed is reduced, requiring a greater exposure to produce the same amount of blackening.

A32–E. Image contrast will likely be higher because gradients of screen/film combinations are generally higher than those of directly exposed films.

A33–D. Because 3,000 eV is converted into light energy and each (blue) light photon has an energy of 3 eV, 1,000 light photons are emitted.

A34–A. Grids attenuate both Compton and coherent scatter but most of the scatter reaching the screen/film receptor is Compton scatter.

A35–A. There is little scatter in extremity radiography because of the use of low kVps and presence of bone, both of which help to ensure that photo-

electric absorption is the dominant mode of interaction (i.e., very little scatter is present).

A36–E. Photocathodes convert light to electrons.

A37–B. 1 μGy/second (100 μR/second) because a typical image intensifier conversion factor is about 20 cd/m² per μGy/second (200 cd/m² per mR/second).

A38–E. Resolution in fluoroscopy is proportional to number of TV lines.

A39–B. Beam hardening gives rise to image artifacts in computed tomography.

A40–D. The dominant source of image noise is quantum mottle, which is reduced by increasing the number of x-ray photons (i.e., exposure level).

A41–A. Tube voltage (kVp) affects the subject contrast, which is the difference in x-ray beam intensities emerging from the patient. The other factors determine how subject contrast is transformed into image contrast.

A42–E. Film contrast is highest at optical density levels of about 1.5 and is lowest in the overexposed or underexposed regions (all other parameters affect subject contrast).

A43–C. Latitude is inversely proportional to contrast, so that a high value for one indicates a low value for the other.

A44–E. Use of thinner screens reduces screen blur. (There is no focal spot blur in *contact* radiography because there is no magnification.)

A45–C. Poor film/screen contact is the only explanation for the *consistent* appearance of this problem in the same region.

A46–E. The TV system is the component with the worst resolution characteristics in an image intensifier based fluoroscopy system.

A47–D. The standard deviation τ is $\sqrt{10,000}$, or 100; 99% of counts lie between the mean ± 3σ or 10,000 ± 300.

A48–B. When the threshold criterion becomes more lax so that the true-positive fraction increases, the false-positive fraction (FPF) also increases, and specificity, which is (1 − FPF), is reduced.

A49–E. Entrance skin exposure values are typically 20 mGy/minute (2 R/minute).

A50–C. The genetically significant dose is an index of potential genetic damage done to the population; it is obtained by combining the estimated gonadal doses and each patient's probability of producing offspring.

A51–C. The CPU performs all the arithmetic and logical operations in a computer.

A52–B. Buffer memory is used for temporary storage.

A53–E. Each image consists of 0.5 MB (0.5 k × 0.5 k × 2), so the total data storage would be 10 MB.

A54–C. The distance along one dimension is 250 mm, which is used for 256 pixels, so each has a linear dimension of about 1 mm.

A55–C. Charged couple devices are used to detect light (not x-rays), as in video camcorders or to replace TV cameras in fluoroscopy systems.

A56–E. CR is a digital modality and does not have a speed per se; any x-ray signal that is detected could be printed (or displayed) to any selected film density.

A57–C. A typical diagnostic monitor has a luminance of about 100 cd/m^2, which is much less than the 1,500 cd/m^2 of a typical light box.

A58–D. The contrast-to-noise ratio relates directly to lesion visibility.

A59–E. A typical matrix size would be 1,024^2, not 256^2.

A60–E. Asynchronous transfer mode can operate at a nominal 600 Mbit/second (see Table 6.2).

A61–A. At the low x-ray energy used in mammography, the interactions are predominately photoelectric, which results in a high contrast between calcium (Z = 20) and tissues (Z = ∼7).

A62–C. The characteristic K x-rays at about 18 are desirable for maximum calcium and soft tissue contrast.

A63–D. Object contrast, which refers to the physical differences between areas of the imaged breast, is not affected by grids.

A64–D. Spatial resolution is not generally affected by grids.

A65–D. The film speed will not significantly affect spatial resolution.

A66–C. Magnification uses a small focal spot, which limits the tube current to only 25 mA; as a result, exposure times will be much longer than in conventional contact mammography.

A67–E. The source-to-image receptor distance (SID) does not affect the average glandular dose per se.

A68–D. kV is checked on an annual basis and requires special kVp meters used by physicists.

A69–D. The spatial resolution of MR (less than 1 lp/mm) is markedly inferior to that of screen/film (15 to 20 lp/mm).

A70–E. Diaphanography does not use ionizing radiation.

A71–D. +50 HU is [1,000 × (μ − μ$_W$)/μ$_W$], where μ is the attenuation coefficient of the material and μ$_W$ is that of water.

A72–E. Filtered back projection is used for image reconstruction in CT.

A73–D. A value of 500 would be the middle (gray), and 1,000 would be white with zero as black; the window width is from zero to 1,000 (i.e., 1,000), and the center is at 500.

A74–E. In plane spacial resolution is mainly determined by the focal spot and detector sizes.

A75–D. Limiting spatial resolution will increase because the pixel size is reduced when the matrix size is increased.

A76–A. Focal spot size affects spatial resolution, but all the other parameters affect image noise, which impacts the ability to detect low-contrast objects.

A77–B. At a higher kVp, attenuation coefficient differences are reduced and subject contrast is decreased.

A78–A. Intravenous contrast increases the density and atomic number of blood and tissues. This increases x-ray attenuation and thereby the resultant Hounsfield unit value.

A79–B. Phase-encoding artifacts occur only on magnetic resonance (MR) images.

A80–E. None of the doses listed is correct. Typical eye lens dose is approximately 40 mGy (4 rad).

A81–C. ^{131}I has a photopeak at 365 keV.

A82–C. There is no need for high-energy gammas in a therapeutic agent such as ^{32}P.

A83–B. Elutions affect only the amount of ^{99m}Tc in the generator, and because the ^{99m}Tc photon energy (140 keV) is very low, this will not contribute significantly to the measured radiation level *outside* the shielded generator.

A84–D. Larger collimator holes allow more primary photons to pass through to the NaI crystal.

A85–B. Photomultiplier tubes convert light to electrons.

A86–A. Spatial resolution decreases with increasing distance from the collimator face.

A87–B. Increasing collimator thickness improves resolution but reduces sensitivity.

A88–D. Pixel values are proportional to the radioisotope concentration.

A89–E. Patient doses in PET and SPECT are similar with effective doses of about 5 mSv (500 mrem).

A90–C. The biological half-life is determined by biological clearance (i.e., no biological clearance corresponds to an infinite biological half-life).

A91–B. The w_R converts dose (Gy or rad) to equivalent dose (Sv or rem); in diagnostic radiology, w_R is generally 1.0, so that absorbed dose and equivalent dose are numerically equal.

A92–C. Lymphocytes are very radiosensitive.

A93–A. 0%. The eye lens dose will be about 160 mGy (16 rad), which is well below the acute threshold dose of 2 Gy (200 rad) for cataract induction.

A94–C. At the low doses normally encountered in diagnostic radiology, the only significant effect will be the production of ionization.

A95–C. The entrance skin dose in fluoroscopy is about 30 mGy/minute (3 rad/minute); for an anterior-posterior projection, the attenuation by soft tissue would likely result in a threefold reduction in dose to the fetus.

A96–E. Only the radiation received from *occupational exposure* is included for regulatory purposes.

A97–E. There are no dose limits for diagnostic x-ray examinations.

A98–E. Doses to workers and members of the public will quadruple.

A99–E. 1 mGy/hour (100 mR/hour) is the current limit for leakage radiation from x-ray tubes.

A100–B. ^{222}Rn is an alpha emitter and therefore emits alpha particles.

A101–E. Metals propagate ultrasound at about 6,000 m/second, which is much higher than air (330 m/second), soft tissue (1,540 m/second), or bone (3300 m/second).

A102–A. The acoustic impedance (Z) is the product of the velocity of sound in the medium (v) and the medium density (p) (i.e., $Z = v \times p$).

A103–E. Attenuation of ultrasound does not depend on the intensity.

A104–E. The largest echoes occur when the difference between the acoustical impedances of the two media is greatest. In this case, the greatest difference is between fat and kidney.

A105–A. Crystal thickness is half the wavelength and therefore determines the frequency.

A106–A. The Q factor has nothing to do with the intensity produced by the transducer.

A107–C. The total distance traveled is 20 cm, and speed of travel is 1,540 m/second; therefore, time is 0.2 m/1,540 m/second, or 130 μsecond.

A108–D. The typical PRF is 3 kHz, not 100 kHz. The penetration depth would be less than 1 cm for a PRF of 100 kHz.

A109–A. Axial resolution is generally equal to half the pulse length.

A110–E. Cavitation is the creation and collapse of tiny bubbles and occurs only at high ultrasound intensities.

A111–E. ^{40}K is radioactive.

A112–B. T2 is the characteristic time that describes loss of phase coherence in the transverse plane in the absence of magnetic-field inhomogeneity effects.

A113–B. Tissue atomic number plays no role in MR.

A114–E. Resistive magnets dissipate large amounts of power in the coils and generally require water cooling; the practical upper magnetic-field strength is about 0.5 T.

A115–B. For biological tissues, T2 is generally independent of magnetic-field strength.

A116–E. Gradients have strengths up to 60 mT/m, not RF coils.

A117–C. Magnetic fields have the potential to displace aneurysm clips.

A118–C. Cerebrospinal fluid has a long T2 value and will appear bright on T2-weighted spin-echo sequences.

A119–C. The image reconstruction technique does not affect the signal-to-noise ratio.

A120–D. Refraction gives rise to artifacts in ultrasound not MR imaging.

B1. Which of the following is *not* an SI unit?

(A) Meter
(B) Kilogram
(C) Second
(D) Rad
(E) Becquerel

B2. Which of the following is *not* a unit of energy?

(A) Erg
(B) Joule
(C) Watt
(D) British thermal unit (BTU)
(E) Electron volt

B3. Which of the following is *false* for a neutral cobalt 60 atom ($Z = 27$)?

(A) 27 protons in the nucleus
(B) 33 neutrons in the nucleus
(C) Outer-shell binding energy levels of several electron volts
(D) A weight about 60 times a hydrogen atom
(E) K-shell binding energy of 90 keV

B4. Outer-shell electrons differ from K-shell electrons by their:

(A) rest mass energy
(B) charge
(C) magnetic moment
(D) binding energy
(E) particulate nature

B5. Which statement is *not* true of electromagnetic radiation?

(A) It travels at the speed of light.
(B) It exhibits particulate properties.
(C) Photon energy is proportional to its frequency.
(D) Wavelength is proportional to the frequency.
(E) It includes radio waves, infrared radiation, and gamma rays.

B6. When neutral atoms are changed to an electrically charged atom it is called:

(A) fission
(B) fusion
(C) ionization
(D) excitation
(E) scintillation

B7. The energy lost per unit length along the track of an alpha particle is a measure of:

(A) ionization
(B) scintillation
(C) linear attenuation coefficient
(D) mass energy absorption
(E) linear energy transfer

B8. Ten millicuries is equal to:

(A) 37 Bq
(B) 370 Bq
(C) 370 MBq
(D) 27 MBq
(E) 270 MBq

B9. Which of the following is *false* of nuclear transformations?

(A) Electron capture decay, Z decreases by one.
(B) Beta-minus decay, A increases by one.
(C) Beta-plus decay, Z is reduced by one.
(D) Isomeric transitions, A and Z remain constant.
(E) Alpha decay, Z decreases by two.

B10. Which of the following is never emitted during radioactive decay?

(A) Alpha particles
(B) Protons
(C) Positrons
(D) Gamma rays
(E) Neutrinos

B11. An alternating electric current will produce:

(A) a static electric field
(B) a static magnetic field
(C) a direct current electric field
(D) an alternating magnetic field
(E) both a static electric and magnetic field

B12. Compared with a single-phase generator, x-rays from three-phase generators have:

(A) higher maximum energies
(B) fewer photons
(C) lower half-value layers
(D) greater heel effect
(E) higher average energies

B13. To produce a bremsstrahlung x-ray, an energetic electron:

(A) collides with an outer shell electron
(B) is slowed down (decelerated) by the nucleus

(C) is absorbed by the nucleus
(D) moves between shells, emitting the excess energy as an x-ray
(E) causes the nucleus to emit x-ray energy

B14. The continuous spectrum obtained from x-ray tubes is due to:

(A) transitions of atomic electrons from higher to lower energy levels
(B) conversion of electrons to electromagnetic energy
(C) deceleration of electrons when they hit the target
(D) target heating
(E) thermionic emission

B15. The average photon energy of an x-ray beam cannot be changed by:

(A) tube current (mA)
(B) beam filtration
(C) tube voltage
(D) voltage waveform
(E) passage through a patient

B16. The average energy of K-shell characteristic x-rays are not:

(A) about 18 keV for molybdenum anodes
(B) dependent on the shell structure of the target atom
(C) about 65 keV for tungsten anodes
(D) independent on x-ray filtration
(E) independent of atomic number (Z)

B17. X-ray beam quality:

(A) is proportional to the tube current (mA)
(B) is reduced by additional aluminum filtration
(C) is measured in millimeters of aluminum
(D) converts dose (Gy) to equivalent dose (Sv)
(E) is independent of the tube voltage

B18. X-ray tube output will not be increased by increasing the:

(A) voltage across the tube (kV)
(B) anode heat capacity (MJ)
(C) target atomic number (Z)
(D) tube current (mA)
(E) exposure time (seconds)

B19. The heel effect results in the greatest x-ray beam intensity transmitted:

(A) at the anode side
(B) at the cathode side
(C) through the collimator
(D) through the x-ray tube housing
(E) 15° from central axis

B20. Radiation leaving an x-ray tube when the collimators are fully closed is known as:

(A) primary radiation
(B) stray radiation
(C) leakage radiation
(D) entrance radiation
(E) backscattered radiation

B21. Following absorption of a single 30 keV photon in a patient:

(A) temperature rises significantly (more than 1°C)
(B) a number of ionization events occur
(C) several scatter photons emerge
(D) internal conversion electrons are emitted
(E) excited nuclei are produced

B22. The energy of the scattered photon in Compton processes depends primarily on the:

(A) atomic number
(B) density
(C) electron density
(D) molecular structure
(E) scattering angle

B23. Soft-tissue contrast in chest radiographs performed at 140 kVp is due primarily to:

(A) coherent interactions
(B) Compton interactions
(C) photoelectric interactions
(D) pair production interactions
(E) photodisintegration interactions

B24. If the linear attenuation coefficient is 0.1 cm^{-1} and the density is 2 g/cm^3, the mass attenuation coefficient is:

(A) 0.2 cm^2/g
(B) 0.05 cm^2/g
(C) 0.05 g/cm^2
(D) 20 g/cm^2
(E) unable to be determined

B25. If the half-value layer (HVL) is 2 cm, the linear attenuation coefficient is:

(A) 0.50 cm^{-1}
(B) 0.35 cm^{-1}
(C) 2.9 cm^{-1}
(D) 0.35 cm
(E) 2.9 cm

B26. The adequacy of the filtration of an x-ray tube may be determined by:

(A) physical inspection
(B) x-ray tube documentation
(C) kVp measurement

(D) x-ray output measurement
(E) half-value layer measurement

B27. Measuring the charge (of either sign) liberated in a specified mass of air by a beam of diagnostic x-rays yields:

(A) absorbed dose
(B) exposure
(C) dose equivalent
(D) energy
(E) effective dose

B28. Which material receives the highest dose after exposure to 10 mGy (1 R) of 80 kVp x-rays?

(A) Air
(B) Fat
(C) Muscle
(D) Bone
(E) Cannot be determined

B29. Which of the following works on the principle of gas ionization?

(A) Screen/film
(B) Sodium iodine (NaI) crystal
(C) Photostimulable phosphor
(D) Image intensifier
(E) Geiger counter

B30. Which of the following cannot detect x-rays?

(A) Ionization chambers
(B) Scintillation detectors
(C) Geiger-Müller counters
(D) Photostimulable phosphors
(E) Photomultiplier tubes

B31. When two 1.5 optical density films are placed together, the fraction of light transmitted is:

(A) less than 0.001
(B) 0.001
(C) 0.003
(D) 0.03
(E) more than 0.03

B32. Conversion efficiencies of calcium tungstate and gadolinium oxysulfide screens are:

(A) 120% and 110%, respectively
(B) 110% and 120%, respectively
(C) 18% and 4%, respectively
(D) 4% and 18%, respectively
(E) the same

B33. Matching the screen K-edge with incident x-ray energy improves the:

(A) conversion efficiency
(B) spatial resolution
(C) quantum mottle

(D) x-ray absorption
(E) film gamma

B34. What is the most important determinant of grid scatter removal efficiency?

(A) Grid ratio
(B) Focus distance
(C) Gap distance
(D) Strip height
(E) Interspace material

B35. The image intensifier output phosphor is made of:

(A) NaI
(B) ZnCdS
(C) BGO
(D) CsI
(E) BaFBr

B36. Reducing the image intensifier conversion gain increases the:

(A) high-contrast resolution
(B) patient dose
(C) patient blurring
(D) vignetting
(E) image distortion

B37. When an image intensifier is switched from 12 to 6 inches, the exposure at the image intensifier input should:

(A) be reduced by 50%
(B) remain the same
(C) be increased by 50%
(D) be doubled
(E) be quadrupled

B38. Fluoroscopy image brightness is affected by all of the following *except:*

(A) kVp
(B) mA
(C) patient thickness
(D) grid ratio
(E) exposure time

B39. Actual vertical resolution achieved with a 525 line television monitor is:

(A) 525 lp
(B) 180 lp
(C) 370 lp
(D) 262 lp
(E) 425 lp

B40. Exact framing:

(A) uses the entire intensifier image
(B) magnifies the image
(C) records 64% of the image

(D) improves spatial resolution
(E) improves contrast

B41. *Subject* contrast is not affected by changes in:

(A) film/screen combination
(B) lesion atomic number
(C) lesion size
(D) lesion density
(E) background composition

B42. A characteristic curve with a gradient of 3.0 would likely result in:

(A) low radiation dose
(B) low density
(C) long processing time
(D) high contrast
(E) high base plus fog

B43. Gastrointestinal tract contrast on film radiographs is *not* normally improved by:

(A) infusion of barium
(B) reducing voltage (kVp)
(C) increasing current (mA)
(D) tighter x-ray beam collimation
(E) increasing the grid ratio

B44. Doubling the screen thickness is likely to increase the:

(A) exposure time
(B) patient dose
(C) fraction of x-ray photons absorbed
(D) film processing time
(E) image noise

B45. Geometric magnification cannot:

(A) require the same radiation at screen/film
(B) improve system spatial resolution
(C) use smaller focal spot sizes
(D) reduce scatter
(E) change screen film speed

B46. The modulation transfer function does *not* generally:

(A) describe the system resolution
(B) compare image to subject contrast
(C) approach one at low spatial frequencies
(D) equal unity for perfect spatial resolution
(E) increase with increasing spatial frequency

B47. Which of the following does *not* affect image noise for a given film density?

(A) Intensifying screen conversion efficiency
(B) Film processor temperature
(C) Film speed

(D) Screen thickness
(E) Developer replenishment

B48. The area under the receiver operator characteristic curve is all of the following except:

(A) a measure of performance
(B) unlikely to be less than 0.5
(C) 0.5 for random guesses
(D) 1.0 for a perfect diagnostic tool
(E) average of sensitivity and specificity

B49. Entrance skin dose for an anterior-posterior abdominal x-ray examinations is typically:

(A) below 1 mGy (100 mrad)
(B) 1 mGy (100 mrad)
(C) 3 mGy (300 mrad)
(D) 10 mGy (1 rad)
(E) above 10 mGy (1 rad)

B50. The effective dose from an x-ray examination does not normally take into account:

(A) individual organ doses
(B) radiation weighting factor
(C) all exposed tissues
(D) organ radiosensitivity
(E) patient age

B51. Computer hardware includes all the following *except:*

(A) JAVA
(B) hard drives
(C) magnetic tapes
(D) central processing units (CPUs)
(E) array processors

B52. How many shades of gray can ultrasound, which uses 8 bits per pixel, display?

(A) 8
(B) 64
(C) 512
(D) 1028
(E) 256

B53. What is the typical matrix size of digital photospot imaging?

(A) 256^2
(B) 512^2
(C) $1,024^2$
(D) $2,048^2$
(E) $>2,048^2$

B54. Which of the following would *not* likely be found in a digital x-ray detector?

(A) Se
(B) CsI
(C) LSO

(D) Gd_2O_2S
(E) $BaF_2Fl:Eu$

B55. Compared with screen/film, digital radiography has all of the following except:

(A) the potential to reduce patient doses
(B) can eliminate film processing
(C) image processing capabilities
(D) the ability to store data digitally
(E) improves spatial resolution

B56. All of the following relate to digital x-ray image acquisition systems *except:*

(A) computed radiography
(B) laser cameras
(C) charged coupled device (CCD)
(D) direct capture
(E) indirect capture

B57. Energy subtraction would normally make use of all of the following except:

(A) low-energy image (60 kVp)
(B) high-energy image (120 kVp)
(C) unsharp masking
(D) bone display
(E) soft-tissue display

B58. The dominant source of image noise in a radiography flat panel detector is most likely:

(A) phosphor structure mottle
(B) electronic noise
(C) digitization noise
(D) quantum mottle
(E) film granularity

B59. The ratio of doses (per frame) of digital photospot to digital fluoroscopy is:

(A) greater than 20:1
(B) 20:1
(C) 10:1
(D) 3:1
(E) less than 3:1

B60. PACS should reduce all of the following *except:*

(A) use of film
(B) lost images
(C) use of view boxes
(D) radiology capital costs
(E) film library clerks

B61. Increasing the kVp in mammography will reduce:

(A) subject contrast
(B) grid transmission
(C) scatter

(D) resolution
(E) film density

B62. Film/screen mammography uses all the following *except:*

(A) half-wave rectification
(B) low kVp (25 to 35)
(C) molybdenum targets
(D) beryllium windows
(E) molybdenum filtration

B63. Film/screen mammography image quality would likely be degraded by all *except:*

(A) use of grids
(B) high kVp
(C) low mAs
(D) aluminum filtration
(E) increased focal spot size

B64. Which is *not* a characteristic of a mammography screen/film system?

(A) Carbon fiber cassette front
(B) Single thin intensifying screen
(C) Single emulsion film
(D) Dye to prevent light crossover in film
(E) 20×24 cm cassette size

B65. Compression in mammography is *not* used to:

(A) make the breast more uniform
(B) allow a lower kVp to be used
(C) reduce focal spot blur
(D) reduce the radiation dose
(E) reduce quantum mottle

B66. To visualize microcalcifications in mammography requires all of the following *except:*

(A) minimal patient motion
(B) small focal spots
(C) thin screens
(D) good screen/film contact
(E) high kVp

B67. The average glandular dose in mammography is *not:*

(A) regulated by the Mammography Quality Standards Act (MQSA)
(B) typically below 2 mGy (200 mrad)
(C) measured annually by a physicist
(D) proportional to kVp
(E) proportional to mAs

B68. Advantages of ultrasound for breast imaging include all of the following *except:*

(A) differentiation of cysts from solids
(B) no ionizing radiation
(C) noninvasive

(D) good visualization of microcalcifications
(E) use of high-frequency transducers

B69. Use of magnetic resonance (MR) breast imaging may include all of the following *except* identification of:

(A) tumor margins
(B) multifocal disease
(C) microcalcification clusters
(D) scar tissue
(E) tumors in patients with silicone implants

B70. All of the following imaging modalities have been used for breast imaging *except:*

(A) thermography
(B) MR imaging
(C) ultrasound
(D) electron microscopy
(E) diaphanography

B71. Hounsfield units for cortical bone, fat, lung, and muscle, respectively, are typically:

(A) 1,600, 30, −600, −100
(B) −600, 30, 1600, −100
(C) 1600, −100, −600, 30
(D) −600, −100, 30, 1600
(E) 1,600, 100, −300, −30

B72. Increasing the width of the computed tomography (CT) image display window will reduce:

(A) displayed contrast
(B) quantum mottle
(C) section thickness
(D) field of view
(E) image brightness

B73. How many slices could a 5 MJ anode heat capacity x-ray tube acquire? (100 kVp; 500 mA; 1 second scans)?

(A) More than 10
(B) More than 20
(A) More than 30
(B) More than 50
(E) More than 100

B74. In helical CT scanning, which of the following does *not* apply?

(A) A continuous slip ring is required for the x-ray tube.
(B) It cannot be performed with bowtie filters.
(C) Higher x-ray tube heat capacity is needed.
(D) Partial volume effects will increase.
(E) Misregistration effects will decrease.

B75. The limiting spatial resolution in CT is affected by all of the following *except:*

(A) field of view
(B) detector aperture size
(C) mA
(D) matrix size
(E) focal spot size

B76. Iodine contrast results in increased CT numbers in reconstructed images because of:

(A) changes in the image display settings
(B) increased photoelectric absorption
(C) dilation of blood vessels
(D) increased blood flow
(E) increased beam hardening

B77. CT is better than screen/film for neuroimaging because CT:

(A) is quicker
(B) has superior spatial resolution
(C) reduces patient doses (radiation risk)
(D) has excellent contrast discrimination
(E) is less expensive

B78. Voxel Hounsfield units can be significantly affected by all of the following *except* the tissue's:

(A) density
(B) electron density
(C) atomic number
(D) homogeneity
(E) temperature

B79. CT beam-hardening artifacts:

(A) reduce CT numbers in the image center
(B) are independent of x-ray beam filtration
(C) reduce all CT numbers
(D) do not occur with fourth-generation scanners
(E) do not occur on multi-slice scanners

B80. The typical dose to the breast from a CT scan of the chest is:

(A) less than 0.02 mGy (20 mrad)
(B) approximately 0.02 mGy (20 mrad)
(C) approximately 0.2 mGy (200 mrad)
(D) approximately 2 mGy (0.2 rad)
(E) approximately 20 mGy (2 rad)

B81. The "ideal" radiopharmaceutical in nuclear medicine imaging studies would have the following except:

(A) a short half-life

(B) no particulate emissions
(C) rapid clearance from the blood stream
(D) photons with an energy of about 150 keV
(E) high number of internal conversion electrons

B82. ^{99m}Tc:

(A) has a half-life of 67 hours
(B) emits a spectrum of electrons
(C) produces a stable daughter product
(D) emits 140 keV photons
(E) results in no auger electrons

B83. Which of the following is *not* true of radioactive equilibrium?

(A) It is secular when the half-life of the parent is greater than the half-life of the daughter.
(B) It requires about four half-lives for secular equilibrium to be established.
(C) It is transient if the half-life of the parent exceeds that of the daughter.
(D) For a ^{99}Mo/^{99m}Tc generator, it can be termed transient.
(E) Number of parent and daughter atoms are equal.

B84. The sodium iodine (NaI) crystals in gamma cameras normally have all of the following except:

(A) thickness of 1 mm
(B) high absorption at 140 keV
(C) 5% of absorbed energy converted to light
(D) intrinsic resolution of 3 mm full-width half maximum (FWHM)
(E) Thallium (Tl) dopant

B85. The pulse height analyzer in a gamma camera system:

(A) increases detector efficiency
(B) analyzes the total energy deposited
(C) corrects for count rate losses
(D) performs coincidence detection
(E) increases the count rate

B86. Using radionuclides with a higher photon energy generally increases:

(A) detector efficiency
(B) septal penetration
(C) amplifier gain setting
(D) image magnification
(E) resolution

B87. For single positron emission computed tomography (SPECT), which of the following is *not* true?

(A) 128 projections are obtained.
(B) It takes about 20 minutes to perform.
(C) Corrections are usually made for patient motion.

(D) Images show relative radioisotope concentrations.
(E) Image quality is affected by scatter.

B88. Positron emission tomography (PET) scanners generally make use of all of the following *except:*

(A) short-lived radionuclides such as ^{15}O
(B) cyclotrons
(C) directly detected positrons
(D) filtered-back projection reconstruction algorithms
(E) solid-state detectors

B89. All of the following are tests done for radio-pharmaceutical quality control except:

(A) radionuclide purity
(B) radiochemical purity
(C) chemical purity
(D) spectral purity
(E) sterility

B90. All of the following affect the organ dose for a radioisotope study *except:*

(A) organ size
(B) organ shape
(C) uptake of isotope
(D) clearance of isotope
(E) gamma camera imaging time

B91. To convert absorbed dose into equivalent dose, it is only necessary to know the:

(A) f-factor
(B) radiation weighting factor
(C) exposure level
(D) distance to the radiation source
(E) composition of absorbing material

B92. The chronic x-ray threshold dose for radiation-induced cataracts is about:

(A) 5 mGy (0.5 rad)
(B) 50 mGy (5 rad)
(C) 0.1 Gy (10 rad)
(D) 1 Gy (100 rad)
(E) 5 Gy (500 rad)

B93. Stochastic effects of radiation exposure include:

(A) epilation (hair loss)
(B) cataract induction
(C) leukemia
(D) skin erythema
(E) permanent sterility

B94. The dose to the fetus for a single-view lateral lumbar spine x-ray is most likely to:

(A) require an abortion
(B) exceed 100 mGy (10 rad)
(C) exceed 10 mGy (1 rad)
(D) be less than 10 mGy (1 rad)
(E) be difficult to assess

B95. A "nonagreement" state is a state that:

(A) has no nuclear power generating facilities
(B) can set its own levels for occupational exposure
(C) has assumed responsibility for regulating radioactive materials
(D) is regulated by the Nuclear Regulatory Commission (NRC)
(E) has no regulation of radioactive materials

B96. The 1 mSv/year (100 mrem/year) limit for members of the public includes doses from:

(A) dental radiographs
(B) high-altitude airplane flight
(C) radioactive elements in the Earth's crust
(D) routine screening radiographs
(E) sitting in a diagnostic waiting room

B97. Lead aprons for radiographers:

(A) should be worn at the control panel
(B) are essential in mammography
(C) are up to 0.50 mm lead
(D) reduce the thyroid dose
(E) reduce exposure from radon

B98. The use factor (U) refers to the fraction of the:

(A) week that the machine is in operation
(B) week during which the area is occupied
(C) time the beam is directed toward the barrier
(D) time the area beyond any barrier is occupied
(E) time patients are in x-ray room

B99. Low-level radioactive wastes in nuclear medicine should:

(A) never be thrown away
(B) be thrown away immediately
(C) be disposed of by a commercial rad-waste service
(D) stored for 3 half lives
(E) stored for 10 half lives

B100. The mean radiation dose to the lungs is highest from:

(A) a chest x-ray
(B) occupational exposure for an x-ray technologist (1 year)

(C) exposure to domestic radon (1 year)
(D) cosmic radiation (1 year)
(E) mammogram

B101. Ultrasound acoustic impedance is:

(A) measured in ohms
(B) independent of density
(C) inversely proportional to velocity
(D) very low for air
(E) very low for bone

B102. Ultrasound attenuated by 3 dB is how much lower than the original signal?

(A) 3%
(B) 30%
(C) 50%
(D) 70%
(E) 90%

B103. The angle of reflection of an ultrasound beam at an interface is equal to the:

(A) ratio of velocities in the two media
(B) ratio of the impedances of the two media
(C) angle of incidence
(D) angle of refraction
(E) sine of the angle of incidence

B104. Refraction of an ultrasound beam refers to the:

(A) change of beam frequency
(B) multiple reflections at two interfaces
(C) loss of signal intensity
(D) change in direction of the beam at an interface
(E) lack of signal behind absorbers

B105. The Q factor of an ultrasound transducer describes the:

(A) crystal resonance frequency
(B) Fresnel zone length
(C) frequency response of the crystal
(D) FWHM value of the beam intensity
(E) power penetration into patient

B106. Which would most likely improve the transmission of ultrasound into the patient?

(A) Quarter-wave matching layer
(B) Time gain compensation (TGC)
(C) High-frequency transducer
(D) Contrast agents
(E) Harmonic imaging

B107. Time gain compensation compensates for tissue attenuation by increasing the:

(A) transducer output
(B) echo intensity

(C) focal zone length
(D) echo velocity
(E) fresnel zone length

B108. Increasing the ultrasound pulse length will generally reduce the:

(A) axial resolution
(B) power deposited in the patient
(C) acoustical impedance
(D) transducer Q factor
(E) lateral resolution

B109. Ultrasound lateral resolution is generally *not* affected by transducer:

(A) frame rate
(B) focusing
(C) diameter
(D) impedence
(E) beam width

B110. Continuous-wave Doppler ultrasound makes use of:

(A) side lobes
(B) pulsed ultrasound
(C) continuous ultrasound
(D) echo amplitude
(E) time of flight

B111.Which of the following has the shortest T1 value?

(A) fat
(B) liver
(C) kidney
(D) white matter
(E) cerebrospinal fluid

B112. Which of the following has the longest T2 value?

(A) fat
(B) liver
(C) kidney
(D) white matter
(E) gray matter

B113. Which coils adjust the uniformity of the magnetic-field strength?

(A) Shim
(B) Quadrature
(C) Saddle
(D) Surface
(E) RF

B114. Which is false for permanent whole body MR magnets?

(A) They have strengths of up to 2 T.

(B) They have small fringe fields.
(C) They are very heavy.
(D) They have good uniformity.
(E) They do not require liquid helium.

B115. Gradient magnetic fields in MR are used principally to:

(A) reduce fringe fields
(B) localize MR signals
(C) eliminate field perturbations
(D) shorten T1
(E) increase signal intensity

B116. All the following can be adversely affected by stray magnetic resonance (MR) magnetic fields except:

(A) cardiac pacemakers
(B) image intensifiers
(C) optical disks
(D) computer displays
(E) floppy disks

B117. A Fourier transform in magnetic resonance (MR) convert the free induction decay (FID) signals into what components?

(A) T1
(B) T2
(C) T2*
(D) Proton spin density
(E) Frequency domain

B118. All the following signals are associated with magnetic resonance (MR), except:

(A) reverberation echo
(B) free induction decay
(C) gradient echo
(D) spin-echo
(E) frequency encoded

B119. Chemical shift artifacts are caused by differences in the:

(A) T1 relaxation time
(B) T2 relaxation time
(C) spin density
(D) Larmor frequency
(E) atomic number

B120. To perform MR spectroscopy generally requires all of the following except:

(A) high magnetic fields
(B) good field uniformity
(C) large voxels (over 1 cm^3)
(D) administration of gadolinium
(E) Fourier analysis

Answers And Explanations

B1–D. One rad = 100 erg/g; the SI unit for dose is the gray (1 rad = 10 mGy)

B2–C. The watt is a unit of power. It is the rate at which energy is used, expressed in joules per second (J/second).

B3–E. K-shell binding energy of cobalt is 8 keV.

B4–D. Binding energy. Inner shell electrons are tightly bound to the nucleus with binding energies of the order of thousands of eV; outer-shell electrons are loosely bound with binding energies of a few electron volts.

B5–D. The product of the wavelength and frequency is the (constant) speed of light; thus, the frequency is *inversely* proportional to the wavelength.

B6–C. Ionization occurs when electrons are ejected from a neutral atom, leaving behind a positively charged atom.

B7–E. The linear energy transfer for alpha particles is high and equal to about 100 keV/μm.

B8–C. 370 MBq, because 1 mCi is equal to 37 MBq.

B9–B. The mass number A does not change in any beta decay process.

B10–B. Protons are *not* emitted during radioactive decay.

B11–D. If another conductor is brought close by, an electric current is induced in the second conductor; this is the principle of induction that is used to increase or decrease the voltage in a transformer.

B12–E. Three phase generators have a much lower voltage ripple, and therefore result in a higher average photon energy.

B13–B. Bremsstrahlung is braking radiation that occurs when electrons are decelerated (lose energy) in the electric field of a nucleus.

B14–C. Bremsstrahlung radiation, which in German means "braking radiation," results from the deceleration of electrons in the target.

B15–A. Beam quality is independent of the tube current (mA), which determines primarily the x-ray beam output (intensity).

B16–E. K-shell binding energy increases with increasing atomic number.

B17–C. Beam quality is the penetrating power measured as the thickness of aluminum required to attenuate the beam exposure by 50%.

B18–B. Output of an x-ray tube has no direct relationship to the anode heat capacity.

B19–B. The highest x-ray beam intensity is at the cathode side. At the anode side, there is significant absorption within the anode itself.

B20–C. Leakage radiation.

B21–B. Energy will be deposited and produce a large number of ionizations as the photoelectron loses energy.

B22–E. When the scattering angle is 180 degrees, the backscattered photon has the lowest energy, and the Compton electron the highest energy.

B23–B. Compton scatter is the primary interaction for soft tissues at high photon energy levels (i.e., more than 25 keV or more than 75 kVp).

B24–B. The mass attenuation coefficient is equal to the linear attenuation coefficient (μ) divided by the density (ρ) (0.1/2 or 0.05 cm^2/g).

B25–B. Linear attenuation coefficient = 0.693/HVL = 0.693/2 cm = 0.35 cm^{-1}.

B26–E. Adequacy of x-ray tube filtration is determined by measuring the half-value layer, usually at 80 kVp, and ensuring it exceeds 2.5 mm Al.

B27–B. Exposure is the charge liberated per unit mass of air (c/kg).

B28–D. Bone will result in the highest dose because it has the highest f-factor (dose in bone will be about 4 rad because the f-factor for bone at 80 kVp is about 4).

B29–E. Geiger-Müller tubes operate on the principle of gas ionization.

B30–E. Photomultiplier tubes detect light *not* x-rays.

B31–B. The total density is 3.0, which transmits only 0.1% of the incident light.

B32–D. The conversion efficiency is the efficiency with which x-ray photon energy deposited in the phosphor is converted into light; it cannot exceed 100%. Rare earth screens became popular partly because they have a conversion efficiency considerably *higher* than that of calcium tungstate.

B33–D. X-ray absorption will be maximized.

B34–A. The grid ratio (strip height divided by gap distance) determines how efficiently the scattered radiation is removed.

B35–B. The output phosphor scintillator is made of zinc cadmium sulfide (ZnCdS).

B36–B. More radiation is required to produce the output brightness because the input phosphor has a reduced efficiency for converting x-ray photons into light photons.

B37–E. The image brightness is proportional to the number of photons absorbed in the input phosphor of the image intensifier, which is proportional to the area of the input phosphor. To maintain the same output brightness, the input dose must quadruple because the input area in magnification mode is only one-fourth of that in normal mode.

B38–E. There is no "exposure time" in fluoroscopy because the x-ray beam is on all the time.

B39–B. We need two lines to produce a line pair; thus the *maximum* resolution would be 262 (525/2) lp; however, this is never achieved (Kell factor = 0.7), which results in an achievable resolution of about 180 lp.

B40–A. In exact framing, the entire circular image intensifier image is recorded and only 80% of the film is used.

B41–A. Screen/film combination will affect image contrast but not subject contrast.

B42–D. A gradient of 3 is a high-contrast film and is likely to result in high image contrast (used in mammography).

B43–C. The mA will not increase image contrast, whereas all the other factors normally increase gastrointestinal tract contrast.

B44–C. Thicker screens will increase the efficiency of x-ray absorption but reduce the spatial resolution performance because of increasing screen blur.

B45–E. The screen/film speed remains the same; improved resolution is achievable only if focal spot blur is minimized by use of a small focal spot.

B46–E. The modulation transfer function generally *decreases* with increasing spatial frequency.

B47–D. Increasing the screen thickness does not change the total number of x-rays absorbed to give a specified film density, and thus image noise will not be affected.

B48–E. Sensitivity and specificity can be defined at a given point on the ROC curve.

B49–C. Three mGy is a good representative value for the skin dose in an anterior-posterior abdominal radiograph.

B50–E. The patient age is not normally taken into account when computing an effective dose; converting the dose into a risk, however, would need to take into account the age.

B51–A. JAVA is a programming language, not computer hardware.

B52–E. With 8 bits per pixel, the maximum number of gray levels is 2^8 or 256.

B53–C. A typical matrix size in digital photospot imaging is $1 k^2$.

B54–C. LSO is an organic scintillator used in positron emission tomography imaging.

B55–E. Spacial resolution using Digital Radiology (CR, flat panel detectors, etc.) is generally worse that that achievable using screen/film.

B56–B. Laser cameras are used to print digital x-rays but are not involved in image acquisition per se.

B57–C. Unsharp masking is an image-processing algorithm for enhancing the visibility of edges; it has no direct relation to energy subtraction.

B58–D. Quantum mottle will be the only significant noise source in any current flat panel detector use for radiography. In fluoroscopy, however, electronic noise could also be a factor.

B59–A. Digital photospot images are used for diagnostic purposes and require about 1 µGy/frame (100 µR/frame), which is about 50 times higher than any (digital) fluoroscopy frame.

B60–D. PACSs are currently very expensive; their justification is in their potential to cut operating costs (e.g., film, clerks).

B61–A. The subject contrast between fibroglandular and malignant tissues decreases with increasing kVp. Note that film density is always constant in screen/film imaging.

B62–A. Dedicated mammography units currently use either three-phase or high-frequency generators. Half-wave rectification would reduce the x-ray tube output and significantly increase exposure times.

B63–A. Use of grids improves image quality by reducing the scatter contribution.

B64–D. A single-screen/single-emulsion film means crossover is not a problem that needs to be reduced.

B65–E. Quantum mottle depends on the number of photons used to make the image and has no connection to compression.

B66–E. Use of high kVps will reduce image contrast and microcalcification visibility.

B67–D. In mammography, there is no simple linear relationship between kVp and average glandular dose.

B68–D. Ultrasound does not visualize microcalcifications.

B69–C. MR does not visualize microcalcifications.

B70–D. Electron microscopy is used for in vitro tissue analysis.

B71–C. Cortical bone is typically about 1,600 HU because it has high density and high atomic number; fat is typically −100 HU because it has lower density; lung is about −600 HU (very low density); and muscle is about 30 HU because it has a slightly higher density than water.

B72–A. Displayed contrast is the only factor affected by the display window width.

B73–E. Each scan deposits $100 \times 500 \times 1$ J in the anode, or 50,000 J. One hundred scans deposit 5 MJ in the anode, but because heat is being continually dissipated, more than 100 scans will be possible.

B74–B. Most modern CT scanners use bowtie filters to equalize the radiation level incident on the x-ray detectors, including helical scanners.

B75–C. The mA determines the intensity of the x-ray beam, hence image noise, but has no direct effect on spatial resolution.

B76–B. Iodinated contrast has a high atomic number ($Z = 53$ for iodine), which increases x-ray absorption and the attenuation coefficient and, therefore, the computed HU value.

B77–D. CT can differentiate between two adjacent tissues that differ in attenuation properties by as little as 5 HU (i.e., 0.5% difference) and thus has excellent contrast discrimination.

B78–E. Patient temperature does not significantly affect the attenuation properties of the tissue relative to water.

B79–A. Beam-hardening artifacts occur because the average photon energy of an x-ray beam increases as it passes through the patient. The preferential loss of lower energy x-rays depresses the CT numbers because of an apparent increase in x-ray beam penetration.

B80–E. Surface doses in body CT are of the order of 20 mGy (2 rad).

B81–E. Increasing the number of internal conversion electrons reduces the number of gamma rays available for imaging and increases the patient dose.

B82–D. ^{99m}Tc emits 140 keV photons. The daughter product (^{99}Tc) is radioactive, with a half-life of 210,000 years.

B83–E. Equilibrium has nothing to do with the number of parent and daughter atoms.

B84–A. A typical NaI crystal will be about 10 mm thick, not 1 mm.

B85–B. The pulse height analyzer measures the total energy deposited in the photon interaction and "accepts" only photopeak interactions that correspond to a photoelectric interaction with the full photon energy.

B86–B. Septal penetration always increases with increasing photon energy.

B87–C. Patient motion correction is not normally performed for SPECT imaging, as is sometimes performed in digital subtraction angiography imaging.

B88–C. The range of the positrons is only 1 mm in soft tissue. PET makes use of the subsequent 511 keV gammas emitted when the positron annihilates with an electron.

B89–D. Spectral purity (monochromatic photon energy) has nothing to do with radiopharmaceutical quality control.

B90–E. Gamma camera imaging time has no effect on organ doses.

B91–B. Equivalent dose (measured in sieverts or rems) is the product of the absorbed dose (measured in gray or rad) and the radiation weighting factor.

B92–E. 5 Gy is the threshold for cataract induction.

B93–C. Leukemia is a stochastic effect, whereas all the other effects listed are deterministic and have a threshold dose below which the effect does not occur.

B94–D. The entrance skin dose for a lateral lumbar spine is about 10 mGy (1 rad) so that the dose to the embryo will likely be 0.5 to 1 mGy (50 to 100 mrad).

B95–D. Nonagreement states are regulated by the NRC, whereas agreement states such as New York have regulatory requirements at least as stringent as those of the NRC.

B96–E. Regulator dose limits to the public explicitly exclude natural background and medical exposure.

B97–C. Most diagnostic radiology lead aprons have a 0.5 mm lead equivalence.

B98–C. Use factor (U) is the fraction of the operating time during which the radiation under consideration is directed toward the particular barrier.

B99–E. After 10 half lives, the activity will be 0.1% of the initial activity–after monitoring to ensure that the contamination is at background levels, it may be disposed of in the regular waste.

B100–C. The average *effective dose* from 1 year of exposure to domestic radon is 2 mSv (200 mrem), and the mean lung dose will be much higher than this.

B101–D. Acoustic impedance is the product of the velocity of sound and the density. For air, both velocity of sound and density are low; therefore, the acoustic impedance of air is very low.

B102–C. Decibel = $10 \times \log_{10}(I/I_0)$, so 3 dB corresponds to a 50% change in intensity.

B103–C. As in the case of light, the angle of reflection is equal to the angle of incidence.

B104–D. Refraction is governed by Snell's law and results in the ultrasound beam changing direction when passing from one medium to another.

B105–C. The Q factor is related to the bandwidth of the frequencies generated by the ultrasound transducer, where a high Q indicates a narrow bandwidth and relatively pure frequency.

B106–A. Quarter-wave matching layers are designed to maximize ultrasound beam transmission into patients.

B107–B. Time gain compensation (TGC) increases the echo intensity with increasing echo time to account for increasing signal attenuation with tissue depth.

B108–A. Axial resolution is equal to half the pulse length; therefore, increasing the pulse length reduces axial resolution.

B109–D. Transducer impedance has no relationship to lateral resolution.

B110–C. Continuous-wave Doppler provides information about flow from the change in ultrasound frequency generated by any moving object.

B111–A. The T1 of fat at 1.5 T is only 260 ms, which is shorter than all the other tissues listed (see table 12.2).

B112–E. Gray matter has a T2 of 100 ms, which is longer than the other tissues listed (see table 12.2).

B113–A. Shim coils are designed to adjust the main magnetic field to increase its homogeneity.

B114–A. Maximum fields are about 0.5 T.

B115–B. Gradients in the x, y, and z orientations are used to define the imaging planes and to localize the MR signal.

B116–C. Optical disks do not contain magnetic media and are not affected by magnetic fields.

B117–E. A Fourier analysis decomposes the time-varying FID signal into frequency components.

B118–A. Reverberation echoes occur in ultrasound imaging not in MR.

B119–D. Chemical shifts arise from the differing Larmor frequencies of nuclei in differing chemical structures, such as protons in water and fat molecules.

B120–D. Spectroscopy is commonly performed on the naturally occurring metabolites of ^{31}P and ^{1}H.

Appendix

APPENDIX I. *Summary of SI and non-SI units for general quantities*

Quantity	SI unit	Non-SI unit
Length	meter (m)	centimeter (cm)
Mass	kilogram (kg)	gram (g)
Time	second (sec)	minute (min)
Electrical current	ampere (A)	electrostatic unit (ESU) per sec
Amount of substance	mole (mol)	—
Frequency	hertz (Hz)	revolutions per min (rpm)
Force	newton (N)	dyne
Energy	joule (J)	erg
Power	watt (W)	erg/sec
Electrical charge	coulomb (C)	ESU
Electrical potential	volt (V)	—
Magnetic field	tesla (T)	gauss (G)

APPENDIX II. *Summary of units for radiologic quantities*

Quantity	SI unit	Non-SI unit	SI to non-SI conversions	Non-SI to SI conversions
Exposure	C/kg	roentgen (R)	1 C/kg = 3876 R	1 R = 2.58×10^{-4} C/kg
Air kerma	gray (J/kg)	roentgen (R)	1 Gy = 115 R	1 R = 8.73 mGy
Absorbed dose	gray (J/kg)	rad (100 erg/g)	1 Gy = 100 rad	1 rad = 10 mGy
Equivalent dose	sievert	rem	1 Sv = 100 rem	1 rem = 10 mSv
Activity	becquerel	curie	1 MBq = 27 μCi	1 mCi = 37 MBq

APPENDIX III. *Summary of units for photometric* quantities*

Quantity	SI unit	Non-SI unit	To convert non-SI units to SI units
Luminance[†] (light scattered or emitted by a surface)	cd/m^2 (nit)	foot-lambert	1 cd/m^2 = foot-lambert $\times$ 3.426
Illuminance[†] (light falling on a surface)	lumen/m^2 (lux)	foot-candles	1 lumen/m^2 = foot-candle $\times$ 10.76

* Photometric units take into account the spectral sensitivity of the eye.
† One lux falling on a perfectly diffusing surface with no absorption produces a luminance of 1/π cd/m^2.

APPENDIX IV. *Approximate luminance values*

Luminance (cd/m^2)	Viewing conditions
>10^7	Causes retinal damage
~3,000	Average mammography viewbox
~1,500	Standard viewbox
~600	Brightest commercial monitor display for use in radiology
60–200	Typical commercial monitor display brightness

APPENDIX V. *Approximate illuminance values*

Illuminance (lux)	Conditions
5,000	Full daylight
500	Overcast day
100–500	Office illumination for reading text
20	X-ray reading room illumination
5	Twilight
0.1	Moonlight
0.001	Starlight

APPENDIX VI. *Summary of prefix names and magnitudes*

Prefix name	Symbol	Magnitude
exa	E	10^{18}
peta	P	10^{15}
tera	T	10^{12}
giga	G	10^{9}
mega	M	10^{6}
kilo	k	10^{3}
deci	d	10^{-1}
centi	c	10^{-2}
milli	m	10^{-3}
micro	μ	10^{-6}
nano	n	10^{-9}
pico	p	10^{-12}
femto	f	10^{-15}
atto	a	10^{-18}

APPENDIX VII. *Selected radiologic physics Web sites*

Organization or publication	URL
American Association of Physicists in Medicine (AAPM)	www.aapm.org
American Board of Radiology (ABR)	www.theabr.org
American College of Radiology (ACR)	www.acr.org
American Institute of Ultrasound in Medicine (AIUM)	www.aium.org
American Journal of Roentgenology (AJR)	www.aarrs.org/ajr
American National Standards Institute (ANSI)	www.ansi.org
American Roentgen Ray Society (ARRS)	www.arrs.org
American Society of Radiologic Technologists (ASRT)	www.asrt.org
British Institute of Radiology (BIR)	www.bir.org.uk
Conference of Radiation Control Program Directors (CRCPD)	www.crcpd.org
Digital Imaging and Communications in Medicine (DICOM)	www.xray.hmc.psu.edu/dicom
Food and Drug Administration	www.fda.gov
Health Physics Society (HPS)	www.hps.org
International Commission on Non-Ionizing Radiation Protection	www.icnirp.de
International Commission on Radiation Units and Measurements (ICRU)	www.icru.org
International Commission on Radiological Protection (ICRP)	www.icrp.org
Joint Commission for Accreditation of Healthcare Organizations	www.jcaho.org
Medical Physics journal	www.medphys.org
National Council on Radiation Protection and Measurements (NCRP)	www.ncrp.com
National Radiological Protection Board (NRPB)	www.nrpb.org.uk
Physics and Astronomy online education	www.physlink.com
Radiation Research Society	www.radres.org
RadioGraphics journal	www.rsnajnls.org
Radiological Society of North America (RSNA)	www.rsna.org
Radiology journal	www.rsnajnls.org
Society for Computer Applications in Radiology (SCAR)	www.scarnet.org
Society of Nuclear Medicine (SNM)	www.snm.org
United States Food and Drug Administration (FDA)	www.fda.gov
United States National Institute of Standards and Technology (NIST)	www.nist.gov
United States Nuclear Regulatory Commission (NRC)	www.nrc.gov

Glossary

90 degree pulse   in magnetic resonance, radiofrequency pulse that rotates the equilibrium magnetization vector through 90 degrees

180 degree pulse   in magnetic resonance, radiofrequency pulse that rotates the equilibrium magnetization vector through 180 degrees

A-mode ultrasound   displays echo strength versus time

absolute risk   model of cancer induction in which radiation induces a given number of cancers

absorbed dose   radiation energy absorbed per unit mass of a medium, measured in gray or rad

absorption efficiency   fraction of incident photons that are absorbed

acoustic enhancement   hyperechoic area distal to object with low attenuation (e.g., fluid-filled cyst)

acoustic impedance   product of density and the velocity of sound in a medium, measured in Rayls

acoustic shadowing   hypoechoic area distal to object due to high attenuation or reflection

activity   number of nuclear transformations per unit of time, measured in becquerels or curies

air gap   gap between a patient and imaging receptor used in magnification examinations

ALARA   *as low as reasonably achievable* is the principle for minimizing all radiation exposures

aliasing   artifact caused by undersampling in all imaging modalities (magnetic resonance, ultrasound, etc.)

alpha decay   emission of an alpha particle by a radionuclide

alpha particle   particle consisting of two neutrons and two protons emitted from the nucleus of a radioisotope

analog-to-digital convertor (ADC)   converts analog signals into discrete digital values

anode   positive side of an electric circuit, such as the x-ray tube that includes the target

antineutrino   particle with no rest mass and no electric charge emitted in beta-minus decay

array processor   hard-wired computer component used for performing rapid calculations

atom   basic constituent of matter, which has a positive nucleus surrounded by electrons

atomic number (Z)   number of protons in the nucleus of an atom

attenuation coefficient (μ)   measure of the x-ray attenuating property of a material, in cm^{-1}

Auger electron   electron (rather than characteristic x-ray) emitted by an energetic atom

automatic brightness control (ABC)   regulates x-ray tube output to maintain a constant brightness at image intensifier output

average glandular dose (AGD)   the average dose to the glandular breast tissue in mammography

axial resolution   ability to separate two objects lying along the axis of the ultrasound beam

B-mode ultrasound   brightness mode that displays a cross-sectional image

background radiation   radiation exposures from naturally occurring radioactivity and extraterrestrial cosmic radiation

bandwidth   range of frequencies that can be satisfactorily transmitted or processed by a system

base plus fog   density of a processed film in the absence of any radiation exposure

beam hardening   increase in mean energy of a polychromatic x-ray beam as lower energy photons are preferentially absorbed by a filter or patient

beam quality   penetrating ability of an x-ray beam, usually expressed as the aluminum thickness that reduces beam exposure by 50%

becquerel   the SI unit of radioactivity (1 Bq = 1 disintegration per second)

BEIR   *B*iological *E*ffects of *I*onizing *R*adiation is a committee of the U.S. National Academy of Sciences

beta-minus decay   nuclear process in which a neutron is converted to a proton with emission of an electron and antineutrino

beta particle   electron or positron emitted from a nucleus during beta decay

beta-plus decay   nuclear process in which a proton is converted to a neutron with emission of a positron and neutrino

biological half-life   time required to biologically clear half of the amount of a stable material in an organ or tissue

bit   *b*inary dig*it,* the smallest unit of computer memory, which holds one of two values, one or zero

blooming   increase in x-ray focal spot size owing to electron spreading by electrostatic repulsion

blur   loss of image detail produced by an imaging system

bowtie filter   beam-shaping filter located in the computed tomography x-ray tube, used to equalize x-ray transmission through different patient body parts

bremsstrahlung radiation   "braking radiation" x-rays produced when electrons lose energy

brightness gain   ratio of the image brightness at the image intensifier output to the brightness produced at the input phosphor

Bucky   device that moves a grid, named after its inventor

Bucky factor   ratio of incident to transmitted radiation for a given grid

byte   unit of computer memory equal to 8 bits

CAD   computer-*a*ided *d*etection (or *d*iagnosis)

candela/m^2   measure of luminance (brightness)

cathode   negative side of an x-ray tube containing the filament

characteristic curve   plot of film density against the logarithm of relative exposure

characteristic radiation   x-ray photon of characteristic energy emitted from an atom when an inner-shell vacancy is filled by an outer-shell electron

charged coupled device (CCD)   two-dimensional electronic array for converting light patterns into electrical signals (charge)

chemical shift artifacts   artifacts in magnetic resonance caused by small differences in resonance frequencies of different chemical compounds (e.g., water and fat)

coherent scatter   photon scattered by an atom without suffering any energy loss; also known as Rayleigh or classical scatter

collimation   restriction of an x-ray beam or gamma rays by use of attenuators

Compton interaction   photon interaction with an outer-shell electron resulting in a scattered electron and photon of lower energy

computed radiography (CR)   digital radiography that uses photostimulable phosphor plates rather than screen/film systems

computed tomography (CT)   x-ray imaging modality showing cross-sectional anatomy

computed tomography dose index (CTDI)   index used to measure doses in computed tomography

contrast   difference in signal intensity between an object and the surrounding background

contrast improvement factor   ratio of image contrast obtained with and without the use of scatter reduction systems such as grids

contrast-to-noise ratio (CNR)   a measure of image quality that compares the contrast of a lesion to the noise level

controlled area   area with potentially high exposure rates that must be supervised by a radiation safety officer

converging collimator   a collimator used to image small organs, resulting in a magnified image

conversion efficiency   the percentage of x-ray energy deposited into a screen converted to light

conversion factor   in image intensifiers, the light output (Cd/m^2) per input exposure rate (mGy/second)

coulomb (C)   unit of electric charge

count density   used in nuclear medicine to specify the number of counts per unit area

cumulative activity   a measure of the total number of radioactive disintegrations obtained by integrating the activity over time (i.e., area under the curve of activity versus time)

curie (Ci)   the non-SI unit of activity (1 Ci = 3.7×10^{10} disintegrations per second)

current   rate of flow of electric charge, measured in amperes

cyclotron   charged particle accelerator used to make radioisotopes

decay constant (λ)   the rate of decay of radionuclides ($\lambda = 0.693/T_{1/2}$, where $T_{1/2}$ is the half-life)

densitometer   device used to measure optical density on film

deterministic effect   biological effect of radiation (e.g., epilation) that has a threshold dose

DICOM   *Digital Imaging and Communications in Medicine*, a standard used for transferring digital images in radiology

digital   quantity specified by discrete numbers, as opposed to analog (continuous)

digital fluoroscopy   fluoroscopic imaging with television signal digitized and processed, in real time

digital photospot imaging   acquisition of a digital diagnostic quality image of the output of an image intensifier

digital radiography   use of a flat-panel detector array or computed radiography system to acquire a digital x-ray image

digital subtraction angiography (DSA)   imaging modality in which digital images made before and after the introduction of iodine contrast are subtracted from each other

directly ionizing radiations   charged particles, such as electrons, that directly ionize atoms

diverging collimator   collimators for large organs (e.g., lungs) that result in a minified image

Doppler shift   change in ultrasound frequency with motion (e.g., flowing blood)

dose   absorbed energy per unit mass, expressed in grays or rads

dose area product   product of the entrance skin dose and cross-sectional area of the x-ray beam

dose calibrator   ionization chamber used in nuclear medicine to measure the amount of radioactivity prior to injection into a patient

dose equivalent   see *equivalent dose*

dynamic range   ratio of the largest to smallest signal intensities

echo planar imaging (EPI)   fast magnetic resonance imaging mode

edge enhancement   enhancement of structure margins (edges) using digital processing techniques

edge packing   nuclear medicine artifact that occurs at the periphery of the gamma camera

effective atomic number   average atomic number obtained from a weighted summation of the atomic constituents of a compound

effective dose   uniform whole-body dose that has the same risk as a given (non-uniform) dose distribution

effective half-life   half-life of a radioactive material in an organ that is also being cleared biologically

electromagnetic radiation   transverse wave in which electric and magnetic fields oscillate perpendicular to wave motion

electron   constituent of matter with 1/1,836 of the mass of a proton and a negative charge

electron beam computed tomography (EBCT)   fifth-generation CT scanner design used in cardiac imaging

electron binding energy   energy that must be supplied to extract a bound atomic electron

electron capture   nuclear process in which a proton is converted to a neutron by capturing an electron from the surrounding shell structure and emitting a neutrino

electron density   number of electrons per unit volume (electrons per cm^3)

electron volt (eV)   unit of energy corresponding to the kinetic energy gained by an electron when accelerated through a potential of 1 V

electrostatic force   force that results from electric charges and that holds atoms together

emulsion   layer of film that contains silver halide grains

energy   ability to do work measured in joule (J)

entrance skin exposure   x-ray exposure incident at the skin surface

equivalent dose   product of the absorbed dose and radiation weighting factor, expressed in sieverts (Sv) or rems (also known as the dose equivalent)

exact framing   the entire circular image of an image intensifier is recorded on the film

excited state   any energy level above the lowest energy ground state in an atom or nucleus

exposure   ability of a source of x-rays to ionize air, measured in C/kg or roentgens (R)

extrinsic flood   gamma camera image obtained of a uniform source of activity

f-factor   factor used to convert exposures into absorbed dose for a specified absorbing medium

faraday cage   radiofrequency copper shielding sheets built into the wall around a magnetic resonance scanner

fast spin-echo (FSE)   magnetic resonance imaging technique that uses multiple spin-echoes to reduce imaging times in comparison to spin-echo imaging

ferromagnetic   material (e.g., iron and nickel) with large intrinsic magnetic fields produced by a regular array of unpaired atomic electrons in a domain

field uniformity   a measure of the uniformity of a nuclear medicine gamma camera

filament   wire on the cathode of an x-ray tube that is heated to emit electrons

file transfer protocol (FTP)   method for transferring files across a computer network

film badge   film used to estimate worker radiation dose from the amount of film blackening

film gamma   the maximum gradient of a film characteristic curve

film latitude   the range of exposure levels over which the film can be used

film mottle   random fluctuations in film density owing to the granular nature of the emulsion

filter   aluminum, copper, or other absorber placed in an x-ray beam to preferentially absorb low-energy x-rays

filtered back projection   computed tomographic image reconstruction technique

flat panel detectors   digital x-ray detector consisting of an x-ray absorber (photoconductor or scintillator) and a two-dimensional readout array

flip angle   the angle through which the net magnetization vector is rotated by an applied radiofrequency pulse

flux gain   number of light photons at the output phosphor of an image intensifier per light photon produced at the input phosphor

focal spot   region in the x-ray tube anode where the x-ray beam is produced

focused transducer   ultrasound transducer that can focus the beam using acoustical lenses

focusing cup   directs electrons leaving the x-ray tube filament

force   directed energy that can change the motion of a mass

Fourier analysis   analysis of time signals that identifies the individual signal frequencies

Fraunhofer zone   the far zone of an ultrasound beam where it diverges and cannot be used for imaging

free induction decay (FID)   decreasing magnetic resonance signal following a 90 degree pulse which decreases in intensity because of the dephasing of nuclear spins

frequency   the number of oscillations per second (i.e., hertz)

frequency encode gradient   magnetic field gradient applied during the acquisition (readout) of a free induction decay signal

Fresnel zone   near zone of an ultrasound beam used for imaging

fringe field   magnetic field at a distance from a magnet

full-width half maximum (FWHM)   a measure of resolution equal to the width of an image of a line source at points where the intensity is reduced to half the maximum

functional imaging   imaging modality that measures changes in regional blood flow arising from mental activity

fusion imaging   combination of two images, such as computed tomography and positron emission tomography

gamma camera   nuclear medicine imaging system that detects gamma rays

gamma decay   nuclear transformation that results in the emission of a gamma ray

gamma rays   high-frequency electromagnetic radiation produced by nuclear processes

Gaussian distribution   a bell-shaped statistical distribution that is symmetrical about the mean value and with spread that is characterized by the standard deviation σ

Geiger-Müller counter   ionization chamber with a high voltage resulting in amplified output following the detection of an ionizing particle

generator   produces radionuclides such as ^{99m}Tc in nuclear medicine

genetically significant dose (GSD)   an estimate of the genetic significance of gonad radiation doses, which takes into account the child expectancy of exposed individuals

geometric unsharpness   image blur resulting from the finite size of the x-ray focal spot

gradient   the average slope of a film characteristic curve

gradient coils   current-carrying coils in magnetic resonance that create small magnetic field gradients superimposed on the large stationary magnetic field

gradient recalled echo (GRE)   magnetic resonance spin-echo created using gradients rather than 180 degree rephasing radiofrequency pulses

gravity   force responsible for attraction between all matter

gray (Gy)   the SI unit of absorbed dose (1 Gy = 1 J/kg)

grid (antiscatter grid)   strips of lead in a radiolucent matrix used to reduce scattered radiation

grid line density   the number of grid lines per centimeter

grid ratio   ratio of height to separation gap of the attenuating strips in a grid

ground state   lowest energy level of an atom or nucleus

gyromagnetic ratio (γ)   a value characteristic of any magnetic nucleus that determines the Larmor precession frequency, f_L, in a given magnetic field B ($f_L = \gamma \times B$)

half-life (physical) ($T_{1/2}$)   time for the activity of a radioisotope to decrease by a factor of two

half-value layer (HVL)   thickness of specified material (e.g., aluminum) needed to reduce the x-ray beam exposure by 50%

heat unit   energy unit for a *single-phase x-ray* system taken as the product of exposure time, peak voltage, and amperage (1 J = 1.35 heat units)

heel effect   the x-ray intensity is greater at the cathode side and lower at the anode side because of absorption in the Tungsten target

Helmholtz coils   coaxial coils used to generate a magnetic field gradient in magnetic resonance

Hertz (Hz)   frequency expressed in cycles per second

Hounsfield unit (HU)   the attenuation coefficient of a material relative to that of water as used in computed tomography

ICRP   *International Commission on Radiological Protection* is an international agency that issues recommendations regarding radiation safety

ICRU—International Commission on Radiological Units and Measurements is an international agency that defines radiation units

image compression   reduction of the space required to store or time required to transfer a digital image

image contrast   difference in intensity of a lesion and the adjacent background tissues

image intensifier   converts incident x-ray pattern to a light image

indirectly ionizing radiation   uncharged radiation that produces ionization via charged particles such as photoelectrons (for x-rays) and recoil protons (for neutrons)

integral dose   a measure of the total amount of energy imparted to a patient during a radiologic examination

intensification factor   ratio of x-ray exposure without and with an intensifying screen to produce a given film density

intensifying screen   phosphor that converts x-rays into light

internal conversion   electron emitted from a nucleus in lieu of a gamma ray

intrinsic flood   gamma camera image of a uniform source of activity obtained *without* a collimator

intrinsic resolution   spatial resolution of a gamma camera *without* a collimator

inverse square law   exposure decreases in proportion to the square of the distance from the source

inversion recovery (IR)   magnetic resonance pulse sequence designed to emphasize T1 differences

ionization   production of electrons and positive ions by the absorption of radiation energy

ionization chamber   gas filled chamber used to measure x-ray exposure by measuring the charge liberated in a given mass of air

ionizing radiation   radiation that can eject bound electrons from atoms

isobar   nuclides with the same total number of neutrons and protons (mass number, A)

isomer   nuclides with an excited nuclear state

isometric state   metastable state that exists for more than 10^{-12} seconds

isotone   nuclides with the same number of neutrons

isotope   nuclides with the same number of protons

joule (J)   SI unit of energy (1 J = 10^7 erg)

K-edge   binding energy of K-shell electrons

Kell factor   correction factor used to determine actual vertical resolution on a television system from the theoretical maximum resolution (70%)

kerma   *k*inetic *e*nergy *r*eleased in the *m*edi*a*, which refers to the transfer of energy from uncharged to charged particles

kinetic energy   energy associated with motion

lag   afterglow of an image on a screen or television camera

Larmor frequency   precession frequency of a magnetic nucleus in an applied magnetic field

lateral resolution   in ultrasound, ability to resolve two laterally adjacent objects

latitude   the range of exposures over which an image recording system can operate

LD$_{50}$ radiation dose that kills 50% of irradiated cells

leakage radiation   radiation emerging from an x-ray unit when the collimators are closed

limiting resolution   highest spatial frequency resolved by an imaging system, measured in line pairs per millimeter (lp/mm)

line density   in ultrasound, the number of lines used to generate an image

line focus principle   result of viewing a sloped surface (x-ray tube anode) at an angle, thus reducing its apparent size

line spread function (LSF)   image of a narrow line, which quantifies the amount of blur produced by an imaging system

linear attenuation coefficient (μ)   the fraction of photons lost from an x-ray beam in traveling a unit of distance, measured in cm^{-1}

linear energy transfer (LET)   energy absorbed by the medium per unit of length traveled, measured in keV/μm

longitudinal magnetization   component of magnetization that is oriented parallel to the main magnetic field in a magnetic resonance scanner

lookup table   used to assign (transform) digital data into image brightness values

luminance   the brightness of a light-emitting source (e.g., view box or computer monitor)

M-mode ultrasound   displays depth versus time and permits motion to be observed

magnetic moment   strength of nuclear or electronic magnetism

magnetic susceptibility   the inherent property of a substance that modifies the local magnetic field when placed in a strong applied (external) field

Mammography Quality Standards Act (MQSA)   act passed into law in the United States in 1992, which requires all mammography facilities to be accredited

mass   resistance to acceleration (inertia) of matter, measured in kilograms (kg)

mass attenuation coefficient   linear attenuation coefficient divided by the physical density, measured in squared centimeters per gram (cm^2/g)

mass number (A)   total number of nucleons (protons and neutrons) in the nucleus of an atom

matching layer   layer of material placed in front of an ultrasound transducer to improve the efficiency of energy transfer into a patient

matrix size   the number of pixels allocated to each linear dimension in a digital image

maximum intensity projection (MIP)   an image processing method used in computed tomography and magnetic resonance

mean   the average value of any distribution of values

median   value of a statistical distribution in which half the distribution is higher and half is lower

metastable state (isomeric state)   transient energy state of an atom with a half-life longer than 10^{-12} seconds

minification gain   ratio of the area of the image intensifier input to area of the output phosphor

modem (modulator/demodulator)   device for sending digital data via a telephone line

modulation transfer function (MTF)   measure of resolution performance of an imaging system; ratio of output to input signal amplitude as a function of spatial frequency

mole   amount of substance (number of atoms) in which 1 gram mole is about 6×10^{23} atoms

monochromatic radiation   radiation in which all photons have the same energy

multiplanar reformatting (MPR)   technique used in 2-dimensional tomographic imaging (computed tomography and magnetic resonance) to generate sagittal, coronal, and oblique views from axial sections

National Committee on Radiological Protection and Measurements (NCRP)   a U.S. agency that advises on radiation protection issues

natural back ground radiation   radiation exposure from cosmic radiation and naturally occurring radionuclides ($\sim$3 mSv/year in the United States)

negative predictive value   probability of not having a disease, given a negative diagnostic test result

neutrino   particle with no rest mass and no charge that is emitted during beta-plus decay and in electron capture

neutrons   uncharged particles found in the atomic nucleus

noise   random fluctuations in image intensity at a contant exposure

nonspecular reflection   diffuse ultrasound reflections (scatter) at irregular (rough) surfaces

Nuclear Regulatory Commission (NRC)   U.S. federal agency responsible for regulating nuclear materials

nucleon   neutron or proton

nuclides   nuclei with differing numbers of protons or neutrons

object contrast   physical differences (density, atomic number, and thickness) of a lesion in comparison to the surrounding tissues

occupancy factor   a factor used in designing radiation shielding that accounts for how long a given location is occupied by a worker or member of the public

occupational dose limit   regulatory dose limits applied to radiation workers (e.g., 50 mSv/year)

optical density (OD)   measure of the degree of film blackening using a logarithmic scale

optical disk   large-capacity digital data storage device used to store digital radiographic images

overframing   capturing a circular image intensifier image with a square film frame with the square circumscribed by the circle

PACS   *p*icture *a*rchiving and *c*ommunications *s*ystem, in which a radiology department replaces film with electronically stored and displayed digital images

pair production   an electron and positron pair produced in an atomic nucleus by a high-energy photon (over 1.022 MeV)

parallel processing   performing several computer tasks simultaneously

paramagnetism   substance with a positive susceptibility, which enhances the local magnetic field due to the presence of unpaired atomic electrons (e.g., gadolinium chelates)

partial volume artifact   an artifact caused by a mixture of tissues with different attenuation coefficients within any given voxel

peak voltage (kV$_p$)   maximum voltage across the x-ray tube

phase encode gradient   magnetic resonance gradient applied perpendicular to the frequency encode gradient

photodisintegration   disintegration of a nucleus after absorbing a high-energy photon (greater than 15 MeV)

photoelectric effect   a photon is absorbed by an atom and a photoelectron is emitted

photomultiplier tube   electronic device that converts light into an electric signal

photon   bundle of electromagnetic radiation that behaves like a particle and that has an energy proportional to frequency

photopeak   signal produced in a gamma camera crystal as a result of a photoelectric interaction in which all the incident gamma ray energy is absorbed by the crystal

photospot film   photograph of the image intensifier output

photostimulable phosphor   barium fluorohalide material used to capture radiographic images in computed radiography systems

phototimer   x-ray detector used to terminate a radiographic exposure

piezoelectric effect   conversion of electric energy into mechanical motion (and vice versa)

pin cushion distortion   image distortion associated with image intensifiers

pinhole collimator   collimator used in nuclear medicine for high-resolution images of small structures

pitch   term used in helical computed tomography; defined as the ratio of table advancement per 360 degree rotation of x-ray tube to detector collimation

pixel   *pi*cture *el*ement constituting the smallest component of a digital image

Poisson distribution   random distribution in which the variance is equal to the mean value

positive predictive value   probability of having a disease given a positive diagnostic test result

positron emission tomography (PET)   nuclear medicine imaging modality that detects the annihilation radiation (511 keV gamma rays) of positron emitters

positron   particles identical to electrons but with a positive electric charge

potential energy   energy associated with the location of a particle at a high-energy potential, such as an electron at a cathode

power   rate of doing work, measured in watts (W)

primary transmission   the fraction of the primary x-ray beam that penetrates a patient or a grid

progressive scan mode   method of television scanning in which all the lines are scanned successively (in interlaced scanning, the odd lines are scanned first and then the even lines).

projection data   attenuation data set acquired in computed tomography with the x-ray tube at one location; about 1,000 projections are required to reconstruct the CT image

proton   positively charged particle found in the nucleus

pulse height analyzer (PHA)   used in a gamma camera to select energies that correspond to the photopeak of the nuclide used to generate the image

pulse repetition frequency (PRF)   the number of ultrasound pulses generated by the transducer each second

pulse sequence   sequence of radio frequency pulses and magnetic gradients used to generate a magnetic resonance image

Q factor   determines the purity of an ultrasound pulse; high Q values correspond to pure frequencies and vice versa

quantum mottle   image noise resulting from the discrete nature of x-ray photons

quenching gas   gas added to Geiger counters and ionization chambers to minimize electronic discharges

rad   *r*adiation *a*bsorbed *d*ose; non-SI unit of absorbed dose (1 rad = 100 erg/g)

radiation weighting factor (w_R)   used to convert absorbed dose into dose equivalent, and normally equal to unity in radiology (also known as the quality factor)

radiochemical purity   a measure of chemical impurity assessed by thin layer chromatography

radiographic mottle   random fluctuations (noise) in a film image with a *uniform* exposure

radioisotope   atoms with unstable nuclei

radionuclide   an unstable nuclide that decays exponentially

radionuclide purity   a measure of radioactive contaminants (other radionuclides)

radiopharmaceutical   chemical or pharmaceutical that is labeled with a radionuclide

radon (^{222}Ra)   radioactive gas produced when naturally occurring radium (^{226}Ra) decays; found at high levels in some home basements

RAID   *r*edundant *a*rray of *i*nexpensive *d*isks; computer data storage medium with rapid image access time and fault tolerance

random access memory (RAM)   volatile computer memory that loses information when the computer power supply is switched off

range   distance traveled by a charged particle before losing all of its energy

rare earth screen   radiographic screen containing rare earth elements

read-only memory (ROM)   permanent memory in computers

real-time ultrasound imaging   cross-sectional image updated 20 to 40 times per second, allowing motion to be followed

receiver operating characteristic (ROC) curve   curve that plots the true-positive fraction versus false-positive fraction, and is used to evaluate imaging performance

reciprocating grid   a grid that moves during a radiographic exposure and smears out the grid lines in the resultant image

rectification   changing an alternating voltage into one polarity (i.e., AC to DC)

refraction   change of direction of any wave when moving from one medium to another

relative risk   model of cancer induction in which radiation exposure increases the natural incidence by a fixed percentage

rem   non-SI unit of equivalent dose

repetition time (TR)   time period over which a basic magnetic resonance pulse sequence is repeated

resolution (see spacial resolution)

reverberation   artifact in ultrasound caused by multiple echoes from parallel tissue interfaces

ring artifact   artifact resembling a ring produced by a defective detector in third-generation computed tomography and single photon emission computed tomography

ring down time   the time an ultrasound transducer requires for a generated pulse intensity to be reduced to a negligible value

roentgen (R)   unit of exposure that measures charge liberated in air

scatter   radiation deflected from its initial direction

scintillator   material that emits light after absorption of radiation

screen mottle   fluctuations in image density produced by random variations in screen thickness

screen unsharpness   blur caused by light diffusion within the intensifying screens

secular equilibrium   occurs after four half-lives of the daughter with a long-lived parent radionuclide

self-rectification   a reference to the fact that electrons cannot flow from the anode to the cathode in an x-ray tube

sensitivity   the ability of a test to detect disease

septal penetration   gamma rays that penetrate the collimator septa

shim coils   current-carrying coils used in magnetic resonance to improve the magnetic field homogeneity

signal-to-noise ratio (SNR)   a measure of image quality that depends on the diagnostic task

slice sensitivity profile   broadening of the computed tomography slice thickness along the patient axis in helical CT

somatic effects   radiation effects such as cancer that occur in the exposed individual, as opposed to genetic effects, which occur in the individual's offspring

space charge   result of an electron cloud around the filament in an x-ray tube

spatial frequency   sinusoidal signal intensity expressed in line pairs or cycles per millimeter

spatial peak temporal average intensity (I_{SPTA})   ultrasound intensity obtained at a single point and averaged over many pulses, which quantifies thermal effects

spatial resolution   ability to discriminate between two adjacent high-contrast objects

specificity   the ability to identify the absence of disease

SPECT   *s*ingle *p*hoton *e*mission *c*omputed *t*omography, which is a tomographic imaging technique in which a gamma camera is rotated around a patient

spectroscopy   magnetic resonance analysis of the chemical species (e.g., ^{31}P may be present as adenosine triphosphate, inorganic phosphor, and so on)

spectrum   display of the number of x-ray photons at each photon energy of polychromatic radiation

specular reflection   ultrasound reflections from large smooth surfaces

spin-echo (SE)   magnetic resonance pulse sequence in which echoes are generated by rephasing spins in the transverse plane using radiofrequency pulses or magnetic field gradients

spot film   radiographic image taken by placing a cassette in front of the image intensifier

standard deviation (SD)   a measure of the spread of a statistical distribution

stochastic effect   radiation effects, such as carcinogenesis, and genetic effects where probability of occurrence depends on the absorbed dose

streak artifacts   computed tomography artifacts caused by patient motion or metallic implants

strong force   force that holds the nucleus of an atom together

subject contrast   difference in x-ray beam intensities emerging from a lesion and adjacent background tissues

superconducting   property of zero electrical resistance when a material is cooled to very low temperatures

superparamagnetism   magnetic property similar to ferromagnetism but occurring in small aggregates of atoms (single domains)

T1   spin lattice or longitudinal relaxation time

T2   spin-spin or transverse relaxation time

T2*   rapid reduction of free induction decay signals due to magnetic field inhomogeneities

TE (time to echo)   time from the initial 90 degree radiofrequency pulse to the echo signal in magnetic resonance spin-echo sequences

tenth-value layer (TVL)   thickness of material needed to reduce an x-ray beam intensity to 10% of its initial value

thermoluminescent dosimeter (TLD)   solid-state dosimeter that, after x-ray exposure, emits light when heated

threshold dose   dose below which deterministic radiation effects do not occur

TI   time to inversion, or the time interval between the initial 180 degree pulse and subsequent 90 degree radiofrequency pulse in an inversion recovery pulse sequence

time gain compensation (TGC)   used in ultrasound to correct for increased attenuation of sound with tissue depth

TR   repetition time in magnetic resonance pulse sequences, corresponding to the time interval before the basic pulse sequence is repeated

transducer   device that converts mechanical energy into electric current and vice versa

transformer   device used to increase or decrease voltages

transient equilibrium   equilibrium between the parent and daughter radionuclides in which the parent half-life is relatively short

transmittance   the fraction of light transmitted by darkened radiographic film

transverse magnetization   magnetization vector oriented in a plane perpendicular to the main external magnetic field in magnetic resonance

UNSCEAR   United Nations Scientific Committee on the Effects of Atomic Radiation, a United Nations body that assesses radiation exposures

unsharp masking   image processing method used to enhance the visibility of edges

use factor   term used in designing x-ray shielding that accounts for the fraction of time an x-ray beam is pointing in any given direction

vignetting   peripheral reduction of light intensity in image intensifiers

veiling glare   loss of contrast due to light scattering in image intensifiers

voxel   vo*lume* el*ement* obtained from the product of pixel area and the image section thickness

watt (W)   unit of power (1 W = 1 J/second)

waveform ripple   temporal variation in voltage across an x-ray tube

wavelength   the distance between two consecutive crests of a wave

weak forces   account for beta-decay processes

window width and center   method for displaying digital images; determines the allocation of stored image data to shades of white, black, and gray in the displayed image

work   product of force and distance, measured in joules

x-rays   high-frequency (energetic) electromagnetic radiation produced using electrons

Bibliography

GENERAL RADIOLOGIC IMAGING (RESIDENTS)

Bushberg JT, Seibert AJ, Leidhodt EM Jr, Boone JM. *The essential physics of medical imaging,* 2nd ed. Philadelphia: Lippincott Williams & Wilkins, 2001.

Curry TS, Dowdey JE, Murray RC Jr. *Christensen's physics of diagnostic radiology,* 4th ed. Philadelphia: Lea & Febiger, 1990.

Dendy PP, Heaton B. *Physics for diagnostic radiology,* 2nd ed. Bristol: Institute of Physics Publishing, 1999.

Dowsett DJ, Kenny PA, Johnston RE. *The physics of diagnostic imaging.* London: Chapman & Hall, 1998.

Farr RF, Allisy-Roberts PJ. *Physics for medical imaging.*Philadelphia: WB Saunders, 1997.

Hendee WR, Ritenour R. *Medical imaging physics,* 4th ed. St Louis: Mosby—Year Book, 2002.

Sprawls P Jr. *Physical principles of medical imaging,* 2nd ed. Madison: Medical Physics Publishing, 1993.

Wolbarst AB. *Physics of radiology.* Madison: Medical Physics Publishing, 1993.

GENERAL RADIOLOGIC IMAGING (TECHNOLOGISTS)

Ball J, Moore AD. *Essential physics for radiographers,* 3rd ed. Oxford: Blackwell Science, 1997.

Bushong SC. *Radiologic science for technologists,* 7th ed. St Louis: Mosby, 2001.

Carlton RR, Adler AM. *Principles of radiographic imaging: an art and a science.* Albany: Delmar Publishing, 1992.

Cullinan AM, Cullinan JE. *Producing quality radiographs,* 2nd ed. Philadelphia: JB Lippincott Co, 1994.

Daniels C. *Fundamentals of diagnostic radiology* [CD-ROM]. Madison: Medical Physics Publishing, 1996.

Graham TG. *Principles of radiological physics,* 3rd ed. New York: Churchill Livingstone, 1996.

Kelsey CA, Fasbinder R. *Essentials of radiologic science.* New York: McGraw-Hill, 2001.

Malott JC, Fodor J III. *The art and science of medical radiography.* St Louis: CV Mosby, 1993.

Selman J. *The fundamentals of imaging physics and radiobiology: for the radiologic technologist,* 9th ed. Springfield: Charles C Thomas Publisher, 2000.

EXAMINATION REVIEW BOOKS

Carlton RR. *Radiography exam review.* Philadelphia: JB Lippincott Co, 1993.

Compilation of radiologic physics examintions (RAPHEX) Vol. 2 Diagnostic, Madison: Advanced Medical Publishing, 1994.

Cummings GR, Meixner E. *Corectec's comprehensive set of review questions for radiography,* 5rd ed. Athens: Corectec, 2000.

Leonard WL. *Examination review: radiography,* 9th ed. JLW Publications, 1997.

Saia DA. *Appleton and Lange's review for the radiography examination,* 4th ed. New York: McGraw-Hill, 2000.

RAPHEX Q & A booklets. Madison: Medical Physics Publishing, 1994.

BREAST IMAGING

American College of Radiology. *Mammography quality control manual.* Reston: American College of Radiology, 1999.

Haus AG, Yaffe MJ, eds. *Syllabus: a categorical course in physics, technical aspects of breast imaging.* Oak Brook: Radiological Society of North America, 1999.

Myers CP. *Mammography quality control: the why and how book.* Madison: Medical Physics Publishing, 1997.

Philpot D, Carlton RR, McLaughlin MJ, Miller PA. *Mammography exam review.* Philadelphia: JB Lippincott Co, 1992.

COMPUTED TOMOGRAPHY

Blanck C. *Understanding helical scanning.* Baltimore: Williams & Wilkins, 1998.

Philpot-Scroggins D, Reddinger W Jr, Carlton R, Shappell A. *Lippincott's computed tomography review.* Philadelphia: JB Lippincott Co, 1995.

Romans LE. *Introduction to computed tomography.* Baltimore: Williams & Wilkins, 1995.
Seeram E. *Computed tomography: physical principles, clinical applications, and quality control,* 2nd ed. Philadelphia: WB Saunders, 2001.

NUCLEAR MEDICINE

Chandra R. *Introductory physics of nuclear medicine,* 5th ed. Philadelphia: Lea & Febiger, 1998.
Mettler FA, Guibertean MJ. *Essentials of nuclear medicine imaging,* 4th ed. Philadelphia: WB Saunders, 1998.
Powsner RA, Powsner ER. *Essentials of nuclear medicine physics.* Oxford: Blackwell Science, 1998.
Saha GB. *Physics and radiobiology of nuclear medicine,* 2nd ed. New York: Springer-Verlag New York, 2000.
Sorensen JA, Phelps ME. *Physics in nuclear medicine,* 2nd ed. Orlando: Grune & Stratton, 1987.

RADIOBIOLOGY AND RADIATION PROTECTION

American College of Radiology. *Radiation risk: a primer.* Reston. American College of Radiology, 1996.
Bushong SC. *Radiation protection.* New York: McGraw-Hill, 1998.
Hall EJ. *Radiobiology for the radiologist,* 5th ed. Philadelphia: Lippincott—Raven Publishers, 2000.
Seeram E. *Radiation protection.* Philadelphia: Lippincott—Raven Publishers, 1997.
Sherer-Statkiewicz MA, Visconti PJ, Ritenour ER. *Radiation protection in medical radiography,* 3rd ed. St Louis: Mosby—Year Book, 1998.
Wagner LK, Lester RG, Saldana LR. *Exposure of the pregnant patient to diagnostic radiations: a guide to medical management,* 2nd ed. Madison: Medical Physics Publishing, 1997.

ULTRASOUND

Evans DH. *Doppler ultrasound: physics, instrumental, and clinical applications,* 2nd ed. New York: John Wiley and Sons, 2000.
Fish P. *Physics and instrumentation of diagnostic medical ultrasound.* Chichester: John Wiley and Sons, 1990.
Hedrick WR, Hykes DL, Starchman DE. *Ultrasound physics and instrumentation,* 3rd ed. St Louis: Mosby, 1995.
Hoskins PR, Thrush A, Whittingham T. *Diagnostic ultrasound: physics and equipment.* London: Greenwich Medical Media, 2002.
Odwin CS, Dubinsky T, Fleischer AC. *Appleton & Lange's review for the ultrasonography examination,* 2nd ed. Norwalk: Appleton & Lange, 1993.
Zagzebski JA. *Essentials of ultrasound physics.* St Louis: Mosby–Year Book, 1996.

MAGNETIC RESONANCE

Bushong SC. *Magnetic resonance imaging: physical and biological principles,* 2nd ed. St Louis: Mosby—Year Book, 1996.
Bushong SC. *Magnetic resonance imaging: study guide and exam review,* St Louis: Mosby—Year Book, 1996.
Faulkner W, Seeram E. *Tech's guide to MRI: basic physics, instrumentation and quality control (Rad Tech Series).* Oxford: Blackwell Science, 2001.
Mitchell DG. *MRI principles.* Philadelphia: WB Saunders, 1999.
Smith HJ, Ranallo FN. *A non-mathematical approach to basic MRI.* Madison: Medical Physics Publishing, 1989.
Sprawls P. *Magnetic resonance imaging: principles, methods and techniques.* Madison: Medical Physics Publishing, 2000.

Subject Index

Page numbers followed by *t* indicate tables. Page numbers followed by *f* indicate figures.

A

Absorption, x-ray, 34–35, 41
Acoustic enhancement, 184
Acoustic impedance, 173–174
Acoustic shadowing, 184
Air gaps, scatter removal, 55
Alpha decay, 11
Alpha particles, 7
American College of Radiology, accreditation requirements, 113*t*
A-mode ultrasound, 180
Amplitude, 6
Analog x-ray imaging, 49–67
   film. *See* Film
   fluoroscopy. *See* Fluoroscopy
   image intensifiers. *See* Image intensifiers
   scatter. *See* Scatter
Angiography, subtraction, 95–96, 96*t*
Artifacts
   computed tomography, 130
   magnetic resonance, 204
   nuclear medicine, 148
   ultrasound, 184
Atomic number
   K-shell binding energy, density of elements, 5*t*
   number of neutrons, relation between, 9*f*
Atoms, 2–3
Attenuation, 34, 38–41
   half-value layer, 39
   linear attenuation coefficient, 38
   mass attenuation coefficient, 39
   ultrasound, 175
Automatic brightness control, fluoroscopy, 61–62

B

Background radiation exposure, 167*t*
Background subtraction, 91
Bandwidth, 97
Base plus fog, 51
Baud rate, 87
Beam hardening, 27, 130
Beta-minus decay, 10
Beta-plus decay, 10
Bias, data analysis, 76

Binding energy, electron, 4–5
Bioeffects, ultrasound, 184
Biological basis of radiation exposure, 156–160, 158*f*
   cellular radiation effects, 156–157
   deterministic effects, 157–158
   dose response curves, 159*f*
   equivalent dose, 157
   linear energy transfer, 157
   stochastic effects, 159–160
   threshold doses, deterministic radiation effects, 159*t*
B-mode ultrasound, 180
Bohr model, atom, 4*f*
Breast cancer
   detection, 104
   diagnosis, 104–106
   incidence, mortality, 105*f*
   microcalcifications, 104
   modern mammography, 104–105
Breast imaging, 115–116
   magnetic resonance, 115
   mammography. *See* Mammography
   nuclear medicine, 115–116
   positron emission tomography, 116
   scintimammography, 116
   ultrasound, 115
Breast tissue, properties of, 105*t*
Bremsstrahlung radiation, 19, 19*f*
Bridge, in radiology, 97

C

Camera types, television, 59–60
Cancer
   breast. *See* Breast cancer
   radiation-induced, 160
Capillary blockade, nuclear medicine, 138
Cell sequestration, nuclear medicine, 138
Cellular radiation effects, 156–157
Chemical shift artifacts, magnetic resonance, 204
Coherent scatter, 34
Collimator, 54, 124–125, 142, 142*f,* 143, 143*t*
Color scanning, Doppler, 187
Compression, mammography, 108
Compton scatter, 34, 37*f,* 37–38